CHANGE YOUR BRAIN
CHANGE YOUR LiFE

The breakthrough programme for conquering anger, anxiety, obsessiveness and depression

Dr. DANIEL G. AMEN

PIATKUS

PIATKUS

First published in Great Britain in 2009 by Piatkus
Previously published in the US in 1998 by Three Rivers Press
Originally published in the US in 1998 by Times Books

A CIP catalogue record for this book
is available from the British Library

ISBN 978-0-7499-4191-8

Text design by Emma Ashby

Typeset in Caecilia by Action Publishing Technology Ltd, Gloucester
Printed and bound in Great Britain by Clays Ltd, St Ives plc

Papers used by Piatkus are natural, renewable and recyclable
products sourced from well-managed forests and certified in
accordance with the rules of the Forest Stewardship Council.

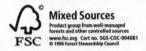

Mixed Sources
Product group from well-managed
forests and other controlled sources
www.fsc.org Cert no. SGS-COC-004081
© 1996 Forest Stewardship Council

FSC

Piatkus
An imprint of
Little, Brown Book Group
100 Victoria Embankment
London EC4Y 0DY

An Hachette UK Company
www.hachette.co.uk

www.piatkus.co.uk

"Cutting edge technology, clinical wisdom, and heartfelt guidance come together to create a 'user's manual for enhancing the human brain.' Dr. Amen offers simple, direct, and immediately applicable prescriptions that can change anyone's life."
—Emmett E. Miller, M.D., author of *Deep Healing: The Essence of Mind/Body Medicine*

"*Change Your Brain, Change Your Life* is a pioneering book. Dr. Amen provides clear and convincing evidence that many behavioral disorders formerly considered psychological actually have a biological basis. Through the lens of exciting new brain imaging techniques, you can see what depression, anxiety, temper, impulsiveness, and obsession actually look like in the brain. He gives many practical suggestions for overcoming these problems, and gives many tools for optimizing the brain and improving life."
—Rob Kohn, D.O., psychiatrist and neurologist,
University of Illinois at Chicago

"Dr. Amen's groundbreaking work will forever change the fields of psychiatry and psychology. A healthy brain is prerequisite to a healthy life. Dr. Amen provides a practical guide."
—Earl Henslin, Ph.D., author of *You Are Your Father's Daughter* and *Man to Man: Helping Fathers Relate to Sons and Sons Relate to Fathers*

"This book is brilliant. Dr. Amen is a pioneer."
—Jonathan Walker, M.D., psychiatrist

"Dr. Amen's exquisite documentation of brain function is a unique contribution to this rapidly developing field. However, he adds a remarkable twist: dozens of 'how to help' suggestions for patients and parents. This book is by far the most complete and specific compendium of suggestions patients and parents may learn and follow to assist their own personal recovery efforts."
—Corydon Clark, M.D., psychiatrist

To Andrew,
who taught me how important it is
to continue to do this work
and to tell the world about it.

Acknowledgments

So many people have been involved in the process of creating this book. I am grateful to my agent, Faith Hamlin, whose wisdom and love helped focus and nourish the book. I also feel blessed to have Betsy Rapoport as my editor at Times Books. She truly understood the significance of this book and helped me present the ideas in a clear, accessible way. Also, I very much appreciate the staff at Times Books, who have been deeply committed to this project.

This book would not have been possible without the staff at the Amen Clinic. From the front-office staff to the staff clinicians I consider these people part of my family and feel grateful to have their love, dedication, knowledge, and wisdom. I am especially grateful to Shelley Bernhard, the clinic manager, who keeps all of us on track; to Lucinda Tilley, my assistant, who prepared all the images in the book and spent many hours in research; to Bob Gessler, who is always willing to help and pitch in; and to the forward-thinking staff physicians and clinical staff, Stanley Yantis, Jennifer Lendl, Jonathan Scott Halverstadt, Ronnette Leonard, Lewis Van Osdel, Cecil Oakes, Matthew Stubblefield, Ed Spencer, Brian Goldman, Jane Massengill, Lloyd King, and Cora Davidson.

In addition, I so much appreciate my friends and colleagues Earl Henslin, Sheila Krystal, and Linda and Leon Webber for reading the manuscript and giving feedback.

Finally, my gratitude and love go to my family, who have lived through my brain research for the past ten years. I know that many times they were tired of listening about the brain and SPECT imaging but nonetheless loved me anyway and gave me the limbic connectedness necessary to live and make a difference in the lives of others.

Contents

Acknowledgments vi

Introduction to the U.K. Edition ix

Introduction 3

1. **For Those Who Have Eyes, Let Them See:** 16
   Images Into the Mind

2. **Carving Knives and Tooth Fairies:** 25
   A Prelude to the Brain and Behavior

3. **Looking Into Love and Depression:** 38
   The Deep Limbic System

4. **Enhancing Positive Thought Patterns and
   Strengthening Connections:** 56
   Deep Limbic System Prescriptions

5. **Looking Into Anxiety and Fear:** 84
   The Basal Ganglia

6. **Mastering Fear:** 100
   Basal Ganglia Prescriptions

7. **Looking Into Inattention and Impulsivity:** 114
   The Prefrontal Cortex

8. **Becoming Focused:** 138
   Prefrontal Cortex Prescriptions

9.   **Looking Into Worry and Obsessiveness:** 155
     The Cingulate System

10. **Getting Unstuck:** 176
     Cingulate System Prescriptions

11. **Looking Into Memory and Temper:** 192
     The Temporal Lobes

12. **Enhancing Experience:** 210
     Temporal Lobe Prescriptions

13. **The Dark Side:** 218
     Violence: A Combination of Problems

14. **Brain Pollution:** 232
     The Impact of Drugs and Alcohol on the Brain

15. **The Missing Links:** 253
     Drugs, Violence, and the Brain

16. **I Love You and I Hate You, Touch Me,
     No, Don't, Whatever:** 265
     Brain Patterns That Interfere with Intimacy

17. **Help!** 290
     When and How to Seek Professional Care

18. **Who Is Andrew Really?** 303
     Questions About the Essence of Our Humanity

19. **Brain Dos and Brain Don'ts:** 307
     A Summary of Ways to Optimize Brain Function
     and Break Bad Brain Habits

     Appendix: Medication Notes 311

     Bibliography 318

     Index 323

     About the Author 338

Introduction to the U.K. Edition

Since *Change Your Brain, Change Your Life* was first published in the United States in 1999 the use of brain imaging has exploded into worldwide consciousness. Virtually every week, major newspapers and magazines are reporting on a brain-imaging study related to some aspect of human behavior, such as our buying tendencies, mating habits, aggressive proclivities and political persuasions. How could it be otherwise? The brain is involved in everything we do and everything we are. Finally, brain-imaging technology is beginning to live up to some of the promises discussed in this book.

Not one to avoid controversy, I wrote a tongue-in-cheek piece for the *Los Angeles Times* in December 2007 on whether or not we should think about performing brain scans on political candidates. The president of the United States is one of the most powerful people on earth, so, before we voted for him or her, shouldn't we want to know whether or not he or she had a brain that works right? I was not really expecting anyone to take me up on the idea, but I was weary of presidents who showed clear brain abnormalities running the country, from Reagan's memory issues, Clinton's impulsivity struggles, and Bush's cognitive rigidity.

Tucker Carlson on American television read the piece and asked to interview me on his show. Towards the end of the interview he said, "This is my key and final question. Where is free will in this? So if you gave Clinton a brain scan and it said this guy is going to have impulse-control and self-control issues it doesn't allow for his own will in the equation. Does it?"

I have been asked about free will and the brain many times. I replied to Mr. Carlson, "If you have low activity in your prefrontal cortex, as many people who have attention deficit hyperactivity disorder (ADHD) who come to our clinics do, you can balance it with either supplements or medication or lifestyle changes, but if you don't know that someone has this kind of problem then you will just judge people who behave inappropriately as bad and say 'Oh, well, they have free will, they chose to do this.'" That kind of attitude is really 17th-century reductionist, Cartesian thinking that separates the mind from the brain. That kind of thinking about the mind and the brain, we now know, is wrong, and it's time we moved the discussion to the next level, which is to look at how the brain works. Can we make it work better? And if it works better won't we be more thoughtful, reliable, predictable, effective people?

If we really want to solve our most pressing problems about human behavior then we have to consider how the brain works. This is the message you will find between the pages of this book—a new way to look at and optimize human behavior. It is time for us to stop looking for the simplistic, "easy-way-out" explanation of bad or sociopathic or anti-social behavior, by saying "We are all responsible," and it's time to start looking at the data, especially brain data, because that will help us generate new, more effective solutions. Here's an example.

Jorge, 17, came to our clinics with extreme mood swings, suicidal and homicidal thoughts, and explosive outbursts. He had dropped out of school because he could never predict his moods. He was also abusing multiple drugs including marijuana, alcohol, ecstasy, and methamphetamine. Since childhood, Jorge had had problems with anger, and could be set off by very minor things; his reaction was almost always out of proportion to the incident. When angry he yelled, became confrontational, threw and broke things and hurt others. He had sudden dark, violent thoughts. When I first met Jorge, he told me that he recently had made a decision to be threatening and intimidating because it enabled him to get what he wants. He had threatened to kill his family if they tried to send him away and stated he would be justified because they would have become his enemy. Jorge's mood was very erratic. There were times when he became profoundly sad and couldn't stop crying and other times when he felt invincible.

Most of my colleagues would have diagnosed Jorge with bipolar disorder and conduct disorder, a prelude to antisocial personality disorder, and placed him on medications to treat bipolar disorder such as lithium or an antiseizure or antipsychotic medication. Through my eighteen years of experience with brain-imaging technology on tens of thousands of patients, however, I knew that we had to do more. Indeed, he might have bipolar disorder and conduct disorder or he may have had a brain injury that had damaged the most human, thoughtful part of his brain, the prefrontal cortex. He also may have had a brain cyst putting pressure on his brain and disrupting the normal circuitry that makes us human. Or he may have been suffering from some form of toxic exposure. How would I ever really know unless I looked at his brain? Yet, every day thousands of children, teenagers and adults are being diagnosed and treated with bipolar disorder, depression, ADHD, or antisocial personality disorder and placed on powerful medications without anyone ever looking at their brains. And when the medications prove ineffective, as in Jorge's case, the doctors and families label these people as bad and send them away to residential treatment programs, or prison, or to the streets as homeless. This societal madness must stop and it will when we start to evaluate brain function as the key to evaluating troubled behavior!

At the Amen Clinics we do brain SPECT (single photon emission computed tomography) studies to look at blood flow and activity patterns to show us how the brain functions. Jorge's scan was severely abnormal (see images below), with a very large cyst occupying nearly 30 percent of the left side of his brain. No amount of psychiatric medication, counseling, or incarceration would likely make him better. The cyst needed to come out first. I was very sensitive to this problem, as thirteen years earlier, as you will read in this book, I had found my first left-sided brain cyst in my nine-year-old nephew, Andrew, after he attacked a little girl on the baseball field for no particular reason. At the time, he had been also drawing pictures of himself shooting other children and committing suicide by hanging from a tree. Without appropriate intervention, Jorge and Andrew may well have become school shooters like Kip Kinkel, the 15-year-old boy in Springfield, Oregon, who in 1998 killed his parents and then shot 25 people at Thurston High School. He also had severe problems in this part of his brain.

The exciting news is that brain-imaging technology is starting to be used more and more by health professionals in clinical practice. Thomas Insel, M.D., Ph.D., Director of the United States National Institute of Mental Health, America's chief psychiatrist, said in a keynote lecture at the American Psychiatric Association's Annual Meeting in 2005

Jorge's SPECT Study

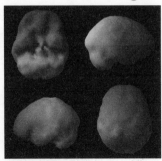

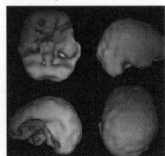

healthy brain
Shows full, even, symmetrical activity

Jorge's brain
Left-sided cyst

that, "Brain imaging in clinical practice is the next major advance in psychiatry. Trial-and-error diagnosis will move to an era where we understand the underlying biology of mental disorders. We are going to have to use neuroimaging to begin to identify the systems' pathology that is distributed in each of these disorders and think of imaging as a biomarker for mental illnesses. The *DSM-IV*, the psychiatrists' diagnostic bible, has 100 percent reliability and 0 percent validity. We need to develop biomarkers, including brain imaging, to develop the validity of these disorders. We need to develop treatments that go after the core pathology, understood by imaging. The end game is to get to an era of individualized care." Dr. Insel believed then that brain imaging in clinical practice would be a reality in five years.

It is clearly time for all of us to change our attitude about healthy brains as well as those that are injured or ill. *Change Your Brain, Change Your Life* will help you understand your own brain and give you many ideas for enhancing the moment-by-moment functioning of your brain to help you become more effective in all aspects of your life. One of my goals for you throughout the book is to help you develop brain envy. I want you to want a better brain, because improved brain function enhances everything in your life. Also, understanding the concepts in the book will not only help you on the road to better brain health, it will also increase your capacity for empathy and enable you to look at those who struggle in a completely new way.

At the Amen Clinics we have seen patients now from 73 countries, many from the United Kingdom. My hope is that you use the information in this book to have a better brain and a better life.

CHANGE YOUR Brain CHANGE YOUR LifE

Introduction

Your brain is the hardware of your soul. It is the hardware of your very essence as a human being. You cannot be who you really want to be unless your brain works right. How your brain works determines how happy you are, how effective you feel, and how well you interact with others. Your brain patterns help you (or hurt you) with your marriage, parenting skills, work, and religious beliefs, along with your experiences of pleasure and pain. If you are anxious, depressed, obsessive-compulsive, prone to anger, or easily distracted, you probably believe these problems are "all in your head." In other words, you believe your problem is purely psychological. However, research that I and others have done shows that the problems are related to the physiology of the brain—and the good news is that we have *proof* that you can change that physiology. You can fix what's wrong for *many* problems.

Until very recently, scientists could only speculate about the brain's role in our personality and decision-making skills. We did not have advanced tools to look at the functioning of the brain and thus made many false assumptions about its impact on our lives. With the advent of sophisticated brain-imaging techniques, we are now answering questions about the brain's role in behavior at a phenomenal pace, questions that have practical applicability to your life, from relationships at home and at work to understanding what makes you unique.

I have been involved in brain-imaging research for the past eighteen years. I first began studying the brain with sophisticated quantitative EEG (brain wave) studies, and in the last sixteen years I've used a nuclear medicine brain study called SPECT (single photon emission computed tomography), which measures cerebral blood flow and meta-bolic activity patterns. These last eighteen years have been both exhil-arating and frustrating. They have been exhilarating because through these studies we now have visual evidence of brain patterns that cor-relate with behavior, such as tendencies toward depression, anxiety, distractability, obsessiveness, and violence. This physical evidence of phenomena mostly thought of as purely "psychological" in origin has revolutionized the way others and I practice psychiatric medicine. We can now show patients and their families the physical "brain" evidence of problems, helping them to be more accepting and compliant with treatment. We have more information to make more effective treat-ment decisions with complex cases than ever before. And we use the information from this research to educate the public on the effects of drug abuse, head injuries, and even "negative thinking" on the brain. This has been truly an amazing time.

It has also been a frustrating time because dissemination of these new insights has been slower than I would like. There is natural resis-tance in the scientific community to dramatic shifts in thinking. Once a scientist uncovers new information, it needs to go through a peer review process that can take years. I'm pleased that the brain-imaging work I and others have pioneered is continuing to gain accept-ance from the medical and scientific community. In the meantime, the knowledge gained from this research is helping people across the world. It can help you too.

Seeing is Believing

I was not a brain-imaging researcher by design. After medical school at Oral Roberts University in Tulsa, Oklahoma, I did my psychiatric intern-ship and residency at Walter Reed Army Medical Center in Washing-ton, D.C. I always believed that there was a strong connection between spiritual health and mental health. Nothing in my training dissuaded me from that idea, but little did I know that the connection could go both ways. I then did a fellowship in child and adolescent psychiatry in Honolulu, Hawaii, where I learned how stressful early beginnings could set up lifelong problems. In Hawaii I began to write about apply-ing mental health principles to everyday life (in relationships, at work, and within ourselves). I wanted to teach large groups of people how to be more effective day to day. On the basis of my work, I was selected as a fellow in the prestigious Group for Advancement of Psychiatry and received a research award from the American Psychiatric Association.

In 1986, 1 wrote a program titled *Breaking Through: How to Be Effective Every Single Day of Your Life*, about identifying and overcoming behaviors that hold people back from success. The program has been extremely helpful for thousands of readers, yet many people needed more. As I worked with groups across the country and patients in my practice, using the principles in the program, many would experience very positive changes (within themselves, their relationships, and their work), but others didn't seem to get the help they needed. These "resistant" cases were very frustrating to me. I continually asked myself, what was the difference between the people who benefited from the program and those who didn't? Were some people ready to change and others not? Were some people just resistant to change because of deep-rooted psychological reasons? Was the program good for only certain personality types and not others? I searched for answers. When the answer hit me, the course I had set for my life changed.

In 1990, I was working in a psychiatric hospital in Fairfield, California (forty miles northeast of San Francisco). I was the director of the dual-diagnosis treatment unit (caring for people with both substance abuse and psychiatric problems) and saw other patients as well. One day at grand rounds, I heard Dr. Jack Paldi, a local nuclear medicine doctor, give a lecture on brain SPECT imaging. SPECT studies are nuclear medicine studies that measure blood flow and activity levels in the brain. Dr. Paldi showed "functional" brain images of people who had problems with dementia, depression, schizophrenia, and head injuries and compared them with the images of normal brains. I wondered if the brain were the missing piece of the puzzle in my resistant patients. Perhaps, I hypothesized, the people who were struggling had brains that could not "run" the new programs I was trying to give them, much like a computer cannot run sophisticated software unless it has enough speed and memory. One of the things that amazed me about Dr. Paldi's lecture was that he showed brain images before and after treatment. Treatment with medication actually changed the physical functioning of the brain! I wanted to know more.

The same week Dr. Paldi gave the lecture, Alan Zametkin, M.D., from the National Institutes of Health published an article in the *New England Journal of Medicine* on the use of PET (positron emission tomography) studies, in adults with attention deficit hyperactivity disorder (ADHD). Since ADHD was one of my specialties, the article really caught my interest. Dr. Zametkin demonstrated that when adults with ADHD try to concentrate, there is decreased activity in the prefrontal cortex, rather than the expected increase seen in normal "control" adults. Here was physical evidence of a problem many people thought was psychological! A third event that week helped me integrate what I'd learned: I met Sally.

Sally, a forty-year-old woman, had been hospitalized under my care for depression, anxiety, and suicidal ideas. In my clinical interview with her, I discovered that she had many adult ADHD symptoms (such as a short attention span, distractibility, disorganization, and restlessness). She had a son with ADHD (a frequent tip to diagnosing ADHD in adults). Despite her IQ of 140, she had never finished college, and she was employed below her ability as a laboratory technician. I decided to order a SPECT study on Sally. Sally's studies were abnormal. At rest, she had good overall brain activity, especially in the prefrontal cortex. But when she was asked to perform maths problems (an exercise to challenge her ability to concentrate), she had marked decreased activity across her whole brain, especially in the prefrontal cortex! With that information, I placed her on a low dose of Ritalin (methylphenidate), a brain stimulant used to treat ADHD in children and adults. She had a wonderful response. Her mood was better, she was less anxious, and she could concentrate for longer periods of time. She eventually went back to school and finished her degree. No longer did she think of herself as an underachiever, but rather as someone who needs treatment for a medical problem. Seeing the SPECT pictures was very powerful for Sally. She said, "Having ADHD is not my fault. It's a medical problem, just like someone who needs glasses." Sally's experience led me to believe that SPECT might have a powerful application in decreasing the stigma many patients feel when they are diagnosed with emotional, learning, or behavior problems. Sally could see that the problem wasn't "all in her head." The scan and her response to medication changed her whole perception of herself.

With Sally's enthusiasm and positive response to treatment fresh in my mind, I ordered more SPECT studies on my most resistant patients. Many patients, previously "treatment failures," began to get better when I identified through SPECT the part of their brain that wasn't working and targeted treatment to that area. After that series of events

Sally's SPECT Studies

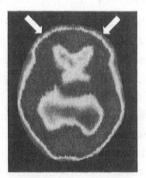

horizontal view at rest

Note good prefrontal activity (arrows).

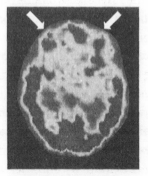

horizontal view during concentration

Note marked decreased activity, especially in the prefrontal cortex.

in 1990, my colleagues and I began to do clinical research with SPECT on a wide variety of patients. Our research confirmed the work of others and expanded the body of knowledge in new directions, especially in the areas of violence, obsessiveness, and "difficult personality temperaments."In doing this research, I have seen with my own eyes the brain SPECT patterns that show abnormalities that interfere with behavior. These brain abnormalities sabotage my patients' efforts to improve their lives and send interrupt signals to the changes they try to make. *I have seen how correcting (normalizing) abnormal brain function can change people's lives, even their very souls.* Person after person who had previously been a treatment failure began to improve through prescriptions targeted at optimizing the brain's physical functioning. This was such a simple concept: *When your brain works right, so can you. When your brain doesn't work right, neither can you.* The implication was profound: Various parts of the brain influence our behavior. Using SPECT studies, I was more effective at pinpointing trouble spots and providing more appropriate interventions. Seeing these scans caused me to challenge many of my basic beliefs about people, character, free will, and good and evil that had been ingrained in me as a Catholic schoolboy.

When the physical functioning of the brain was optimized through the use of medications, nutrition, and targeted psychological exercises, people who had previously been unable to change developed a capacity for new skills and behaviors. They developed more access to productive brain activity and more ability to make changes (even though they had always had the will to change). A major shift occurred in my thinking, uncovering new possibilities for the patients who had been "left behind."

Over the next eight years, I conducted more than five thousand brain studies. The lessons from the brain taught me that without optimal brain function, it is hard to be successful in any aspect of life, whether it is in relationships, work, schooling, feelings about yourself, or even your feelings about God—no matter how hard you try. Indeed, the first step to being successful is to understand and optimize the working patterns of the brain. By enhancing the physical functioning of the brain I also enhance my patients' potential for success in every area of their lives. First, optimize the hardware and circuitry of the brain; then put in new programs. The brain-imaging work provided insights that have revolutionized the way I understand and treat patients. These insights are the foundation of this book.

I am one of only a handful of psychiatrists in the world who are licensed in nuclear brain imaging. Currently, I am the medical director of Amen Clinics, Inc. We now have four clinics, three on the west coast of the United States and one outside of Washington D.C. We run the most active brain imaging centers in the world and see well over a thousand patients a month. We see patients from around the globe, and we are recognized as experts in the fields of attention deficit hyperactivity disorder, learning disabilities, head trauma, violence, and obsessive-compulsive disorder. Even though I am a rarity among psychiatrists, I believe what I do will be more commonplace in the years to come. It is just too helpful and too exciting to be confined to only a few clinics.

Focus of the Book

The aim of this book is to explain how the brain works, what happens when things go wrong, and how to optimize brain function. You will be introduced to five of the brain systems that are most intimately involved with our behavior and make up much of what is uniquely human.

You'll learn that the **deep limbic system,** at the center of the brain, is the bonding and mood control center. Being connected to others is essential to humanity, yet when this part of the brain is off kilter, people struggle with moodiness and negativity. You'll learn how certain smells and clear thinking soothe the activity in this part of the brain, and why spending time with positive people is essential to deep limbic health.

The **basal ganglia,** large structures deep within the brain, control the body's idling speed. When this part of the brain works too hard, anxiety, panic, fearfulness, and conflict avoidance are often the result. As I describe in the book, I inherited overactive basal ganglia, which leave me vulnerable to anxiety and nervousness. I know personally that anxiety is no fun and will give you plenty of ideas on how to settle down this part of the brain. When it is underactive, people often struggle with concentration and fine motor control problems.

The **prefrontal cortex,** at the front tip of the brain, is your supervisor, the part of the brain that helps you stay focused, make plans, control impulses, and make good (or bad) decisions. When this part of the brain is underactive, people have problems supervising themselves and also have significant problems with attention span, focus, organization, and follow-through. Learning how to activate the prefrontal cortex in a positive way leads to better internal supervision.

The **cingulate** (pronounced *sing-u-lat*), a part of the brain that runs longitudinally through the middle part of the frontal lobes, is the part of the brain I call your "gear shifter." It allows you to shift attention from thought to thought and between behaviors. When this part of the brain is overactive, people have problems getting stuck in certain loops of thoughts or behaviors. Understanding its function will help you deal with repetitive worries. Dealing with worry, rigidity, and "overfocused" behavior in yourself or others will be easier after reading this book.

Lastly, the **temporal lobes,** underneath the temples and behind the eyes, are involved with memory, understanding language, facial recognition, and temper control. When there are problems, especially in the left temporal lobe, people are more prone to temper flare-ups, rapid mood shifts, and memory and learning problems. Optimizing this part of the brain may help you experience inner peace for the first time in your life.

It is important to note that none of these brain systems exists in a vacuum. They are intricately interconnected. Whenever you affect one system, you're likely to affect the others as well. Also, some brain researchers would separate the systems differently than I lay them out in this book, placing the cingulate system and deep temporal lobes within the limbic system. I am presenting the system we use in my clinic, which has worked so well for our patients.

Presenting and defining these five terms—prefrontal cortex, cingulate system, deep limbic system, basal ganglia, and temporal lobes—is about as technical as the book gets. Mastering these systems will give you a whole new view about why you do what you do and what you can do about it.

After I describe each brain system, I'll offer targeted behavioral, cognitive, medicinal, and nutritional prescriptions to optimize its function. These prescriptions are practical, simple, and effective. They are based on my experience with more than a hundred thousand patient visits to my clinic over the past eighteen years, as well as the experiences and research of my colleagues.

Some people might wonder if readers should be the ones identifying and changing brain problems. My answer is an emphatic yes! I believe it benefits almost everyone to know as much about how his or her own brain works as possible. Most of the problems discussed in this book, such as moodiness, anxiety, irritability, inflexibility, and worrying, are faced by large numbers of the population. Most do not require professional help, but rather effective, brain-based prescriptions to optimize the brain's effectiveness. Since the brain controls our behavior, optimizing its function can help nearly anyone's ability to be more effective in life.

This book will also make it clear that if your ability to function in everyday life is significantly impaired (at school, at work, or in relationships), it is important to seek appropriate help from a competent professional. Letting problems fester untreated can ruin a life. But given the fact that there are hundreds of different kinds of psychological therapies available, seeking the right help can be complicated and downright confusing. In this book I will provide guidance and resources on how to seek appropriate help when it's needed.

Researching the brain has been my greatest personal challenge. In 1993, when I first started to talk at medical meetings about the discoveries we were making at our clinic, some colleagues severely criticized us, saying we could not infer behavioral patterns from brain patterns. Their lack of enthusiasm over this exciting technology bothered me, but it did not dissuade me from work. What I was seeing in the brain was real and changed the lives of many patients. But I did not like the adversarial environment of those meetings and decided to keep a low profile, expecting others would do the research. Then nine-year-old Andrew came into my clinic.

Andrew is a very special child. He is my godson and nephew. Until about a year and a half before he came to my clinic as a patient, he had been happy and active. But then his personality changed. He appeared depressed. He had serious aggressive outbursts and he complained to his mother of suicidal and homicidal thoughts (very abnormal for a nine-year-old). He drew pictures of himself hanging from a tree. He drew pictures of himself shooting other children. When he attacked a little girl on the baseball field for no particular reason, his mother called me late at night in tears. I told Sherrie to bring Andrew to see me the next day. His parents drove straight to my clinic, which was eight hours from their home in southern California.

As I sat with Andrew's parents and then with Andrew I knew something wasn't right. I had never seen him look so angry or so sad. He had no explanations for his behavior. He did not report any form of abuse. Other children were not bullying him. There was no family history of serious psychiatric illnesses. He had not sustained a recent head injury. Unlike in most clinical situations, I knew firsthand that he had a wonderful family. Andrew's parents were loving, caring, pleasant people. What was the matter?

The vast majority of my psychiatric colleagues would have placed Andrew on some sort of medication and had him see a counselor for psychotherapy. Having performed more than one thousand SPECT studies by that time, I first wanted a picture of Andrew's brain. I wanted to know what we were dealing with. But with the hostility from my colleagues fresh in my mind, I wondered whether Andew's problem wasn't completely psychological. Perhaps there was a family problem that I just didn't know about. Maybe Andrew was acting out because his older brother was a "perfect" child who did well in school and was very athletic. Maybe Andrew had these thoughts and behaviors to ward off feelings of insecurity related to being the second son in a Lebanese family (I had personal knowledge of this scenario). Maybe Andrew wanted to feel powerful and these behaviors were associated with issues of control. Then logic took over my mind. Nine-year-old children do not normally think about suicide or homicide. I needed to scan his brain. If it was normal, then we would look further for underlying emotional problems.

I went with Andrew to the imaging center and held his hand while he had the study performed. Andrew sat in a chair while the technician placed a small intravenous needle in his arm. Several minutes later a very small dose of a radioisotope was injected through the needle while Andrew played a concentration game on a laptop computer. Shortly thereafter, the needle was taken out of his arm and he went into the imaging room next door. He climbed onto the SPECT table and lay on his back. The imaging camera took fifteen minutes to rotate slowly around his head. As his brain appeared on the computer screen, I thought there had been a mistake in performing the procedure. Andrew had *no* left temporal lobe! Upon quick examination of the complete study, I realized the quality of the scan was fine. He was indeed missing his left temporal lobe. Did he have a cyst, a tumor, a prior stroke? A part of me felt scared for him as I was looking at the monitor. Another part of me felt relieved that we had some explanation for his aggressive behavior. My research and the research of others had implicated the left temporal lobe in aggression. The next day Andrew had an MRI (an anatomical brain study) which showed a cyst (a fluid-filled sac) about the size of a golf ball occupying the space where his left temporal lobe should have been. I knew the cyst had to be removed. Getting someone to take this seriously proved frustrating, however.

Andrew's Missing Left Temporal Lobe

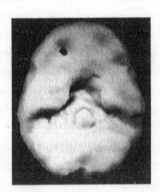

3-D underside surface view

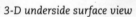

Normal study

Andrew's brain
Missing left temporal lobe

That day I called Andrew's pediatrician and informed him of the clinical situation and brain findings. I told him to find the best person possible to take this thing out of Andrew's head. He contacted three pediatric neurologists. All of them said that Andrew's negative behavior was probably not in any way related to the cyst in his brain and they would not recommend operating on him until he had "real symptoms." When the pediatrician relayed this information, I became furious. *Real symptoms!* I had a child with homicidal and suicidal thoughts who was losing control over his behavior and attacking people. I contacted a pediatric neurologist in San Francisco, who told me the same thing. I then called a friend of mine at Harvard Medical School, also a pediatric neurologist, who told me yet again the same thing. She even used the words "real symptoms." I practically jumped down her throat; how more real could Andrew's symptoms be? "Oh, Dr. Amen," the neurologist replied, "when I say 'real symptoms,' I mean symptoms like seizures or speech problems." Could the medical profession really not connect the brain to behavior? I was appalled! But I wasn't going to wait until this child killed himself or someone else. I called pediatric neurosurgeon Jorge Lazareff at UCLA and told him about Andrew. He told me that he had operated on three other children with left temporal lobe cysts who had all been aggressive. He wondered if it was related. Thankfully, after evaluating Andrew, he agreed to remove the cyst.

When Andrew woke up from the surgery, he smiled at his mother. It was the first time in a year that he had smiled. His aggressive thoughts were gone, and his temperament changed back to that of the sweet child he had been before the age of seven. Andrew was lucky. He had someone who loved him paying attention to his brain when his behavior was off. With this very personal experience in my heart, I decided that I had to share our SPECT work with a larger audience, no matter how much criticism came my way. There were too many children, teenagers, and adults like Andrew who had clear brain abnormalities whom society was just writing off as bad human beings.

Now, only a few years later, the situation has come full circle. I have presented the information in this book to thousands of medical and mental health professionals across North America: in medical schools, at national medical meetings, and even at the prestigious National Institutes of Health. I have published much of this research in chapters in medical books and in journal articles. In 1996 I was invited to give the State of the Art Lecture in Medicine to the Society of Developmental Pediatrics. Clearly there is much more research to do, but many of my colleagues are beginning to see that this work can change our understanding of why people do what they do and give guidance for a new way of thinking about and healing people hurting from detectable and correctable brain abnormalities.

This book will teach you that human behavior is more complex than society's damning labels would have us believe. We are far too quick to attribute people's actions to a bad character when the source of their actions may not be their choice at all, but a problem with brain physiology. One teenage boy, for example, who was brought in to see me for both suicidal and violent tendencies, had a temporal lobe problem that responded positively to antiseizure medication. He was not a "bad kid" after all. As he told his mother later, "I always wanted to be polite, but my brain wouldn't let me." How many "bad kids" sitting in young offenders' institutions would prove to be perfectly nice people with the right treatment? Sometimes people aren't being loving, industrious, cheerful, peaceful, obedient, or kind not because they wouldn't like to be, but because something is wrong with their brain, something that is potentially fixable.

When a person gets treatment that doesn't work, either because the diagnosis is wrong or the operating theory of the therapist is outdated, things get worse. People wonder, "What is wrong with me? Am I not trying hard enough? Am I not good enough? Am I not meant to be happy or well? I am even a failure at getting help for myself." I have found that most people indeed want to be better. When they struggle, it is most often not for a lack of trying, thinking, or motivation. For many people, we as professionals just didn't have the right answers.

Until recently, scientists had no sophisticated tools for evaluating a working brain. Standard brain MRI (magnetic resonance imaging) scans and CAT (computerized axial tomography) scans, available since the 1970s, are anatomical studies, and although they can evaluate what a brain looks like physically, they cannot provide information on how well the brain works. EEGs (electroencephalograms) help in some cases by measuring electrical activity in the brain, but this information provides little sophisticated information on the workings of the deep structures in the brain. SPECT studies, on the other hand, show very nicely what happens in various parts of the brain when you try to activate them. With this tool, I and my colleagues in the United States have been able to correlate over- and under-functioning of different brain parts with certain abnormal behaviors in patients. Also available at this time are two other sophisticated brain studies that are also very useful for studying brain function, functional MRI (fMRI) and PET (positron emission tomography). Each one has its advantages and disadvantages. At this time, in my opinion, due to cost, ease of use, and availability, SPECT is our diagnostic tool of choice.

It is important to note that having an abnormal SPECT scan is not an excuse for "bad behavior." SPECT adds to our knowledge about and understanding of behavior, but it does not provide all the answers. Many people who have difficulties in their brains never do anything harmful or destructive to others. These scans need to be interpreted in the context of each clinical situation.

Not all scientists will agree with every finding in this book. The information here is based largely on extensive clinical experience and research. The Brain Imaging Division of the Amen Clinic for Behavioral Medicine has done more brain SPECT studies for psychiatric reasons than any other clinic I know of in the world. Experience is one of the best teachers in medicine. Second, I have had the privilege of working closely with a nuclear medicine doctor, Jack Paldi, who has a passion for applying his knowledge to psychiatry. Third, we have had the use of one of the best SPECT cameras available, which provides more and better information than older cameras.

The purpose of this book is not to encourage readers to go out and get their brains scanned. You don't need a SPECT scan to benefit from this book. In fact, if you go to a medical center that has little experience with SPECT, the results are not likely to mean much to your doctor. My goal is to help explain a wide variety of human behaviors, both aberrant and normal, by showing the images of the brain that SPECT provides. These images make it plain that many problems long thought of as psychiatric in nature—depression, panic disorders, attention deficit hyperactivity disorders—are actually medical problems that can be treated using a medical model, along with the traditional psychological and sociological models. I hope that by providing new insights into how the brain works, you'll gain a deeper understanding of your own feelings and behavior and the feelings and behaviors of others. And I hope you'll use the specific brain-based "prescriptions" to optimize the patterns in the brain to help you be more effective in your day-to-day life.

1

For Those Who Have Eyes,
Let Them See:

Images into the Mind

What is SPECT? An acronym for single *photon* emission computerized tomography, it is a sophisticated nuclear medicine study that "looks" directly at cerebral blood flow and indirectly at brain activity (or metabolism). In this study, a radioactive isotope (which, as we will see, is akin to myriad beacons of energy or light) is bound to a substance that is readily taken up by the cells in the brain.

A small amount of this compound is injected into the patient's vein, where it runs through the bloodstream and is taken up by certain receptor sites in the brain. The radiation exposure is similar to that of a head CT or an abdominal X-ray. The patient then lies on a table for about fifteen minutes while a SPECT "gamma" camera rotates slowly around his head. The camera has special crystals that detect where the compound (signaled by the radioisotope acting like a beacon of light) has gone. A supercomputer then reconstructs offline images of brain activity levels. The elegant brain snapshots that result offer us a sophisticated bloodflow/metabolism brain map. With these maps, doctors have been able to identify certain patterns of brain activity that correlate with psychiatric and neurological illnesses.

SPECT studies belong to a branch of medicine called nuclear medicine. Nuclear (refers to the nucleus of an unstable or radioactive atom) medicine uses radioactively tagged compounds (radiopharmaceuticals). The unstable atoms emit gamma rays as they decay, with each gamma ray acting like a beacon of light. Scientists can detect those gamma rays with film or special crystals and can record an accumulation of the number of beacons that have decayed in each area of the brain. These unstable atoms are essentially tracking devices—they track which cells are most active and have the most blood flow and those that are least active and have the least blood flow. SPECT studies actually show which parts of the brain are activated when we concentrate, laugh, sing, cry, visualize, or perform other functions.

Nuclear medicine studies measure the physiological functioning of the body, and they can be used to diagnose a multitude of medical conditions: heart disease, certain forms of infection, the spread of cancer, and bone and thyroid disease. My own area of expertise in nuclear medicine, the brain, uses SPECT studies to help in the diagnosis of head trauma, dementia, atypical or unresponsive mood disorders, strokes, seizures, the impact of drug abuse on brain function, and atypical or unresponsive aggressive behavior.

During the late 1970s and 1980s SPECT studies were replaced in many cases by the sophisticated anatomical CAT and later MRI studies. The resolution of those studies was far superior to SPECT's in delineating tumors, cysts, and blood clots. In fact, they nearly eliminated the use of SPECT studies altogether. Yet despite their clarity, CAT scans and MRIs could offer only images of a static brain and its anatomy; they gave little or no information on the activity in a working brain. It was analogous to looking at the parts of a car's engine without being able to turn it on. In the last decade, it has become increasingly recognized that many neurological and psychiatric disorders are not disorders of the brain's anatomy, but problems in how it functions.

Two technological advancements have encouraged the use, once again, of SPECT studies. Initially, the SPECT cameras were single-headed, and they took a long time—up to an hour—to scan a person's brain. People had trouble holding still that long, and the images were fuzzy, hard to read (earning nuclear medicine the nickname "unclear medicine"), and did not give much information about the functioning deep within the brain. Then multiheaded cameras were developed that could image the brain much faster and with enhanced resolution. The advancement of computer technology also allowed for improved data acquisition from the multiheaded systems. The higher-resolution SPECT studies of today can see into the deeper areas of the brain with far greater clarity and show what CAT scans and MRIs cannot—how the brain actually functions.

SPECT studies can be displayed in a variety of different ways. Traditionally the brain is examined in three different planes: horizontally (cut from top to bottom), coronally (cut from front to back), and sagittally (cut from side to side). What do doctors see when they look at a SPECT study? We examine it for symmetry and activity levels, indicated by shades of color (in different color scales selected depending on the doctor's preference, including gray scales), and compare it to what we know a normal brain looks like. The black-and-white images in this book are mostly two kinds of three-dimensional (3–D) images of the brain.

One kind is a **3–D surface image,** looking at the blood flow of the brain's cortical surface. These images are helpful for picking up areas of good activity as well as underactive areas. They are helpful when investigating, for instance, strokes, brain trauma, and the effects of drug abuse. A normal 3–D surface scan shows good, full, symmetrical activity across the brain's cortical surface.

The **3–D active brain image** compares average brain activity to the hottest 15 percent of activity. These images are helpful for picking up areas of overactivity, as seen, for instance, in active seizures, obsessive-compulsive disorder, anxiety problems, and certain forms of depression. A normal 3–D active scan shows increased activity (seen by the light color) in the back of the brain (the cerebellum and visual or occipital cortex) and average activity everywhere else (shown by the background grid).

Doctors are usually alerted that something is wrong in one of three ways: they see too much activity in a certain area; they see too little activity in a certain area; or they see asymmetrical areas of activity that ought to be symmetrical.

In the rest of the book, I will go into greater detail about how this remarkable technology has touched people's lives. For now, however, I will simply offer a sample of five common ways in which SPECT studies are utilized in medicine.

1. *To make early intervention possible.* Ellen, sixty-three, was suddenly paralyzed on the right side of her body. Unable even to speak, she was in a panic and her family was extremely concerned. As drastic as these symptoms were, two hours after the event, her CAT scan was still normal. Suspecting a stroke, the emergency room doctor ordered a brain SPECT study that showed a hole of activity in her left frontal lobe caused by a clot that had choked off the blood supply to this part of the brain. From this information, it was clear that Ellen had had a stroke, and her doctors were able to take measures to limit the extent of the damage. CAT scans are generally not abnormal until twenty-four hours after a stroke.

Normal 3–D Brain SPECT Studies

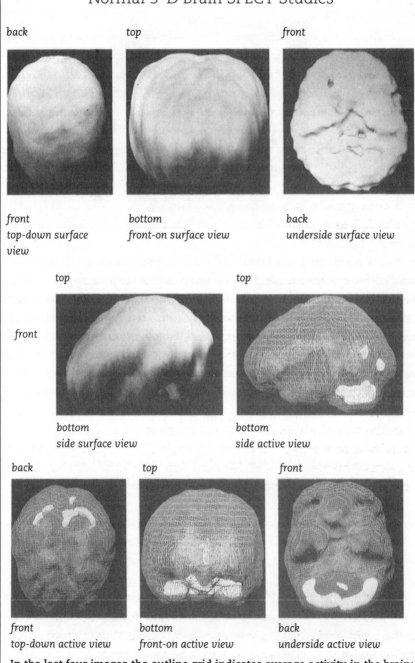

back

top

front

front
top-down surface
view

bottom
front-on surface view

back
underside surface view

top

top

front

bottom
side surface view

bottom
side active view

back

top

front

front
top-down active view

bottom
front-on active view

back
underside active view

In the last four images the outline grid indicates average activity in the brain; the light color indicates the most active 15 percent of the brain. The back of the brain is normally the most active part.

Ellen's Stroke-Affected Brain

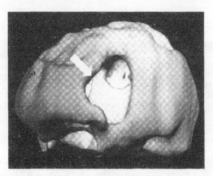

3–D left-side surface view
Notice the large hole, which indicates a left frontal lobe stroke.

2. *To evaluate the patient accurately so that future illness can be prevented.* Nancy was a fifty-nine-year-old woman suffering from severe depression that had been nonresponsive to treatment. She was admitted to a psychiatric hospital, where a SPECT study was done to evaluate her condition. Since she had not experienced any symptoms that would point to this, I was surprised to see that she had had two large strokes. Nearly immediately her nonresponsive depression made more sense to me. Sixty percent of the people who have frontal lobe strokes experience severe depression within a year. As a result of the SPECT study, I

Nancy's Brain, Affected by Two Strokes

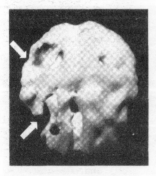
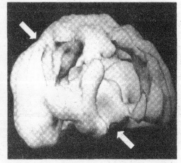

3-D top-down surface view   *3-D right-side surface view*
Notice the two large holes, which indicate two right-brain strokes.

sought immediate consultation with a neurologist, who evaluated her for the possible causes of the stroke, such as plaques in the arteries of the neck or abnormal heart rhythms. He felt the stroke had come from a blood clot and placed her on blood-thinning medication to prevent further strokes.

3. *To help the doctor elicit understanding and compassion from the patient's family.* When Frank, a wealthy, well-educated man, entered his seventies, he began to grow forgetful. At first it was over small things, but as time went on, the lapses of memory progressed to the point where he often forgot essential facts of his life: where he lived, his wife's name, and even his own name. His wife and children, not understanding his change in behavior, were annoyed with his absentmindedness and often angry at him for it. Frank's SPECT study showed a marked suppression across the entire brain, but especially in the frontal lobes, parietal lobes, and temporal lobes. This was a classic Alzheimer's disease pattern. By showing the family these images and pointing out the physiological cause of Frank's forgetfulness in living images, I helped them understand that he was not trying to be annoying, but had a serious medical problem.

Consequently, instead of blaming him for his memory lapses, Frank's family began to show compassion toward him, and they developed strategies to deal more effectively with the problems of living with a person who has Alzheimer's disease. In addition, I placed Frank

Frank's Brain, Affected by Alzheimer's Disease

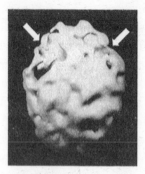 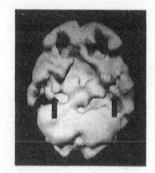

3-D top-down surface view *3-D underside surface view*

Notice marked overall suppression, especially in the parietal lobes (arrows, left image) and temporal lobes (arrows, right image).

on new treatments for Alzheimer's disease that seemed to slow the progression of the illness.

4. *To differentiate between two problems with similar symptoms.* I first met Margaret when she was sixty-eight years old. Her appearance was ragged and unkempt. She lived alone, and her family was worried because she appeared to have symptoms of serious dementia. They finally admitted her to the psychiatric hospital where I worked after she nearly burned the house down by leaving a stove burner on. When I consulted with the family, I also found out that Margaret often forgot the names of her own children and frequently got lost when driving her car. Her driving habits deteriorated to the point where the Department of Motor Vehicles (DMV) had to take away her license after four minor accidents in a six-month period. At the time when Margaret's family saw me, some members had had enough and were ready to put her into a supervised living situation. Other family members, however, were against the idea and wanted her hospitalized for further evaluation.

While at first glance it may have appeared that Margaret was suffering from Alzheimer's disease, the results of her SPECT study showed full activity in her parietal and temporal lobes. If she had Alzheimer's, there should have been evidence of decreased blood flow in those areas. Instead, the only abnormal activity shown on Margaret's SPECT was in the deep limbic system at the center of the brain, where the activity was increased. Often, this is a finding in people suffering from depression. Sometimes in the elderly it can be difficult to distinguish between Alzheimer's disease and depression because the symptoms can be similar. Yet with pseudodementia (depression masquerading as dementia), a person may appear demented, yet not be at all. This is an important distinction, because a diagnosis of Alzheimer's disease would lead to prescribing a set of coping strategies to the family and possibly new medications, whereas a diagnosis of some form of depression would lead to prescribing an aggressive treatment of antidepressant medication for the patient along with psychotherapy.

The results of Margaret's SPECT study convinced me that she should try the antidepressant Zyban (bupropion). After three weeks, she was talkative, well groomed, and eager to socialize with the other patients. After a month in the hospital she was released to go home. Before discharge she asked if I would write a letter to the DMV to help her get her driver's license back. Since I drive on the same highways she

Margaret's Pseudodementia-Affected Brain

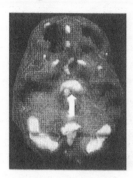 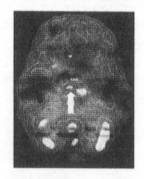

3-D underside active view
before treatment

3-D underside active view
after treatment

Before treatment notice good overall activity, with increased deep limbic system activity (center arrow); after treatment with Zyban the deep limbic system normalizes.

does, I was a bit hesitant. I told her that if in six months she remained improved and she was compliant with treatment, I would write to the DMV for her. Six months later she remained markedly improved. I repeated her SPECT study. It was completely normal. I wrote the letter to the DMV, and it gave her back her license!

5. *To discern when a problem is the result of abuse and remove the patient from a dangerous environment.* Betty was the most beautiful eighty-eight-year-old woman I had ever met. She was very proper and very proud. When she was young she had emigrated from England after marrying an American soldier. It was not her ninety-year-old husband who brought her to the hospital to see me, however, it was her sister. Her husband, far from being supportive, angrily denied that his wife was suffering from serious cognitive problems. Yet during the evaluation process it was clear that Betty had severe memory problems; she did not know where she lived, her phone number, or her husband's name. I ordered a SPECT study that showed a dent in the right side of Betty's frontal lobe. It was obvious to me that she had at some point suffered a significant head injury. When I asked her about it, all she could do was look down and cry; she could not give me details of the event. When I asked her sister, she reported that Betty and her husband had a stormy relationship and that he was abusive toward her. Sometimes he would

Betty's Trauma-Affected Brain

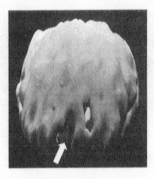

3-D front-on surface view

Notice the areas of decreased activity in the right frontal cortex.

grab her by the hair and slam her head into the wall. The sister wanted Betty to go to the police, but Betty had said it would only make things worse.

Shortly after Betty was hospitalized, her husband began pressuring me to send her home. He kept protesting that there was nothing wrong with her, yet I knew that Betty needed to be removed from her home environment, so I contacted Adult Protective Services. At Betty's hearing, I used her SPECT studies to convince the judge that her home held potential danger. He then ordered her to have a conservator, and she went to live with her sister.

It will be clear from these and many other stories in this book that a doctor who can give an accurate diagnosis can be the greatest friend a patient can have. By now, you may be starting to understand why this technology has so forcefully grabbed my attention.

2

Carving Knives and Tooth Fairies:

A Prelude to the Brain and Behavior

When I first started my brain-imaging research, I decided to study the brain patterns of my own family, including my mother, my aunt, my wife, all three of my children, and myself. I wanted to see if the patterns I was seeing correlated with those of the people of whom I had the most intimate knowledge. I quickly learned that getting my own brain scanned was not an easy experience. Even with all that I have accomplished in my life, I was still very anxious about going through the procedure. What if something was wrong with my brain? What if my brain showed the pattern of a murderer? What if nothing was there at all? I never felt more naked than after my scan, when my own brain activity was projected onto a computer screen in front of my colleagues. At that moment, I would have rather been without clothes than without the covering of my skull. I was relieved to see very good activity in nearly all of my brain. I saw an area of overactivity, however, that stood out like a red Christmas tree light in the right side of my basal ganglia (a deep brain structure that controls the body's anxiety level). It was working too hard. Of note, my mother (who tends to be a bit anxious) and my aunt (who has been clinically diagnosed with a panic disorder) both had the same pattern (increased activity in the right side of the basal ganglia). As we have discovered, these problems often run in families.

The little Christmas tree light made sense to me. Even though I do not have a clinical disorder, my whole life I have struggled with minor issues of anxiety. I used to bite my nails and sometimes still do when I feel anxious. I used to find it very difficult to ask for payments from patients after therapy sessions. I also had a terrible time speaking in front of large groups (which I now love). My first appearance on television was terrible. My hands sweated so much that I unknowingly rubbed them on my trousers throughout the interview. Right before my second television interview, on the nationally syndicated *Sonya Live* on CNN, I nearly had a panic attack. While I was sitting in the greenroom in the CNN studio in Los Angeles waiting to go on the air, my mind flooded with negative thoughts. I started to predict disaster for myself: I might say something stupid. Stumble over my words. Basically make an idiot of myself in front of two million people. Thankfully, in time I recognized what was happening to me. I reminded myself, "I treat people who have this problem. Breathe with your belly. Think good thoughts. Remember the times when you were most competent. Relax; after the show is over most people are going to go back to thinking about themselves and not you anyway, no matter how good or how bad you are." I used the "Basal Ganglia Prescriptions," which I will give in chapter 6, to successfully deal with my anxiety. The interview was a delight.

I also hate conflict. This isn't surprising; any situation that triggers uncomfortable feelings, such as anxiety, causes a person with basal ganglia problems to avoid the situation. Conflict avoidance has had a negative impact on my life, and left me unable to deal with some difficult situations at school or in my professional life. As I thought about

Dr. A.'s Anxiety-Affected Brain

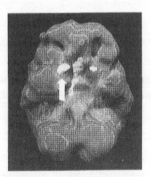

3-D underside active view
Notice increased activity in right basal ganglia area (arrow).

the increased activity in the right side of my basal ganglia, I realized it was a hereditary pattern (my mother and aunt had this same SPECT pattern). Knowing this has helped me to develop and *use* basal ganglia prescriptions to overcome the biological brain pattern that was subjecting me to anxiety.

Michelle

Sometimes these patterns are subtle, and sometimes they are more pronounced. Here are four more examples that highlight the connection between the brain and behavior. On three separate occasions, Michelle, a thirty-five-year-old nurse, left her husband. Each time she left him within the ten days before the onset of her menstrual period. The third time her irritability, anger, and irrational behavior escalated to the point where she attacked him with a knife over a minor disagreement. The next morning, her husband was on the phone to my office. When I first met Michelle, it was several days after her menstrual period had started and things had significantly settled down. The severe temper outbursts were usually over by the third day after her period started. In my office, she appeared to be a gentle, soft-spoken woman. It was hard for me to imagine that this woman had only days before gone after her husband with a carving knife. Because her actions were so serious, I decided to perform two brain SPECT studies on her. The first one was done four days before the onset of her next period—during the roughest time in her cycle—and the second one was done eleven days later—during the calmest time of her cycle.

My colleagues and I have observed that left-side brain problems often correspond with a tendency toward significant irritability, even violence. On Michelle's brain study before the onset of her period, her deep limbic system (the mood control center) near the center of her brain was significantly overactive, especially on the left side. This "focal" deep limbic finding (on one side as opposed to both sides) often correlates with cyclical tendencies toward depression and irritability. There was a dramatic change in her second scan taken eleven days later when Michelle was feeling better. The deep limbic system was normal!

Contrary to the beliefs of some naysayers, PMS, or premenstrual syndrome, is real. Women with PMS are *not* imagining things; the chemistry of their brain is genuinely altered and produces reactions they cannot control. The deep limbic system has a higher density of estrogen receptors than other parts of the brain, making it more vulnerable, in some women, to the estrogen changes that occur at puberty, before the onset of menses, after a baby is born, or during menopause. Sometimes these changes can produce dramatic effects. For women like Michelle, PMS can be debilitating or even dangerous—and thus we must pay attention to it. I have seen the same general pattern in other couples I have counseled whom I saw with Michelle and her husband. During the best time of the woman's cycle, the two people get along. During the worst time, there is fighting and alienation.

I often prescribe an antiseizure medication called Depakote (valproate semisodium) for people who have cyclic mood disorders like manic-depressive disorder. Because Michelle's SPECT findings showed an area of focal intensity in the left side of her deep limbic system (a finding I often see in someone who has a cyclic mood disorder), I put her on Depakote. It evened out her moods very nicely. We tried taking her off the Depakote after nine months, but her symptoms returned quickly. Her husband and best friend called me within the month to beg me to put her back on it. Two years on Depakote seemed to be the magic number. It was only then that Michelle was able to gradually stop taking the medication without relapse.

Michelle's PMS-Affected Brain (Before and After)

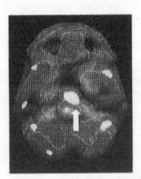 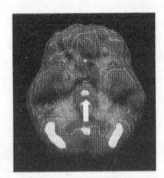

3-D underside active view

Left picture is four days before onset of period; notice increased deep limbic activity (arrow). Right picture is seven days after onset of period; notice normal deep limbic activity (arrow).

Brian

Brian, age six, was very excited the night he lost his first tooth. His tooth was secure under his pillow in a special pouch for the tooth fairy. The next morning Brian was ecstatic when he found money in the pouch. All day long he thought and thought and thought about the tooth fairy. He was so happy, in fact, that he secretly pulled out another tooth after school. His mother, who was surprised by the other tooth, went through the tooth fairy ritual again. Two days later Brian pulled out a third tooth. His mother started to worry when she saw Brian tugging at a tooth she knew wasn't loose. She told him that the tooth fairy doesn't come if you pull out your own teeth. She told him not to do it anymore. There was no tooth fairy that night. Over the next month, however, Brian couldn't get the thought of the tooth fairy out of his head and he pulled out three more teeth. His mother brought him to me for an evaluation.

In Brian's family there was a history of alcohol abuse, depression, and obsessive-compulsive disorder. Behavioral interventions were not successful in keeping Brian's hands out of his mouth. Additionally Brian was oppositional and had trouble at school. The teacher said he "always got stuck on certain thoughts" and could not pay attention to his classwork. After several months, individual therapy was not progressing. I ordered a brain SPECT study to better understand the functional pattern of Brian's brain. His study revealed marked increased activity in the top middle portion of his frontal lobes (the cingulate

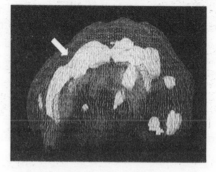

Brian's Brain

3-D side active view

Note markedly increased cingulate activity.

area, with which you will become very familiar). This part of the brain allows you to shift your attention from one thing to another. When it is overactive, people may end up getting "stuck" on certain thoughts and behaviors. Given the intense level of overactivity in this part of his brain, I put Brian on a low dose of Lustral (sertraline—an antiobsessive antidepressant that is known to cool down this part of the brain). Within several weeks the compulsive teeth-pulling disappeared and Brian was more attentive in class.

Marriage and the Brain

The Bentleys

The Bentley family came to see me because their two children were having problems in school. Ten-year-old Wendy was talking too much in class, not finishing her work, and frequently distracted. Seven-year-old Charles was often out of his seat, aggressive with the other boys, off task, poorly organized, and seemingly loved to be in the middle of trouble. The teachers had been telling the parents, Bob and Betsy, to seek help for Charles since preschool. During the evaluation, the parents told me they had a solid marriage with little conflict.

The children were both diagnosed with a condition known as attention deficit hyperactivity disorder (ADHD), a genetic, neurobiological disorder that affects approximately 5 percent of children in the United States and approximately 1.7 percent of the U.K. population. It is characterized by a short attention span, distractibility, disorganization, and often, although not always, hyperactivity and impulse-control problems. The parents and children were educated about ADHD, the teachers were involved in discussions about the children, medication was prescribed, and the parents took a parent training class to become more effective in dealing with the children at home.

After several weeks, Wendy had a very positive response to treatment. She was doing better in school, she got her homework done more quickly and accurately, and she was better able to manage her behavior in the classroom. Charles was a different story. He continued to have problems with his behavior at school and home; nothing seemed to help. During several individual sessions with Charles, I found that he was under severe stress. Despite what his parents had initially told me about themselves, they fought nearly every night and he was very worried they would get divorced. Charles told me about the yelling matches, slamming doors, and threats of leaving. "I can't think of doing my schoolwork when I'm so worried about my parents getting a divorce." I discussed this information with his parents. They readily agreed that there was a lot of tension between them, but they didn't think it had anything to do with the children's problems. They had no idea how much it was bothering Charles. They agreed to come for marriage counseling once a week.

I have two couches in my office. I can tell a lot about a couple by where they sit. If they sit on the same couch there is a willingness to be close, less so if they are on different couches. This couple sat on the opposite end of each couch, as far away from each other as possible. I usually have fun when I do marriage counseling. I find it satisfying to see couples and families become closer and more loving. I help them clarify their goals in the relationship and teach them the skills they need to reach those goals. Working with Bob and Betsy, however, was anything but fun. The fury between them was often so intense that others in my clinic knew when they were in my office. For nearly nine months they talked about divorce at every session. Despite the therapy, they fought nearly every night. I wondered what kept them together.

Without clear structure and interventions from me, the sessions would take on a pattern. After they told me about the traumatic fights of the week, Betsy would bring up an issue from the past and go over and over and over it, despite my attempts to encourage her in a more constructive direction. She had severe problems letting go of prior events or disappointments. She held on to grudges from many years ago, with Bob and others, and she continually brought up the same problems. Bob, on the other hand, never really seemed to pay attention. As soon as Betsy started to talk, he would look away, as if he were off in some distant place. I found myself frequently having to bring him back to the therapy session. When he entered the conversation, it was often with some snide remark. Then his attention would wander again. He reminded me of a hit-and-run driver: Cause a problem, then leave the scene.

After nine months of "marital therapy" going nowhere, Charles was getting worse. One day after seeing him for an individual session, I called his parents into my office. "Look," I said, "both of you are trying really hard to make this work. Yet it is *not* working. The tension at home is damaging your kids, especially Charles. Either you should get an amicable divorce and give yourselves and these kids some peace, or let me scan your brains and see if I'm not missing a biological piece to your marriage puzzle." They agreed to get the set of brain studies.

As I looked at their brain scans with the experience of seeing them as a couple for nine months, the results made perfect clinical sense to me. In fact, I was irritated with myself that I hadn't done it earlier. The cingulate part of Betsy's brain was extremely overactive, causing her to be unable to shift her attention and to become tenaciously locked on to certain thoughts or ideas. Her brain was causing her to go over and over the same material. Bob, on the other hand, had a normal brain pattern at rest, but when he performed a concentration task, the front part of his brain, which should increase in activity during concentration, completely shut down. This meant that the harder he tried to pay attention to Betsy, the more his attention wandered. He often sought conflict as a way to stimulate his own brain. Bob's symptoms and his brain study clearly indicated he had ADHD like his kids (ADHD is usually a genetic disorder).

It was now clear to me that this couple's problems existed, at least in part, on a biological level. I needed to optimize their brain biology if the therapy was going to do any good at all. I placed Betsy on Prozac (fluoxetine). Prozac, like Lustral, decreases overactivity of the cingulate and allows people to shift their attention more freely between topics

Betsy's Overfocused Brain

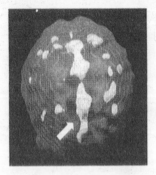

3-D top-down active view
Note markedly increased cingulate activity.

and become less stuck on thoughts and behaviors. I think of these medications as "lubricants" for the brain's shifting mechanism. I put Bob on Ritalin, which is a stimulant medication that helps children and adults with ADHD concentrate, stay on task, and be less impulsive. I'm sure there are some people who would strongly object to marital therapy through the use of medication, but in this case I believed it was essential.

Three weeks after they were on medication, there was a dramatic shift in the couple's relationship. My first clue came when they sat on the same couch, next to each other. The second clue was that Betsy had her hand on Bob's leg (a very hopeful sign). They reported that the medications had made a big difference. Betsy stopped nagging and "beating ideas to death." Bob started to pay more attention and be less conflict-driven. There were no more hit and runs. He became more thoughtful. To my delight, with their brains working in more normal ways, they were able to utilize our marital therapy. They spent regular time together, agreed on their parenting strategies together, and even resumed making love on a more regular basis. As Betsy and Bob did better, so did Charles. How many marriages end in divorce or chronic unhappiness because of brain patterns that interfere with intimacy? Later I'll devote a whole chapter to relationships and the brain.

Bob's ADHD-Affected Brain

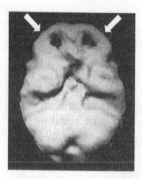 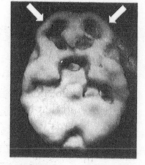

3-D underside surface view

At rest; note good prefrontal activity (arrows).

During concentration; note marked drop-off of prefrontal activity.

Willie

Willie was the kind of guy who got along with everyone. An A student, he had a college scholarship waiting for him, and his future seemed altogether promising—until his head collided with the dashboard when his car accidentally hit a guardrail. Although Willie felt dazed, he seemed to be okay by the next day. Three months later he got into another accident when he swerved to avoid hitting a dog that had run out into the street. His head hit the windshield very hard, and this time he had to be sent to hospital. After examining Willie, the doctor told him he had nothing to worry about; he had only a minor concussion. In the months that followed, however, Willie found that the "minor concussion" was wreaking havoc with his life. Normally a friendly person, he found himself suddenly losing his temper at the smallest things. His whole attitude and demeanor began to change. Where he had once been patient, he now had a short fuse. Where he had once been amiable and calm, he was now always angry. His irritability and constant flares of temper began to alienate his friends and family.

The brunt of his anger came to rest on his college roommate and strangely began to center around food. Inexplicably, Willie's appetite was changing. In just three months, he had put on seventy pounds, and he was hungry all the time. He seemed to be devouring every morsel of food in the house. When his roommate finally got fed up with Willie eating all the groceries and asked Willie to eat only the food he bought himself, Willie felt that by depriving him of the food needed, his roommate was trying to hurt him. Willie was consumed with negative, paranoid thoughts about this person who was "trying to take the food out of his mouth." In his mind, the only way to protect himself against this enemy was to hurt the enemy. One afternoon he took a huge meat cleaver and a butcher knife and waited at the front door for the man who used to be his friend. "He was going to be instantaneously dissolved," Willie later told me.

Yet even as he was gripped by paranoia, some part of Willie's mind was still sane. He saw himself, as if from above, standing behind the door and holding these weapons. He knew he was out of control and that he had to stop himself before it was too late. He went to the telephone and called a friend, who gave him my telephone number, and the immediate crisis was averted.

Willie described for me his two accidents and the severity of his personality changes. I immediately ordered a brain study. As I expected, the study showed abnormalities. Two areas were working too hard: One was in his left temporal lobe, where dysfunction is often associated with paranoia and violence. The second was the top, middle section of the frontal lobes (cingulate area), again, the part of the brain that allows a person to shift attention freely from one thing to another. When this part of the brain is overactive, people get stuck in thought spirals. The minute I saw Willie's brain study, it clearly explained for me the changes that had been occurring in his personality: paranoia, fiery temper, and negative thoughts about his roommate, which he couldn't turn off.

The next step was clear. I prescribed medication to alleviate his symptoms: an antiseizure medication for the temporal lobe abnormality and an antiobsessive antidepressant to help him get "unstuck" from negative thoughts. After several weeks of treatment, the results were dramatic. Willie began to regain his sense of humor and to reconnect with his friends and family. At the time of this writing, it has been six years since his two accidents. Now on medication to control the trauma-induced brain problems, he is one of the nicest human beings you will ever meet.

The brain is the seat of feelings and behavior. Your brain creates your world—a radical statement about ordinary thinking. Yet it is your brain

Willie's Brain, Affected by Head Trauma

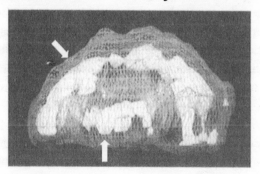

3-D side active view
Note markedly increased cingulate and left temporal lobe activity (arrows).

that perceives and experiences. Everything begins and ends in the brain. How our brains work determines the very quality of our lives: how happy we will be, how well we'll get along with others, how successful we will be in our profession. The brain probably influences how close or how distant we feel from God. The patterns of our brain predispose what kind of husband or wife we will be, whether we will fail in school, be irritable with our children, or have the ambition to strive toward our goals.

Most of us are not a short fuse on a stick of dynamite like Willie before treatment or Michelle during the worst time of her cycle. We do not use meat cleavers or carving knives to deal with others who irritate us. Most of us are warm, kind, reasonable people who want to form meaningful relationships and be successful in our day-to-day lives. When our brain patterns are normal and balanced, we are generally able to do all these things. When behavior becomes abnormal, however, as in the cases mentioned above, often there is something the matter with the patterns in the body's computer—the brain. These case histories demonstrate that *the actual physical patterns of our brain have a dramatic impact on how we think, feel, and behave from moment to moment.* Only recently have we discovered how to recognize those patterns and how to treat them with both behavioral and medical prescriptions.

Unfortunately, there are many professionals who lack sophisticated information on how the brain actually works. They believe the behavior of their patients is primarily the result of environmental stress or conditioning and do not consider the possibility that it may be based on abnormal brain physiology. Willie, for example, could have talked to a therapist about his toilet training until the end of the millennium and it would not have helped him. I believe that we need a more holistic approach to psychotherapy. I believe that we need to understand the role of brain physiology along with other factors such as stress or conditioning before we can design successful treatments for people.

In chapters 3, 5, 7, 9, and 11 I am going to teach you about five different brain systems. Understanding these brain systems will help you understand yourself and others in a totally new way. The activity in these systems provides the basis for much of the behaviors we call human. Each of these chapters will begin with a description of the functions and general locations of each part of the brain. I'll then discuss how each area contributes to everyday behavior as well as to certain medical disorders, such as depression or anxiety. Each of these five chapters will close with a checklist to help you identify yourself or loved ones who may fit into certain categories. In chapters 4, 6, 8, 10, and 12, I'll discuss specific healing and optimization prescriptions.

3

Looking Into Love and Depression:
The Deep Limbic System

FUNCTIONS OF THE DEEP LIMBIC SYSTEM

- *sets the emotional tone of the mind*
- *filters external events through internal states (creates emotional coloring)*
- *tags events as internally important*
- *stores highly charged emotional memories*
- *modulates motivation*
- *controls appetite and sleep cycles*
- *promotes bonding*
- *directly processes the sense of smell*
- *modulates libido*

The deep limbic system lies near the center of the brain. Considering its size—about that of a walnut—it is power-packed with functions, all of which are critical for human behavior and survival.* From an evolutionary standpoint, this is an "older" part of the mammalian brain that enabled animals to experience and express emotions. It freed them from the stereotypical behavior and actions dictated by the brain

* I use the term "deep limbic system" to differentiate it from the classic term "limbic system," which also incorporates the cingulate gyrus and deep temporal lobes, which will be covered in separate chapters. In this definition, the deep limbic system includes the thalamic structures, and hypothalamus, along with the immediate surrounding structures. As I mentioned in the introduction, I have simplified the five brain systems discussed in the book. All of these systems are much more complex and interconnected than presented. Clinically, we have found these divisions helpful to explain much of the behavior we have seen.

The Deep Limbic System

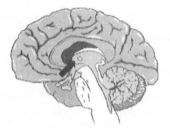

side view

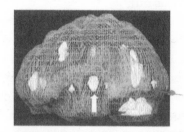

3-D side active view

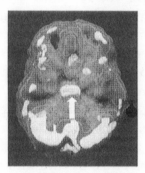

3-D underside active view

stem, found in the older "reptilian" brain. The subsequent evolution of the surrounding cerebral cortex in higher animals, especially humans, gave us the capacity for problem solving, planning, organization, and rational thought. Yet in order for these functions to have an effect in the world, one must have passion, emotion, and the desire to make something happen. The deep limbic system adds the emotional spice, if you will, in both positive and negative ways.

This part of the brain is involved in setting emotional tone. When the deep limbic system is less active, there is generally a positive, more hopeful state of mind. When it is heated up, or overactive, negativity can take over. This finding actually surprised my colleagues at the clinic and me at first. We thought that excessive activity in the part of the brain that controlled emotion might correlate with enhanced feelings of all kinds, not solely negative ones. Yet we noticed, again and again, that when this area was overactive on SPECT, it correlated with the subject's depression and negativity. It seems that when the deep limbic system is inflamed, painful emotional shading results. New research on depression from other laboratories around the world has borne this out.

The emotional shading provided by the deep limbic system is the filter through which you interpret the events of the day. It colors events depending on your emotional state of mind. When you are sad (with an overactive deep limbic system), you are likely to interpret neutral events through a negative filter. For example, if you have a neutral or even positive conversation with someone whose deep limbic system is overactive or "negatively set," he or she is likely to interpret the conversation in a negative way. When this part of the brain is "cool" or functions properly, a neutral or positive interpretation of events is more likely to occur. Emotional tagging of events is critical to survival. The valence or charge we give to certain events in our lives drives us to action (such as approaching a desired mate) or causes avoidance behavior (withdrawing from someone who has hurt us in the past).

PMS, discussed in the last chapter, is a classic example of this emotional shading principle. As mentioned, in our study of PMS within five to ten days before the onset of menstruation, the deep limbic system becomes inflamed or more active with the drop in hormones. This deep limbic activation colors events in a more negative way. A friend's wife has a fairly severe case of PMS. He tells me that during the first week of her cycle, she looks at him with love and affection, and almost anything he does seems to be right. She is more loving and affectionate. Ten days before her period, things are dramatically different. She doesn't want to be touched. She "has a different look," which he describes as a combination of a scowl and a "don't mess with me" look. Little he does is right. She emotionally colors most events in a negative way. Then, a few days after her cycle starts, she's back to being more positive, loving, and affectionate.

The deep limbic system, along with the deep temporal lobes, has also been reported to be involved in storing highly charged emotional memories, both positive and negative. If you have been traumatized by a dramatic event, such as being in a car accident or watching your house burn down, or if you have been abused by a parent or a spouse, the emotional component of the memory is stored in the deep limbic system of the brain. And if you have won the lottery, graduated with distinction, or watched your child's birth, those emotional memories are stored here as well. The total experience of our emotional memories is responsible, in part, for the emotional tone of our mind. The more stable, positive experiences we have, the more positive we are likely to feel; the more trauma in our lives, the more emotionally set we become in a negative way. These emotional memories are intimately involved in the emotional tagging we impose on the day's events.

The deep limbic system also affects motivation and drive. It helps get you going in the morning and encourages you to move throughout the day. Overactivity in this area, in our experience, is associated with lowered motivation and drive, which is often seen in depression. The deep limbic system, especially the hypothalamus, controls the sleep and appetite cycles of the body. Healthy sleep and appetite are essential to maintaining a proper internal milieu. Both of these components are often a problem with limbic abnormalities.

The deep limbic structures are also intimately involved with bonding and social connectedness. When the deep limbic system of animals is damaged, they do not properly bond with their young. In one study of rats, when the deep limbic structures were damaged, mothers would not feed and nurture the young but would drag them around the cage as if they were inanimate objects. The deep limbic system affects the bonding mechanism that enables you to connect socially with other people; your ability to do this successfully in turn influences your moods. We are social animals. When we are bonded to people in a positive way, we feel better about ourselves and our lives. This capacity to bond then plays a significant role in the tone and quality of our moods.

The deep limbic system also directly processes the sense of smell. The olfactory system is the only one of the five sensory systems that goes from the sensory organ to directly where it is processed in the brain. The messages from all the other senses (sight, hearing, touch, and taste) are sent to a "relay station" before they are sent to their final destination in different parts of the brain. Because your sense of smell goes directly to the deep limbic system, it is easy to see why smells can have such a powerful impact on our feeling states. The multibillion-dollar perfume and deodorant industries count on this fact: beautiful smells evoke pleasant feelings and draw people toward you; unpleasant smells repel them.

I learned about the limbic-smell connection firsthand when I was sixteen years old and dating the woman who became my wife. She was a good Catholic girl. As a typical hot-blooded teenager, I was extremely interested in physical affection. One night I ran out of aftershave and borrowed my brother's English Leather. When I picked her up for our date, I noticed a difference. I had a car with a bench seat in front. Usually she sat in the part of the seat nearest to the passenger door. That night she sat in the middle part, next to me. She took my hand before I reached for hers. She came close to me before I moved toward her. She was cuddlier and more affectionate than before. Needless to say, from then on English Leather was the only scent I wore.

Bonding, smells, sexuality, and the deep limbic system are intimately connected. Napoleon once wrote to Josephine to ask her not to bathe for two weeks before he came home from a battle. He wanted her scent to be powerful, because it excited him sexually. It is likely that positive, sexual smells cool the limbic system and intensify our mood for love. Deep limbic overactivity, often associated with depression, frequently results in decreased sexual interest. For many years, I have hypothesized that decreased sexual activity is associated with increased deep limbic activity and more vulnerability to depression.

I studied this phenomenon in an adult male who had problems with depression and increased activity in his deep limbic systems on SPECT. I asked him to make passionate love with his wife. I then rescanned him within an hour. His limbic activity was significantly decreased. Orgasm has been described as a mini-seizure of the limbic system and tends to release or lessen deep limbic activity. Sexuality is good for the bonded human brain.

Whenever a person is sexually involved with another person, neurochemical changes occur in both their brains that encourage limbic, emotional bonding. Yet limbic bonding is the reason casual sex doesn't really work for most people on a whole mind and body level. Two people may decide to have sex "just for the fun of it," yet something is occurring on another level they might not have decided on at all: Sex is enhancing an emotional bond between them whether they want it or not. One person, often the woman, is bound to form an attachment and will be hurt when a casual affair ends. One reason it is usually the woman who is hurt most is that the female limbic system is larger than the male's. One likely consequence is that she will become more limbically connected.

I once treated a patient named Renee who had a high sex drive. She was not sexually satisfied by her husband. For years, other men flirted with her and she remained faithful, until one day she decided, out of pure frustration, to have an affair with a coworker. From the outset, they agreed that they were going to have friendly sex, just for fun, just for the pleasure, and in the first two months that seemed to work. Then Renee felt herself wanting to see him more often. She tried to get him to meet with her twice a week instead of once a week, as they had originally agreed. Instead of responding positively, her lover pulled away. The more attached she became, the more detached he became. Although Renee and her lover had been on the same wavelength in the beginning, in the end she had changed and he hadn't, and she felt used. It is important to understand how your body and psyche work. In this case, Renee would have been wise to realize that her limbic system was not quite as open to casual sex as she wanted to be. She would have been better off to stay with her husband and work things out sexually with him, rather than to pick a casual acquaintance for a sexual liaison.

As mentioned above, current research has demonstrated that females, on average, have a larger deep limbic system than males. This gives females several advantages and disadvantages. Because of their larger deep limbic brain, women are more in touch with their feelings, and they are generally better able to express their feelings than men. They have an increased ability to bond and be connected to others (which is why women are the primary caretakers of children—there is no society on earth where men are primary caretakers of children). Females have a more acute sense of smell, which is likely to have developed from an evolutionary need for the mother to recognize her young. Having a larger deep limbic system leaves a female somewhat more susceptible to depression, especially at times of significant hormonal changes such as the onset of puberty, before menses, after the birth of a child, and at menopause. Women attempt suicide three times more often than men. Yet men's suicide attempts are sucessful three times more often than women's, in part because they use more violent means (women tend to use overdoses with pills while men tend to either shoot or hang themselves), and men are generally less connected to others than are women. Disconnection from others increases the risk of completed suicides.

The deep limbic system, especially the hypothalamus at the base of the brain, is responsible for translating our emotional state into physical feelings of relaxation or tension. The front half of the hypothalamus sends calming signals to the body through the parasympathetic nervous system. The back half of the hypothalamus sends stimulating or fear signals to the body through the sympathetic nervous system. The back half of the hypothalamus, when stimulated, is responsible for the fight-or-flight response, a primitive state that gets us ready to fight or flee when we are threatened or scared. This "hardwired response" happens immediately upon activation, such as seeing or experiencing an emotional or physical threat: The heart beats faster, breathing rate and blood pressure increases, the hands and feet become cooler to shunt blood from the extremities to the big muscles (to fight or run away), and the pupils dilate (to see better). This deep limbic translation of emotion is powerful and immediate. It happens with overt physical threats and also with more covert emotional threats. This part of the brain is intimately connected to the prefrontal cortex and seems to act as a switching station between running on emotion (the deep limbic system) and rational thought and problem solving using our cortex. When the limbic system is turned on, emotions tend to take over. When it is cooled down, more activation is possible in the cortex. Current research shows a correlation between depression and increased deep limbic system activity and shutdown in the prefrontal cortex, especially on the left side.

PROBLEMS IN THE DEEP LIMBIC SYSTEM

- *moodiness, irritability, clinical depression*
- *increased negative thinking*
- *negative perception of events*
- *decreased motivation*
- *flood of negative emotions*
- *appetite and sleep problems*
- *decreased or increased sexual responsiveness*
- *social isolation*

The problems in the deep limbic system (as in all the other systems) generally correspond to their functions. Do you know people who see every situation in a bad light? That pessimism actually could be a deep limbic system problem because, as mentioned, when this part of the brain is working too hard, the emotional filter is colored by negativity. One person could walk away from an interaction that ten others would have labeled as positive, but which he or she considers negative. And since the deep limbic system affects motivation, people sometimes develop an "I don't care" attitude about life and work; they don't have the energy to care. Because they feel hopeless about the outcome, they have little willpower to follow through with tasks.

Since the sleep and appetite centers are in the deep limbic system, disruption can lead to changes, which may mean an inclination toward too much or too little of either. For example, in typical depressive episodes people have been known to lose their appetites and to have trouble sleeping despite being chronically tired, and yet in atypical depression they will sleep and eat excessively.

There are three problems caused by abnormalities of the deep limbic system that warrant their own sections: bonding disruption, mood disorders, and PMS.

Bonding Disruption

Bonding and limbic problems often go hand in hand. One of the most fundamental bonds in the human universe is the mother-infant bond. Hormonal changes shortly after childbirth, however, can cause limbic or emotional problems in the mother. They are called the "baby blues" when they are mild, and postnatal depression or psychosis when they are severe. When these problems arise, the deep limbic system of the mother's brain shows abnormal activity. (The phenomenon has been detected in animals as well as humans.) In turn, significant bonding problems may occur. The mother may emotionally withdraw from the baby, preventing the baby from developing normally. Babies who experience "failure to thrive," for instance, or who have low weight or delayed development, often have mothers who are unattached emotionally.

In such cases, the abnormal activity of the mother's deep limbic system causes developmental problems for the baby. Conversely, problems in the deep limbic system can be caused by outside events that disrupt the human bonding process. This can occur at any stage in life. Here are three of the most common.

Death

The death of a parent, spouse, or child causes intense sadness and grief. In these familial relationships, there is often a tight neurochemical bond (from the myriad of stored emotional memories and experiences). When it is broken, the activity of the deep limbic system is disrupted. Many who experience grief say the pain actually feels physical. This sensation is not imaginary. Grief often activates the pain centers in the brain, which are housed near the deep limbic system.

It is interesting to note that the people who had a good relationship with the person who died often heal their grief much more easily than those whose relationship with the deceased was filled with turmoil, bitterness, or disappointment. The reason is that a positive relationship is associated with good memories, and remembering and reprocessing these memories helps in the healing process. When people who had a bad relationship think back on it, they have to relive the pain. In their mind, they are still trying to fix what was wrong, to heal the wound, but they can't. In addition, the guilt they carry with them impairs the healing process. Donna is a case in point. Donna and her mother had had a stormy relationship, fighting constantly over things that seemed insignificant in and of themselves. Yet in spite of their problems, the year after her mother's death was the hardest of Donna's life. Her husband could not understand the force of her grief; all he had ever heard her do was complain that her mother was selfish and uninterested in her. What he failed to understand was that Donna had to grieve not only over her mother's death, but also over the fact that now she would never have the mother-daughter bond she had always wanted. Death had ended all her hopes.

Losing a spouse or lover is traumatic in a different way from losing any other loved one. Once you have made love with a person on a regular basis, death can be extraordinarily painful because the deep limbic connection has been broken. The spouse has become part of the chemical bond of that part of the brain, and it takes time for that bond to dissolve. Your deep limbic system misses the person's touch, voice, and smell.

Deep limbic connection doesn't depend only on sexual intimacy. Another often-overlooked "deep limbic loss" is the loss of a family pet. Many people become as attached to their pets as they do to the significant people in their lives. Pets often give unconditional love and connect with our innermost caring selves. I have often felt that holding one of my cats or petting my dog during a scan would have a positive "limbic cooling" effect. Unfortunately, while I was writing this chapter my dog, Samantha, died of cancer. The sadness in my family was great, with many tears, especially from my daughters and wife. We all had problems sleeping, no one felt like eating, and anything that reminded us of Samantha would quickly bring up tears and feelings of intense sadness and loss. I have known some pet owners who became so depressed after a pet died that they felt suicidal and even paranoid. Appreciating this significant grief is often necessary to healing.

Divorce

Divorce can be a source of the most severe kind of stress it is possible for a human being to experience. For many, it actually causes more anguish to lose a spouse through divorce than it does through death. As stated above, people who are "limbically connected" have a very powerful bond, and I believe this phenomenon may be one of the major reasons women cannot leave abusive men. They have had their children with these men, shared their beds and their homes with them. To break that bond, which is at the core of their brain, causes a severe rupture that can make the woman feel fragmented, as if she were not quite whole without the man. She may be plagued by sleep and appetite problems, depression, irritability, and social isolation. I once treated a woman who was married to a controlling, angry man whom she could never please. On the day he told her he was leaving her for another woman (causing her a severe limbic injury), she became so depressed that she put her head in the oven and turned on the gas. Fortunately she was rescued and taken to the hospital. It wasn't until her deep limbic system began to heal and she could feel her own autonomy that she realized she didn't even like her husband, and in any case, it certainly wasn't worth killing herself over a man who cheated on her.

Even the one who initiates a separation suffers distress and often goes through a period of depression, because the "chemical limbic bonds" break for everyone involved in the separation. The one who is walking out the door may fail to realize this and not anticipate the grief period that will likely follow. For some, divorce is so devastating that it can trigger enormous anger and vengefulness. In fact, I have never seen two people more cruel to each other than those going through a messy divorce. They lose all sense of fairness and rationality and do everything possible to hurt each other. What ignites such negative responses? Breaking the chemical connection activates the deep limbic system. People become not only depressed and negative but also oversensitive, taking every little thing the wrong way. Anger quickly follows. They know they have to separate, and unconsciously they use the anger and aggression as a way to do it.

The Empty Nest Syndrome

When children leave home, parents often feel intensely sad and bereft. Many lose their appetites and have trouble sleeping. Something is missing. This may be confusing because the parents remember how arduous it was struggling through the growing pains of their offsprings' adolescence, and they assumed it would be a relief when the teenagers were finally out of the house and off to their own lives. (It has been suggested that the discordant nature of the parent-child relationship during adolescence may be nature's way of helping parents and teens make the transition from the close bond of childhood to the total independence of young adulthood.) Yet no matter how difficult those adolescent years were for both sides, a tremendous bond still exists, and breaking it is stressful.

I once treated a man who developed a clinical depression after his only daughter left home for college. Even though he was happily married, enjoyed his work, and was otherwise healthy, he felt sad, cried easily, had trouble sleeping, became more irritable, and had concentration problems—all symptoms of depression. Another woman I treated whose two sons went off to college one year after the other became so depressed and felt so lonely and unimportant that she resorted to having an affair as a way to deal with her pain. She lost her marriage over the affair, became suicidal, and almost lost her life.

Depression

Lack of bonding and depression are often related. People who are depressed often do not feel like being around others and consequently isolate themselves. The social isolation tends to perpetuate itself: The more isolated a person becomes, the less bonding activity occurs. This worsens the depression and increases the likelihood of further isolation.

Depression is known to be caused by a deficit of certain neurochemicals or neurotransmitters, especially noradrenaline and serotonin. In my experience, this deficit can cause increased metabolism or inflammation in the deep limbic system, which in turn causes many of the problems associated with depression. You may have noticed in this chapter how, along with all the other symptoms of deep limbic system disruption, depression seems to be a common factor. Because the deep limbic system is intimately tied to moods, when it is overactive the ensuing problems with depression snowball and affect all the other deep limbic system functions.

Ariel came to see me because she had been experiencing symptoms of depression for over two years. She was tired, suffered from sleeplessness and negative thinking, had no motivation, and had begun to have suicidal thoughts. The symptom that was most difficult for her husband, however, was her complete loss of interest in sex. He was ready to leave her because he thought she wasn't interested in him anymore as a man. Why else, he thought, had it been such a long time since she had wanted to touch him?

After I had her brain scanned, I was not surprised to find that her deep limbic system was on double time. Giving this information to her husband was a powerful tool in helping him to view the situation objectively: His wife was neglecting him not because she didn't like him but because something was off balance in the chemistry of her brain. Most important of all, the problem was rectifiable.

Increased activity in the deep limbic system is part of a pattern that is often responsive to antidepressants, but sometimes people are averse to being put on medication. Ariel was one of them. She had become caught up in the media blitz of 1991, when the hair-raising topic of the news and the talk shows was that Prozac was a dangerous drug that could cause criminally aberrant behavior. It was even reported that it could cause you to kill your mother! I believe this sensationalism was completely irresponsible, especially since it scared many people who suffered from depression, a very treatable illness, and prevented some of them from seeking the help they needed. The fact that medication can cause side effects should not be a blanket deterrent to its use; in many, many cases, the pluses far outweigh the minuses. If you are skeptical about this, consider the following fact: People on antidepressants may experience constipation or an upset stomach, but suicide (often the result of untreated depression) is the eighth leading cause of death in the United States and accounts for one in 100 deaths in the U.K.

Ariel decided against the use of medication. She followed the deep limbic prescriptions (behavioral changes that affect the chemistry of the brain) offered in the next chapter, which I developed specifically to treat depression. Through them she was successful in overcoming her depression. However, the nonmedication prescriptions do not work for everyone and some people may need medication. Let me emphasize the point: Depression is treatable. Please seek help from a qualified professional if you are suffering. Help is out there for you.

Leigh Anne

Here is another example of deep limbic dysfunction. Leigh Anne came to see me fifteen months after the birth of her first child. Several weeks after her child was born, she began experiencing symptoms of nausea, social withdrawal, crying spells, and depression. Three months later she sought help through psychotherapy. But her condition did not improve. Her depression progressed to the point where she became unable to care for her daughter. Desperate to function as the good mother she wanted to be to her child, she came to see me. After diagnosing her with major depression I placed her on Prozac and began seeing her in psychotherapy. Her symptoms remitted after several weeks, and after several months Leigh Anne wanted to discontinue treatment. She associated taking Prozac with a course of action for "a depressed person." She did not want to see herself in that light or be stigmatized by that label. For several months after stopping she had no adverse reaction. Then her symptoms returned.

When she came to see me again, Leigh Anne still didn't want to believe that anything was "wrong" with her, and was still resistant to going back on medication. After I ordered a brain study to evaluate her deep limbic system, I was able to point out to her the marked increase in activity in that area of her brain. It provided me with the evidence needed to convince her to go back on Prozac for a while longer.

Leigh Anne's Depression-Affected Brain

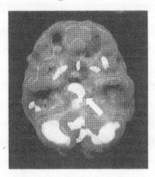

3-D underside active view

Notice increased limbic activity (arrow).

This case illustrates an important point: It has been my experience as well as that of many other psychiatrists that a patient does not necessarily have to stay on medication forever just because he or she has started it. However, with certain medications, like Prozac, a minimum period of treatment is necessary before it can successfully be terminated. If a depressed patient is willing to stay on the medication for long enough, about two years in this case (the time period varies from person to person), there is a greater chance that it can be discontinued with no return of symptoms.

Manic-Depressive Disorder

Sarah

Sarah was fifty-three years old when she was admitted to the hospital under my care. The month before, her family had had her committed to another psychiatric hospital for delusional thinking and bizarre behavior—she had actually ripped out all the electrical wiring in her home because she heard voices coming from the walls. In addition to the above symptoms, she was barely getting any sleep, her thoughts raced wildly, and she was irritable. Her doctor had diagnosed manic-depressive disorder (a cyclical mood disorder) and placed her on lithium (an antimanic medication) and an antianxiety medication. After responding well, she was sent home. But Sarah, like Leigh Anne, did not want to believe that anything was wrong with her, and she stopped taking both medications. Her position was actually fortified by some members of her family who openly told her she didn't need pills, that doctors prescribe them only to force patients into numerous follow-up visits. Yet their advice was ill advised, for within weeks of stopping the treatment, Sarah's bizarre behavior returned. This was when her family brought her to the hospital where I worked. When I first saw Sarah, she was extremely paranoid. Believing that everyone was trying to hurt her, she was always looking for ways to escape from the hospital. Again her thoughts were delusional; she believed she had special powers and that others were trying to take them from her. At times, she also appeared very "spacy." In an attempt to understand what was going on with her for myself, and to convince her that at least part of her problems were biological, I ordered a SPECT study.

Carrying this out did not prove easy. Our clinic tried to scan her on three separate occasions. The first two times she ripped out the intravenous line, saying we were trying to poison her. The third time was a success because her sister stayed with her and calmed her down by talking her through the experience. While the study revealed an overall increase in activity in the deep limbic system, I found more intensity

Sarah's Manic-Depression-Affected Brain

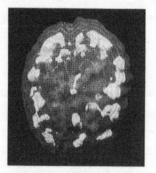

3-D top-down active view

Note patchy uptake throughout the cortex.

on the left side of her scan (focal increased deep limbic uptake) and a markedly patchy uptake across the cortex. In other words, some areas showed increased activity and some showed decreased. My experience told me that cyclic mood disorders often correlate with focal areas of increased activity in the deep limbic system specifically as well as a patchy uptake across the surface of the brain in general.

For Sarah's family, this was powerful evidence that her problems were biological, so that when she refused medication, they were now willing to encourage her to take it. After she accepted their advice, her behavior normalized again. Once I knew she was feeling better, more in control, I showed her the brain studies. Through a better understanding of the problem she was able to agree to follow-up visits and to stay on her medication.

Sometimes I'll rescan a patient several months after the first time to see what difference the medication has made on the physiology of his or her brain. Although Sarah's new study showed a vast improvement from her earlier one, I still noticed an area of increased activity in the left temporal lobe, and Sarah was still complaining of symptoms of spaciness. I changed her medication to Depakote, which is primarily used as an antiseizure medication but has also been used for manic-depressive disorder. Not only did her psychotic symptoms remain in remission, but the spaciness disappeared as well. Five years later, a small dose of Depakote helps Sarah lead a normal life.

Sarah's case illustrates one of the most clinically significant problems in people diagnosed with manic-depressive illness. This disorder is usually quite responsive to medication. The problem is that when people afflicted by the disorder improve, many feel so normal they do not believe they ever had a problem to begin with. It is difficult for people to accept that they have to keep taking medication when they think they no longer have a problem. Yet as we have seen, prematurely stopping medication actually increases the chances of relapsing. Through the use of brain studies I have been able to decrease the relapse rate of my patients by demonstrating graphically the biological nature of their disorders and the need to treat them as such—a great asset in encouraging patients to cooperate in their own healing. In addition to that, brain studies have helped me persuade patients to stop blaming themselves for their symptoms.

PMS

In the last chapter I discussed Michelle's case of clear (and dangerous) PMS. It was a deep limbic problem. Over the past years we have scanned many women with PMS just before the onset of their period, during the most difficult time of their cycle, and then again a week after the onset of their period. Most often when PMS is present we see dramatic differences between the scans. When a woman feels good, her deep limbic system is calm and cool. When she feels bad right before her period, her deep limbic system most often is hot!

I have seen two PMS patterns, clinically and on SPECT, that respond to different treatments. One pattern is focal increased deep limbic activity that correlates with cyclic mood changes. Hotter activity on the left side of the deep limbic system is often associated with anger, irritability, and expressed negative emotion. Increased activity on the right side of the deep limbic system is often associated with sadness, emotional withdrawal, anxiety, and repressed negative emotion. Left-side abnormalities are more a problem for people with whom the woman interacts (because of her outwardly directed anger and irritability), while right-side overactivity is more an internal problem. Focal deep limbic findings, worse during the premenstrual period, often respond best to lithium or anticonvulsant medications, such as Depakote, Neurontin (gabapentin), Lamictal (lamotrigine), or Tegretol (carbamazepine). These medications tend to even out moods, calm inner tension, decrease irritability, and help people feel more comfortable in their own skin.

The second PMS pattern that I have noted is increased deep limbic activity in conjunction with increased cingulate gyrus activity. The cingulate, as we will see, is the part of the brain associated with shifting attention. Women with this pattern often complain of increased sadness, worrying, repetitive negative thoughts and verbalizations (nagging), and cognitive inflexibility. This pattern usually responds much better to medications that enhance serotonin availability in the brain, such as Lustral, Seroxat (paroxetine), or Prozac (see cingulate medications in chapter 10, "Cingulate System Prescriptions").

Deep Limbic Checklist

Please read this list of behaviors and rate yourself (or the person you are evaluating) on each behavior listed. Use the following scale and place the appropriate number next to the item. Five or more symptoms marked 3 or 4 indicate a high likelihood of deep limbic problems.

0 = *never*
1 = *rarely*
2 = *occasionally*
3 = *frequently*
4 = *very frequently*

1........ Feelings of sadness
2........ Moodiness
3........ Negativity
4........ Low energy
5........ Irritability
6........ Decreased interest in others
7........ Feelings of hopelessness about the future
8........ Feelings of helplessness or powerlessness
9........ Feeling dissatisfied or bored
10........ Excessive guilt
11........ Suicidal feelings
12........ Crying
13........ Lowered interest in things usually considered fun
14........ Sleep changes (too much or too little)
15........ Appetite changes (too much or too little)
16........ Low self-esteem
17........ Decreased interest in sex
18........ Negative sensitivity to smells/odors
19........ Forgetfulness
20........ Poor concentration

4

Enhancing Positive Thought Patterns and Strengthening Connections:

Deep Limbic System Prescriptions

Finally, brethren, whatever is true, whatever is
honorable, whatever is right, whatever is pure, whatever
is lovely, whatever is of good repute, if there is any
excellence and if there is anything worthy of praise, let
your mind dwell on these things.

PHILIPPIANS 4:8

As discussed in chapter 3, the deep limbic system processes our sense
of smell, stores highly charged emotional memories, and affects sleep
and appetite cycles, moods, sexuality, and bonding. To heal deep limbic
system problems, we need to focus on a number of diverse prescriptions: accurate thinking, the proper management of memories, the
connection between pleasant smells and moods, and building positive
bonds between oneself and others. The following prescriptions, geared
toward healing deep limbic system problems, are based on my own
personal clinical experience with patients, as well as general knowledge about how the mind/body works.

DL PRESCRIPTION 1:
KILL THE ANTS

Our overall state of mind has a certain tone or flavor based largely on the types of thoughts we think. When the deep limbic system is over-active, it sets the mind's filter on "negative." People who are depressed have one dispiriting thought following another. When they look at the past, they feel regret. When they look at the future, they feel anxiety and pessimism. In the present moment, they're bound to find something unsatisfactory. The lens through which they see themselves, others, and the world has a dim grayness. They are suffering from *automatic negative thoughts*, or ANTs. ANTs are cynical, gloomy, and complaining thoughts that just seem to keep marching in all by themselves.

ANTs can cause people to be depressed and fatalistic. "I know I won't pass that test on Tuesday." This kind of thinking makes for a self-fulfilling prophecy: If someone has already convinced himself that he won't pass, he probably won't study very hard and he won't pass the test. If you are depressed all the time, you don't expect good things to happen, so you don't try very hard to make them happen. The inter-nal distress caused by melancholy thinking can make you behave in ways that alienate others, thus causing you to isolate yourself further. On the other hand, positive thoughts and a positive attitude will help you radiate a sense of wellbeing, making it easier for others to connect with you. Positive thoughts will also help you be more effective in your life. As you can see, what goes on in your mind all day long can deter-mine whether your behavior is self-defeating or self-promoting.

Here are some other examples of typical ANTs:

"*You never listen to me.*"

"*Just because we had a good year in business doesn't mean anything.*"

"*You don't like me.*"

"*This situation is not going to work out. I know something bad will happen.*"

"*I feel as though you don't care about me.*"

"*I should have done much better. I'm a failure.*"

"*You're arrogant.*"

"*You're late because you don't care.*"

"*It's your fault.*"

Healing the deep limbic system requires healing moment-to-moment thought patterns. Unfortunately, there is no formal place where we are taught to think much about our thoughts or to challenge the notions that go through our head, even though our thoughts are always with us. Most people do not understand how important thoughts are and leave the development of thought patterns to chance. Did you know that every thought you have sends electrical signals throughout your brain? Thoughts have actual physical properties. They are real! They have significant influence on every cell in your body. When your mind is burdened with many negative thoughts, it affects your deep limbic system and causes deep limbic problems (irritability, moodiness, depression, etc.). Teaching yourself to control and direct thoughts in a positive way is one of the most effective ways to feel better.

Here are the actual step-by-step "thinking" principles that I use in my psychotherapy practice to help my patients heal their deep limbic systems.

Step 1

Realize that your thoughts are real:
- *You have a thought.*
- *Your brain releases chemicals.*
- *An electrical transmission goes across your brain.*
- *You become aware of what you're thinking.*

Thoughts are real, and they have a real impact on how you feel and how you behave.

Step 2

Notice how negative thoughts affect your body.

Every time you have an angry thought, an unkind thought, a sad thought, or a cranky thought, your brain releases chemicals that make your body feel bad (and activate your deep limbic system). Think about the last time you were angry. How did your body feel? When most people are angry, their muscles become tense, their hearts beat faster, their hands start to sweat, and they may even begin to feel a little dizzy. Your body reacts to every negative thought you have.

Mark George, M.D., from the U.S. National Institute of Mental Health, demonstrated this phenomenon in an elegant study of brain function. He observed the activity of the brain in ten normal women under three different conditions: when they were thinking happy thoughts, neutral thoughts, and sad thoughts. During the happy thoughts, the women demonstrated a cooling of the deep limbic system. During the sad thoughts, he noticed a significant increase in deep limbic system activity—powerful evidence that your thoughts matter!

Step 3

Notice how positive thoughts affect your body.

Every time you have a good thought, a happy thought, a hopeful thought, or a kind thought, your brain releases chemicals that make your body feel good (and cool your deep limbic system). Think about the last time you had a really happy thought. How did your body feel? When most people are happy, their muscles relax, their hearts beat more slowly, their hands become dry, and they breathe more slowly. Your body also reacts to your good thoughts.

Step 4

Notice how your body reacts to every thought you have.

We know from polygraphs or lie detector tests, too, that your body reacts to your thoughts. During a lie detector test, a person is hooked up to equipment that measures hand temperature, heart rate, blood pressure, breathing rate, muscle tension, and how much the hands sweat.

The tester asks questions, like "Did you steal that car?" If the person did steal the car, his body is likely to exhibit a "stress" response. His hands get colder, his heart goes faster, his blood pressure goes up, his breathing gets faster, his muscles get tight, and his hands sweat more.

The reactions take place almost immediately, whether he says anything or not. Remember, the deep limbic system is responsible for translating our emotional state into physical feelings of relaxation or tension. Now the opposite is also true. If the subject did not steal the car, it is likely that his body will experience a "relaxation" response. His hands will become warmer, his heart rate will slow, his blood pressure will go down, his breathing will become slower and deeper, his muscles will relax, and his hands will become drier.

Again, almost immediately, his body has reacted to his thoughts. This happens not only when you're asked about telling the truth—your body reacts to *every* thought you have, whether about work, friends, family, or anything else.

Step 5

Think of bad thoughts as pollution.

Thoughts are very powerful. They can make your mind and your body feel good, or they can make you feel bad. Every cell in your body is affected by every thought you have. That is why when people get emotionally upset, they frequently develop physical symptoms, such as headaches or stomachaches. Some doctors think that people who have a lot of negative thoughts are more likely to get cancer. If you can think about good things, you will feel better.

A negative thought is like pollution to your system. Just as pollution affects everyone who goes outside, so, too, do negative thoughts pollute your deep limbic system, your mind, and your body.

Step 6

Understand that your automatic thoughts don't always tell the truth.

Unless you think about your thoughts, they are automatic; "they just happen." But even if your thoughts just happen, they are not necessarily correct. Your thoughts do not always tell the whole truth. Sometimes they even lie to you. I once treated a college student who thought he was stupid because he didn't do well on tests. When his IQ was tested, however, we discovered that he was close to a genius! You don't have to believe every thought that goes through your head. It's important to think about your thoughts to see if they help you or hurt you. Unfortunately, if you never challenge your thoughts, you just "believe them" as if they were true.

Step 7

Talk back to ANTs.

You can train your thoughts to be positive and hopeful, or you can allow them to be negative and upset you. Once you learn about your thoughts, you can choose to think good thoughts and feel better, or you can choose to think bad thoughts and feel lousy. That's right, it's up to you! You can learn how to change your thoughts, and you can learn to change the way you feel.

One way to learn how to change your thoughts is to notice them when they are negative and talk back to them, as I'll explain below. When you just think a negative thought without challenging it, your mind believes it and your body reacts to it. When you correct negative thoughts, you take away their power over you.

Step 8

Exterminate the ANTs.

Think of these negative thoughts that invade your mind like ants that bother you at a picnic. One negative thought, like one ant at a picnic, is not a big problem. Two or three negative thoughts, like two or three ants at a picnic, become more irritating. Ten or twenty negative thoughts, like ten or twenty ants at a picnic, may cause you to pick up and leave. Whenever you notice these automatic negative thoughts, or ANTs, you need to crush them or they'll ruin your relationships, your self-esteem, and your personal power. One way to crush these ANTs is to write them down and talk back to them. For example, if you catch yourself thinking, "My husband never listens to me," write it down. Then write down a rational response, something like "He's not listening to me now, maybe he's distracted by something else. He often listens to me." When you write down negative thoughts and talk back to them, you take away their power and help yourself feel better. Some people tell me they have trouble talking back to these negative thoughts because they feel that they are lying to themselves. Initially they believe that the thoughts that go through their mind are the truth. Remember, thoughts sometimes lie to you. It's important to check them out before you just believe them!

Here are nine different ways that your thoughts lie to you to make situations seem worse than they really are. Think of these nine ways as different species or types of ANTs. When you can identify the type of ANT, you begin to take away the power it has over you. I have designated some of these ANTs as red, because they are particularly harmful. Notice and exterminate ANTs whenever possible.

ANT 1: "Always/never" thinking. This happens when you think something that happened will "always" repeat itself, or that you'll "never" get what you want. For example, if your partner is irritable and she gets upset, you might think to yourself, "She's always yelling at me," even though in reality she yells only once in a while. But just the thought "She's always yelling at me" is so negative that it makes you feel sad and upset. It activates your limbic system. All-or-nothing words like *always, never, no one, every one, every time, everything* are usually wrong. Here are some examples of "always/never" thinking:

"He's always putting me down."

"No one will ever call me."

"I'll never get a raise."

"Everyone takes advantage of me."

"You turn away every time I touch you."

"My children never listen to me."

"Always/never thinking" ANTs are very common. If you catch yourself thinking in these absolutes, stop and make yourself recall examples that disprove your all-or-nothing attitude.

ANT 2 (red ant): Focusing on the negative. This occurs when your thoughts reflect only the bad in a situation and ignore any of the good. For example, I have treated several professional speakers for depression. After their presentations, they had the audience fill out an evaluation form. If one hundred forms were returned and two of them were terrible but ninety were outstanding, which ones do you think the speakers focused on? Only the negative ones! I taught them to focus on the ones they liked a lot more than the ones they didn't like. It's important to learn from others, but in a balanced, positive way.

Your deep limbic system can learn a powerful lesson from Eleanor Porter's book *Pollyanna*. In the book, Pollyanna went to live with her aunt after her missionary parents died. Even though she had lost her parents, she was able to help many "negative people" with her attitude. She introduced them to the "Glad Game," looking for things to be glad about in any situation. Her father had taught her this game after she experienced a disappointment. She had always wanted a doll, but her parents never had enough money to buy it for her. Her father sent a request for a secondhand doll to his missionary sponsors. By mistake, they sent her a pair of crutches. "What is there to be glad about crutches?" they thought. Then they decided they could be glad because they didn't have to use them. This very simple game changed the attitudes and lives of many people in the book. Pollyanna especially affected the minister. Before she came to town he preached hell-fire and damnation, and he did not seem to be very happy. Pollyanna told him that her father said that the Bible had eight hundred "Glad Passages," and that if God mentioned being glad that many times, it must be because He wants us to think that way. Focusing solely on the negative in situations will make you feel bad. Playing the Glad Game—looking for the positive—will help you feel better. I'm not suggesting you view the world through rose-colored glasses, only that you actively seek to find the positive to give more balance and optimism to a world you experience too often as negative.

ANT 3 (red ant): Fortune-telling. This is where you predict the worst possible outcome to a situation. For example, before you discuss an important issue with your partner, you predict that he or she won't be interested in what you have to say. Just having this thought will make you feel tense. I call fortune-telling a red ANT because when you predict bad things, you help make them happen. Say you are driving home from work and you predict that the house will be a wreck and no one will be interested in seeing you. By the time you get home you're waiting for a fight. When you see one thing out of place or no one comes running to the door, you're more likely to explode and ruin the rest of the evening. Fortune-telling ANTs really damage your chances for feeling good. Remind yourself that if you could see the future, you'd be a lottery billionaire by now.

ANT 4 (red ant): Mind reading. This happens when you believe that you know what other people are thinking even when they haven't told you. Mind reading is a common cause of trouble between people. I tell people, "Please don't read my mind, I have enough trouble reading it myself!" You know that you are mind reading when you have thoughts such as "She's mad at me." "He doesn't like me." "They were talking about me." I tell people that a negative look from someone else may mean nothing more than that he or she is constipated! You can't read anyone else's mind. You never know what others are really thinking unless they tell you. Even in intimate relationships, you cannot read your partner's mind. When there are things you don't understand, ask about them to clarify them. Stay away from mind-reading ANTs. They are very infectious.

ANT 5: Thinking with your feelings. This occurs when you believe your negative feelings without ever questioning them. You tell yourself, "I feel this way, so it must be so." Feelings are very complex and often based on powerful memories from the past. Feelings sometimes lie to you. Feelings are not always about truth. They are just feelings. But many people believe their feelings even though they have no evidence for them. "Thinking with your feelings" thoughts usually start with the words "I feel." For example: "I feel as if you don't love me." "I feel stupid." "I feel like a failure." "I feel nobody will ever trust me." Whenever you have a strong negative feeling, check it out. Look for the evidence behind the feeling. Do you have real reasons to feel that way? Or are your feelings based on events or things from the past? What's true, and what's just a feeling?

ANT 6: Guilt beating. Guilt is not a helpful emotion, especially for your deep limbic system. In fact, guilt often causes you to do things you don't want to do. Guilt beatings happen when you think with words like *should, must, ought,* or *have to.* Here are some examples: "I ought to spend more time at home." "I must spend more time with my kids." "I should have sex more often." "I have to organize my office." Because of human nature, whenever we think that we *must* do something, no matter what it is, we often don't want to do it. It is better to replace "guilt beatings" with phrases like "I want to do ..." "It fits with my goals to do ..." "It would be helpful to do ..." So in the examples above, it would be helpful to change those phrases to "I want to spend more time at home." "It's in our best interests for my kids and me to spend more time together." "I want to please my spouse by making wonderful love with him (or her) because he (or she) is important to me." "It's in my best interest to organize my office." Guilt isn't productive. Get rid of this unnecessary emotional turbulence that holds you back from achieving the goals you want.

ANT 7: Labeling. Whenever you attach a negative label to yourself or to someone else, you stop your ability to take a clear look at the situation. Some examples of negative labels are "jerk," "frigid," "arrogant," and "irresponsible." Negative labels are very harmful, because whenever you call yourself or someone else a jerk or arrogant, you lump that person in your mind with all of the "jerks" or "arrogant people" that you've ever known and you become unable to deal with him reasonably as a unique individual. Stay away from negative labels.

ANT 8: Personalizing. Personalizing occurs when you invest innocuous events with personal meaning: "My boss didn't talk to me this morning. She must be mad at me." Or "My son got into an accident with the car. I should have spent more time teaching him to drive. It must be my fault." There are many other reasons for others' behavior besides the negative explanations an abnormal limbic system picks out. For example, your boss may not have talked to you because she was preoccupied, upset, or in a hurry. You never fully know why people do what they do. Try not to personalize the behavior of others.

ANT 9 (the most poisonous red ant): Blaming. Blame is very harmful. When you blame something or someone else for the problems in your life, you become a passive victim of circumstances and you make it very difficult to do anything to change your situation. Many relationships are ruined by people who blame their partners when things go wrong. They take little responsibility for their problems. When something goes wrong at home or at work, they try to find someone to blame. They rarely admit their own problems. Typically, you'll hear from them statements like:

"It wasn't my fault that …

"That wouldn't have happened if you had …

"How was I supposed to know …

"It's your fault that …"

The bottom-line thinking in the "blame game" goes something like this: "If only you had done something differently, I wouldn't be in the predicament I'm in. It's your fault, and I'm not responsible."

Whenever you blame someone else for the problems in your life, you become powerless to change anything. The "blame game" hurts your personal sense of power. Stay away from blaming thoughts. You have to take personal responsibility for your problems before you can hope to change them.

Summary of ANT Species

1. **"Always/never" thinking:** *thinking in words life* always, never, no one, everyone, every time, everything
2. **Focusing on the negative:** *seeing only the bad in a situation*

3. **Fortune-telling:** *predicting the worst possible outcome to a situation*
4. **Mind reading:** *believing that you know what others are thinking, even though they haven't told you*
5. **Thinking with your feelings:** *believing negative feelings without ever questioning them*
6. **Guilt beating:** *thinking in words like* should, must, ought, *or* have to
7. **Labeling:** *attaching a negative label to yourself or to someone else*
8. **Personalizing:** *investing innocuous events with personal meaning*
9. **Blaming:** *blaming someone else for your own problems*

DL PRESCRIPTION 2:
KILL THE ANTS/
FEED YOUR ANTEATER

Your thoughts really matter. They can either help or hurt your deep limbic system. Left unchecked, ANTs will cause an infection in your whole bodily system. Whenever you notice ANTs, you need to crush them or they'll affect your relationships, your work, and your entire life. First you need to notice them. If you can catch them at the moment they occur and correct them, you take away the power they have over you. When a negative thought goes unchallenged, your mind believes it and your body reacts to it.

ANTs have an illogical logic. By bringing them into the open and examining them on a conscious level, you can see for yourself how little sense it really makes to think these kinds of things to yourself. You take back control over your own life instead of leaving your fate to hyperactive limbic-conditioned negative thought patterns.

Sometimes people have trouble talking back to these grossly unpleasant thoughts because they feel that such obvious age-old "truisms" simply must be real. They think that if they don't continue to believe these thoughts, they are lying to themselves. Once again, remember that to know what is true and what is not, you have to be conscious of the thoughts and have an intelligent perspective on them. Most negative thinking is automatic and goes unnoticed. You're not really choosing how to respond to your situation, it's being chosen for you by bad brain habits. To find out what is really true and what is not, you need to question it. Don't believe everything you hear—even in your own mind!

I often ask my patients about their ANT population. Is it high? Low? Dwindling? Or increasing? Keep control over the ANTs in order to maintain a healthy deep limbic environment.

Whenever you notice an ANT entering your mind, train yourself to recognize it and write it down. When you write down automatic negative thoughts (ANTs) and talk back to them, you begin to take away their power and gain control over your moods. Kill the ANTs by feeding your emotional anteater.

The "kill the ANTs/feed your anteater" exercise is for whenever you feel anxious, nervous, depressed, or frazzled.

Here are some examples of ways to kill these ANTs:

ANT	SPECIES OF ANT	KILL THE ANT
You never listen to me.	"Always/Never" Thinking	I get frustrated when you don't listen to me, but I know you have listened to me and will again.
The boss doesn't like me.	Mind Reading	I don't know that. Maybe she's just having a bad day. Bosses are people, too.
The whole class will laugh at me.	Fortune-telling	I don't know that. Maybe they'll really like my speech.
I'm stupid.	Labeling	Sometimes I do things that aren't too smart, but I'm not stupid.
It's your fault we have these marital problems.	Blaming	I need to look at my part of the problem and look for ways I can make the situation better.

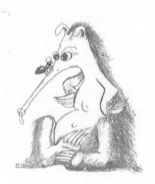

Your turn:

EVENT: Write out the event that is associated with your thoughts and feelings.

_____

_____

_____

_____

ANT	SPECIES	KILL THE ANT
(write out the automatic negative thoughts)	(identify the type of irrational thought)	(talk back to the irrational thoughts)
_____	_____	_____
_____	_____	_____
_____	_____	_____
_____	_____	_____
_____	_____	_____
_____	_____	_____
_____	_____	_____
_____	_____	_____
_____	_____	_____
_____	_____	_____
_____	_____	_____

DL PRESCRIPTION 3:
SURROUND YOURSELF WITH PEOPLE WHO PROVIDE POSITIVE BONDING

Have you ever picked up a container that had ants crawling on it? Within seconds they've crawled onto your body and you are hurriedly trying to brush them off. If you spend a lot of time with negative people, the same thing will happen. You may walk into a room in a buoyant mood, but before long their ANTs are going to rub off on you. Their ANTs will hang out with your ANTs and mate! That's not what you want—so surround yourself with positive people as much as possible.

Look at your life as it is now. What kind of people are around you? Do they believe in you and make you feel good about yourself, or are they constantly putting you down and denigrating your ideas, hopes, and dreams? List the ten people you spend the most time with. Make a note of how much they support you and the ways in which you would like to be supported more.

In my second year of college I got the bright idea that I wanted to go to medical school. I was on the speech team, and one day I told my speech coach about my dream to become a doctor. The first thing out of her mouth was that she had a brother at Michigan State who hadn't made it into medical school. "And," she added, "he was much smarter than you are." The message was clear: You don't have a chance. Making a big decision like that was hard enough to do with encouragement; the disheartening comment from the coach was a blow to my confidence I did not need. I went home with my spirits considerably dampened. Later that evening when I told my father what had happened, he just shook his head and said, "Listen, you can do whatever you put your mind to. And if I were you, I wouldn't spend much time with that coach."

If you think of life as an obstacle course, it is easy to see that the fewer obstacles in the road, the better. Negative people present unnecessary obstacles for you to overcome because you have to push your will to succeed over their doubts and objections and cynicism. Spending time with people who believe you'll never really amount to anything will dampen your enthusiasm for pursuing your goals and make it difficult to move through life in the direction you want to go. On the other hand, people who instill confidence in you with a can-do attitude, people whose spirits are uplifting, will help breathe life into your plans and dreams.

It cannot be overemphasized how contagious the attitudes of others are and how much hidden influence they can exert. The reason so many people feel good about attending a positive-thinking seminar is that they have been in a room full of people who were all reaffirming the best in one another. But let one of those people go home and walk into a house where someone makes fun of his efforts and says he's wasting his time and will never get anywhere anyway, and watch how fast the positive efforts of the seminar wear off!

When you spend a lot of time with people, you bond with them in certain ways, and as I mentioned earlier, the moods and thoughts of others directly affect your deep limbic system. If you go out with someone for dinner and after the first half hour you're beginning to feel bad about yourself, and then you remember that you always feel bad about yourself when you have dinner with this person, you are not imagining it; your deep limbic system is actually being affected by him or her. Deciding that you don't want to spend time with people who are going to have an adverse effect on you doesn't mean you have to blame them for the way they are. It simply means that you have the right to choose a better life for yourself.

I believe that limbic bonding is one of the key principles behind the success of support groups like Alcoholics Anonymous. For years, clinicians have known that one of the best ways to help people with serious problems like alcoholism is to get them to connect with others who have the same problem. By seeing how others have learned from their experiences and got through tough times in positive ways, alcoholics can find the way out of their own plight. While gaining information about their disease is helpful, forming new relationships and connections with others may be the critical link in the chain of recovery. The same can be said about people with other diseases, such as cancer. Stanford psychiatrist David Spiegel demonstrated the effectiveness of support groups for women with breast cancer. Those who participated in a support group had survival rates significantly higher than those who didn't. How our deep limbic system functions is essential to life itself. Spend time with people who enhance the quality of your limbic system rather than those who cause it to become inflamed.

DL PRESCRIPTION 4:
PROTECT YOUR CHILDREN
WITH LIMBIC BONDING

In a study published in *The Journal of the American Medical Association* in 1997, researcher Michael Resnick, Ph.D., and colleagues at the University of Minnesota reported that teenagers who felt loved and connected to their parents had a significantly lower incidence of teenage pregnancy, drug use, violence, and suicide. So important is the bonding between children and parents that it overrides other factors traditionally linked to problem behavior, such as living in a single-parent home or spending less time with a child. The article concluded that the degree of connection (limbic bonding) that teenagers feel with parents and teachers is the most important determinant of whether they will engage in risky sexual activity, substance abuse, violence, or suicidal behavior.

A study published in *USA Today* in the late 1980s reported that "on average, parents spend less than seven minutes a week talking with their children." It is not possible to "limbically bond" and have much of a relationship in such little time. Children need actual physical time with their parents. Think about the times your parents spent positive one-on-one time with you. Did that make you feel important, special?

Some parents complain that their children are too busy or are not interested in spending time with them. When this happens, I recommend that parents force the issue with their kids, telling them that they're important to them and that they need to spend time with them. Of course, the way in which you spend time with them is critical. If you spend the time lecturing or interrogating them, neither of you will find it very enjoyable and both of you will look for ways to avoid contact in the future.

Here is an exercise that I've found extremely powerful in improving the quality of time you have with your child. The exercise is called "special time." Special time works. It will improve the quality of your relationship with your child in a very short period of time. Here are the directions for special time.

1. *Spend twenty minutes a day with the child doing something that he or she would like to do. It's important to approach the child in a positive way and say something like "I feel we have not had enough*

time together and you are important to me. Let's spend some special time together every day. What would you like to do?" It's important to remember that the purpose of this time is to build the limbic bond and relationship with your child. Keep it as positive as possible.

2. During special time there are to be no parental commands, no questions, and no directions. This is very important. This is a time to build the relationship, not discipline difficult behavior. If, for example, you're playing a game and the child starts to cheat, you can reframe her behavior. You can say something like "I see you've changed the rules of the game, and I'll play by your rules." Remember, the goal of special time is to improve the relationship between you and your child, not to teach. Of course, at other times, if the child cheats it is important to deal straightforwardly with it.

3. Notice as many positive behaviors as you can. Noticing the good is much more effective in shaping behavior than noticing the bad.

4. Do much more listening than talking.

I once received a phone call from a friend of mine who complained that his eighteen-month-old daughter did not want anything to do with him when he came home from work. He told me that he thought it must be "one of those mother-daughter things" and that she'd probably grow out of it. I told him that it probably meant he wasn't spending enough time with his daughter and that if he did special time with his daughter she would become much more open and affectionate with him. My friend took my advice. He spent twenty minutes a day doing something that his daughter chose (usually playing with blocks in her room). He spent the time listening to her and feeding back what he heard her say. Within three weeks, his daughter's behavior dramatically changed. Whenever my friend would come home from work, his daughter would run to hug him, and she would hang on his leg all evening.

Remember, spending actual physical daily time with your child will have a powerfully positive effect on your relationship and protect your child from many of the problems in life.

DL PRESCRIPTION 5:
BUILD PEOPLE SKILLS TO
ENHANCE LIMBIC BONDS

It has been shown that enhancing emotional bonds between people will help heal the limbic system. In one large study in which patients were treated for major depression, the U.S. National Institutes of Health compared three approaches: antidepressant medication, cognitive therapy (similar to my ANT therapy), and interpersonal psychotherapy (enhancing relationship skills). Researchers were surprised to find that each of the treatments was equally effective in treating depression; many people in the medical community think that the benefits of medication far outweigh the benefits of therapy. Not surprising was the fact that combining all three treatments had an even more powerful effect. So not only were pharmaceuticals and professional therapists helpful, but patients played a significant role in helping each other. How you get along with other people can either help or hurt your limbic system! The better you get along with those around you, the better you will feel.

I teach my patients the following ten relational principles to help keep their deep limbic systems (and the limbic systems of those they love) healthy and rewarding:

1. Take responsibility for keeping the relationship strong. Don't be a person who blames his or her partner or friends for the relationship problems. Take responsibility for the relationship and look for what you can do to improve it. You'll feel empowered, and the relationship is likely to improve almost immediately.

2. Never take the relationship for granted. In order for relationships to be special, they need constant nurturing. Relationships suffer when they get put low on the priority list of time and attention. Focusing on what you want in a relationship is essential to making it happen.

3. Protect your relationship. A surefire way to doom a relationship is to discount, belittle, or degrade the other person. Protect your relationships by building up the other person.

4. Assume the best. Whenever there is a question of motivation or intention, assume the best about the other person. This will help his or her behavior to actually be more positive.

5. Keep the relationship fresh. When relationships become stale or

boring, they become vulnerable to erosion. Stay away from "the same old thing" by looking for new and different ways to add life to your relationships.

6. Notice the good. It's very easy to notice what you do not like about a relationship. That's almost our nature. It takes real effort to notice what you like. When you spend more time noticing the positive aspects of the relationship, you're more likely to see an increase in positive behavior.

7. Communicate clearly. I'm convinced most of the fights people have stem from some form of miscommunication. Take time to really listen and understand what other people say to you. Don't react to what you think people mean; ask them what they mean and then formulate a response.

8. Maintain and protect trust. So many relationships fall apart after there has been a major violation of trust, such as an affair or other form of dishonesty. Often hurts in the present, even minor ones, remind us of major traumas in the past and we blow them way out of proportion. Once a violation of trust has occurred, try to understand why it happened.

9. Deal with difficult issues. Whenever you give in to another person to avoid a fight, you give away a little of your power. If you do this over time, you give away a lot of power and begin to resent the relationship. Avoiding conflict in the short run often has devastating long-term effects. In a firm but kind way, stick up for what you think is right. It will help keep the relationship balanced.

10. Make time for each other. In our busy lives, time is often the first thing to suffer in our important relationships. Relationships require real time in order to function. Many couples who both work and have children often find themselves growing further apart because they have no time together. When they do spend time together, they often realize how much they really do like each other. Making your special relationships a "time investment" will pay dividends for years to come.

DL PRESCRIPTION 6:
RECOGNIZE THE IMPORTANCE OF
PHYSICAL CONTACT

The deep limbic system not only is involved in emotional bonding, it is also involved in physical bonding. Actual physical touching is essential to good health. It would probably surprise some people to know that there are couples who can go for ten years and longer without touching each other. I have seen them in my practice, and they invariably show such deep limbic system problems as irritability and depression. It is only after I help them correct their nontouching behavior that their depressive symptoms improve.

Physical connection is also a critical element in the parent-infant bonding process. The caressing, kissing, sweet words, and eye contact from the mother and father give the baby the pleasure, love, trust, and security it needs to develop healthy deep limbic pathways. Then a bond or connectedness between the parents and the baby can begin to grow. Without love and affection, the baby does not develop appropriate deep limbic connectedness and thus never learns to trust or connect. He feels lonely and insecure, and becomes irritable and unresponsive.

Touch is critical to life itself. In a barbaric thirteenth-century experiment, German Emperor Frederick II wanted to know what language and words children would speak if they were raised without hearing any words at all. He took a number of infants from their homes and put them with people who fed them but had strict instructions not to touch, cuddle, or talk to them. The babies never spoke a word. They all died before they could speak. Even though the language experiment was a failure, it resulted in an important discovery: Touch is essential to life. Salimbene, a historian of the time, wrote of the experiment in 1248, "They could not live without petting." This powerful finding has been rediscovered over and over, most recently in the early 1990s in Romania, where thousands of warehoused infants went without touch for sometimes years at a time. PET studies (similar to SPECT studies) of a number of these deprived infants have shown marked overall decreased activity across the whole brain.

Bonding is a two-way street. A naturally unresponsive baby may inadvertently receive less love from its parents. The mother and father, misreading their baby's naturally reserved behavior, may feel hurt and rejected and therefore less encouraged to lavish care and affection on their child. A classic example of this problem is illustrated by autistic children. Psychiatrists used to label the mothers of autistic children "cold"; they believed the mother's lack of responsiveness caused the autism. In recent times, however, it has been shown in numerous research studies that autism is biological and preceded any relationship. The mothers of autistic children in their studies started out warm, but actually became more reserved when they did not get positive feedback from their children. The kind of love that is critical to making the parent-infant bond work is reciprocal.

Love between adults is similar. For proper bonding to occur, couples need to hold and kiss each other, say sweet words, and make affectionate eye contact. It is not enough for one side to give and the other to passively receive. Physical manifestations of love need to be reciprocated or the other partner feels hurt and rejected, which ultimately causes the bond to erode.

Intimate relationships require physical love in order to flourish. The entire relationship cannot consist of two people sitting in their respective corners having a lively conversation about the stock market (even if they both adore the stock market). An intimate relationship is missing something essential for human beings if there is not enough physical contact. Without that element, eventually love will sour, causing one person to withdraw and perhaps look for love elsewhere.

Reporting in a *Life* magazine cover story on touch, writers George Howe Colt and Anne Hollister cite numerous incidents of the healing power of touch: "Studies have shown massage to have positive effects on conditions from colic to hyperactivity to diabetes to migraines, in fact, every malady TRI [Touch Research Institute, in Miami, Florida] has studied thus far." They report that "Massage, it seems, helps asthmatics breathe easier, boosts immune function in HIV-positive patients, improves autistic children's ability to concentrate, lowers anxiety in depressed adolescents, and reduces apprehension in burn victims about to undergo debridement ... Even in the elderly, elders exhibited less depression, lower stress hormones, and less loneliness. They had fewer doctor visits, drank less coffee, and made more social phone calls."

Touch is essential to our humanity. Yet, in our standoffish, litigious society, touch is becoming less and less frequent. Touch your children, your spouse, your loved ones regularly. Giving and receiving massages on a regular basis will enhance limbic health and limbic bonding.

DL PRESCRIPTION 7:
SURROUND YOURSELF WITH GREAT SMELLS

Your deep limbic system is the part of your brain that directly processes your sense of smell. That is why perfumes and wonderful-smelling soaps are attractive and unpleasant body odors are repellent.

In *The Lancet,* a study was reported on the benefits of aromatherapy using the oil from lavender flowers. When used properly, lavender oil aroma helped people to feel less stressed and less depressed. It also enhanced sleep. In aromatherapy, special fragrances are used in a steam machine, in the bath, on the pillow, and in potpourris. These fragrances can have an appreciable effect on people's moods. However, there is a difference between ingesting the substance and smelling it. When you ingest something, it goes to the stomach and is processed by the digestive system. (Moreover, many essential oils, including lavender, are dangerous if ingested.) A smell, however, activates the olfactory nerves, which go directly to the deep limbic system.

Consider cinnamon, used for cooking in a number of countries throughout the world. Being of Lebanese descent, my mother used to put cinnamon in many dishes she would bring to the table, including stuffed vine leaves, one of my favorites. When I recently told her that the scent of cooked cinnamon is considered a natural aphrodisiac for men, she put her hand on her forehead and said, "That's why I have seven kids, your father would never leave me alone."

Many people have noticed that certain smells sometimes bring up very strong, clear memories, as if the whole feeling and sense of the original event were coming back to them. There is a good reason for that: Smell and memory are processed in the same area of the brain. Because smells activate neurocircuits in the deep limbic system, they bring about a more complete recall of events, which gives one access to details of the past with great clarity.

Smells have an effect on moods. The right smells probably cool the deep limbic system. Pleasing fragrances are like an anti-inflammatory. By surrounding yourself with flowers, sweet fragrances, and other pleasant smells, you affect the working of your brain in a powerful and positive way.

DL PRESCRIPTION 8:
BUILD A LIBRARY OF WONDERFUL MEMORIES

Because the deep limbic system stores highly charged emotional memories, some of the memories are bound to be disturbing. One common tool for therapists has been to get clients to scan the past for negative memories so they can reprocess them. Unfortunately this form of treatment can be misguided, especially for people who are truly depressed. Depressed people have selective memories. They tend to recall only things that are consistent with their mood. Because they have inflamed deep limbic systems, their mood is negative, and everything they remember is negative. The whole process of recollection makes their lives look like one long bad dream and convinces them that they are justified in being depressed. Therapists sometimes recognize this tendency in clients and interpret it to mean that the patient is somehow invested in being miserable. But there is another explanation that has to do with how the mind/body works.

Whenever you remember a particular event, your brain releases chemicals similar to those released when you originally input impressions of the event. Consequently, remembering brings back a similar mood and feelings. If the memory is of your puppy getting hit by a car, it will put you in a melancholy mood. People whose bonding with their parents was tentative at best, or who had a lot of painful childhood experiences, already have a chemical imprint on the brain that is negative. They will tend to take in new events in a negative way. Whenever someone looks at them the wrong way, it triggers the same chemical patterns in the brain that are common to their early experience. They also tend to dismiss someone smiling at them and not see it as a positive expression because positive information is not consistent with their experience.

This pattern is difficult to change because it sets up a whole way of viewing life: The early patterns continually predispose the people toward taking things in such a way as to prove to themselves that they live in a negative universe. To change the pattern, they actually have to change their brain chemistry by remembering positive things. By calling up pleasant memories, they can tune in to mental states that are healthier. The brain then takes on the same chemical patterns that were inputted at the time the healthy events occurred. Because doing this is such a healing process, I encourage those who have lost a loved one to practice it. When someone dies, recalling the fights and the power struggles keeps the pain going because it sets up a negative mood that is self-perpetuating. By continually remembering the bad things, the emotional filter gets set to actually keep out the good memories. This tends to focus us on the unfinished business instead of the real love that we shared for many years.

For those of us who do not have to battle depression on a daily basis, we may still find ourselves in states more negative than our lives actually warrant. When unfortunate things do happen, we might go on thinking about them for longer than is helpful to solve the problem. In order to balance the bad memories and heal the deep limbic part of our brain, it is important to remember the times of our life that were charged with positive emotions.

Make a list of the ten happiest times in your life. Describe them for yourself in detail, using as many of the five senses as possible. What colors do you remember? What smells were in the air? Was there music? Try to make the picture come alive. In a metaphorical sense you are going through the library shelves of daily experience and looking for the right book.

If you have been involved in a long-term relationship with someone, recollecting the history of your happy times together will enhance the bond between you. Positive memory traces actually encourage behavior that strengthens the bonds. Encouraging affirming thoughts in yourself—in other words, by recalling your partner's caress, how he or she was helpful to you this week, a look or gesture that was particularly touching—will tune you in to a positive feeling, which in turn will dispose you to act lovingly. It might remind you to call your wife during the day, or to remember what special gift you could give your husband on his birthday that will make him especially happy, or help both of you be supportive when times are tough.

DL PRESCRIPTION 9:
CONSIDER LIMBIC MEDICATIONS

Clinical depression, manic-depressive disorder, and severe PMS are more difficult problems than the garden variety most people experience in the form of bad moods. The deep limbic prescriptions I have mentioned so far may not be effective enough to help the more seriously affected person live a happy, functional life. For complete healing to take place, the addition of antidepressant medication or appropriate herbal treatment may be needed. A sure sign that the prescribed medications are really treating the depression is that the deep limbic system activity normalizes. Whenever limbic activity normalizes, there is a corresponding decrease in the patient's symptoms.

In recent years, new antidepressants have entered the market that have a wider application and often have fewer side effects than the original antidepressants. Some of the new pharmaceuticals have the additional benefit of affecting the subclinical patterns the rest of us are more likely to experience at some time in our lives, such as moodiness and negativity. The appendix contains information on current anti-depressant medications that include the brand name, generic name, and dosage range. In treating clinical depression, it is important to use enough medication for a long enough period of time. Often, antidepres-sants take from two to four weeks to become effective. It is essential to work closely with your doctor on this; stopping medication suddenly can have serious repercussions.

St John's wort is an herbal treatment that has also been shown to have a positive impact on depression and a cooling influence on deep limbic structures. It has been used for many years and it is the most commonly prescribed antidepressant with the fewest side effects. For adults I recommend 500 milligrams two times a day of St John's wort, containing 0.3% hypericin. Even though St John's wort has fewer side effects than traditional antidepressants, it is not without side effects altogether. Some people become sun-sensitive and become more easily sunburned. Some get acne. Also, I had one patient who developed a seriously slow heart rate after taking it for a month. I believe if you are taking St John's wort for depression, you should do it under the super-vision of a psychiatrist.

For the best results with all my patients, however, I often combine the use of medications with the deep limbic prescriptions described in this chapter.

DL PRESCRIPTION 10:
TRY PHYSICAL EXERCISE

Physical exercise can be very healing to the deep limbic system. It releases endorphins that induce a sense of wellbeing. The deep limbic system has many endorphin receptors. Exercise also increases blood flow through-out the brain, which nourishes it so that it can function properly. Think about what blood flow and nourishment do for the rest of your body. A body that is constricted or emaciated doesn't feel good. The same is true for the brain. Good blood flow resets the deep limbic system to a healthy level, which in turn favorably affects the person's mood.

People who exercise regularly report a general sense of wellbeing that those who lead a sedentary lifestyle do not experience. They have increased energy and a healthy appetite, they sleep more soundly and are usually in a better mood. Over the years I have found it useful to prescribe physical exercise to depressed patients. This is even more important for people who are unable to tolerate antidepressant medication. Instead of taking medication, some are able to treat themselves, under their doctor's supervision, with a program of strenuous exercise, which makes them feel just as good as something from the pharmacy.

In the fast pace of modern life—long work hours, rush-hour commutes, two-parent working families—it is important to remember how essential exercise and personal care are to good health; don't let them be left out. Technology has worked against us in some ways because many of the advances in the past twenty years have reduced and even eliminated physical activity and exertion from our daily lives. In the movie L.A. Story, Steve Martin runs out of his house, jumps in his car, drives ten yards to his neighbor's house, hops back out, and knocks at his neighbor's door. A bit of an exaggeration, perhaps, but think of how many times we could walk to the newsagent to get a newspaper but instead decide to save time and drive. This inactive lifestyle is causing our bodies to lose their efficiency; in other words, they don't burn fat as they should. Experts in nutrition, physiology, and medicine all agree that a program of physical exertion on a continuing basis is required to maintain low body fat, a strong and healthy heart, and well-toned muscles.

A good exercise program will pay limbic dividends as well:

1. Exercise gives you more energy and keeps you from feeling lethargic.

2. Exercise increases metabolism, will help keep your appetite in check, and will therefore keep your weight down.

3. Exercise helps to normalize melatonin production in your brain and enhances the sleep cycle.

4. Exercise allows more of the natural amino acid tryptophan to enter the brain, enhancing mood. Tryptophan is the precursor to the neurotransmitter serotonin, which has been found to be low in many depressed patients. Tryptophan is a relatively small amino acid, and it often has to compete with larger amino acids to cross the blood

channels into the brain. With exercise, the muscles of the body utilize the larger amino acids and decrease the competition for tryptophan to enter the brain. Exercise makes you feel better.

A lot of people grumble and complain when they're told to get more exercise. They find exercise time-consuming and boring. My advice is to keep trying different activities until you find the one that suits you. Find out what you like best. But make sure you get some form of regular workout (walking, running, cycling) on a daily basis, and an aerobic workout (which increases your heart rate and the flow of oxygen to your muscles) three times a week for at least twenty minutes at a time. Many people make the mistake of thinking that the sport they play as a hobby fulfills their exercise quota, yet the truth is that it depends on the sport. I once treated an obese man by outlining a nutrition and exercise program for him. Several weeks into it, he complained he wasn't losing any weight. When I asked what kind of workout he was getting, he told me he played two whole rounds of golf a week. I had to point out to him that walking around a golf course would not give him the level of activity he needed because it wasn't continuous—a golfer has to keep stopping to hit the ball. With a surprised look on his face, he said, "Wait a minute, Doc. I don't walk and stop to hit the ball. I get out of the cart, hit the ball, and then get back in the cart. That's a lot of activity, hopping in and out of that cart!"

DL PRESCRIPTION 11:
WATCH YOUR LIMBIC NUTRITION

Over the past decade there has been significant research on food, nutrients, and depression. The results surprise many people. We have been inundated by nutritional experts and news reporters who tell us we should eat low-fat, high-carbohydrate diets. "Low fat" is everywhere. Unfortunately, low fat is not the complete answer. In two studies in the *American Journal of Psychiatry*, men who had the highest suicide rates had the lowest cholesterol levels. Our deep limbic system needs fat in order to operate properly. Certainly, some fats are better for us than others, such as the omega-3 fatty acids found most prevalently in fish. Protein is also essential to a healthy "deep limbic diet." Proteins are the building blocks of brain neurotransmitters. Low levels of dopamine, serotonin, and noradrenaline have all been implicated in depression and mood disorders. It is essential to eat enough protein in balanced amounts with fats and carbohydrates. Too much protein for some people may actually restrict the amount of "brain proteins" that cross into the brain. Not enough protein will leave you with a brain protein deficit. The richest sources of protein are lean fish, cheese, beans, and nuts.

Low serotonin levels are often associated with worrying, moodiness, emotional rigidity, and irritability (a combination of deep limbic and cingulate problems). To enhance serotonin levels, eat balanced meals with complex carbohydrate snacks (such as wholegrain crackers or bread). Exercise can be a tremendous help along with nutritional supplementation. The amino acid l-tryptophan, which was recently reapproved by the Food and Drug Administration, is an option. L-tryptophan is a naturally occurring amino acid found in milk, meat, and eggs. I have found it very helpful for patients to improve sleep, decrease aggressiveness, and improve mood control. In addition, it does not have side effects, which gives it a real advantage over the antidepressants. L-tryptophan was taken off the market a number of years ago because one contaminated batch from one manufacturer caused a rare disease and a number of deaths. The l-tryptophan itself actually had nothing to do with the deaths. I recommend l-tryptophan in doses of 1,000–3,000 milligrams taken at bedtime. There have been some recent studies with inositol, from the B vitamin family, which you can get from a health food store. In doses of 12–20 milligrams a day it has been shown to decrease moodiness and depression. Check with your doctor before taking these or any other supplements.

Low noradrenaline and dopamine levels are often associated with depression, lethargy, trouble focusing, negativity, and mental fuzziness. To enhance noradrenaline and dopamine levels, it is better to have protein snacks (such as meat, eggs, or cheese) and to avoid simple carbohydrates, such as bread, pasta, cakes, and sweets. Also, I often have my patients take natural amino acids such as tyrosine (1,000–1,500 milligrams a day) for energy, focus, and impulsivity control, and dl-phenylalanine (400 milligrams three times a day on an empty stomach) for moodiness and irritability. Again, check with your doctor if you want to try these supplements.

5

Looking Into Anxiety and Fear:
The Basal Ganglia

FUNCTIONS OF THE BASAL GANGLIA SYSTEM

- *integrates feeling and movement*
- *shifts and smoothes fine motor behavior*
- *suppresses unwanted motor behaviors*
- *sets the body's idle speed or anxiety level*
- *enhances motivation*
- *mediates pleasure/ecstasy*

The basal ganglia are a set of large structures toward the center of the brain that surround the deep limbic system. The basal ganglia are involved with integrating feelings, thoughts, and movement, along with helping to shift and smooth motor behavior. In our clinic we have noticed that the basal ganglia are involved with setting the body's "idle speed," or anxiety level. In addition, they help to modulate motivation and are likely to be involved with feelings of pleasure and ecstasy. Let's look at each of these functions in more depth.

The integration of feelings, thoughts, and movement occurs in the basal ganglia. This is why you jump when you're excited, tremble when you're nervous, freeze when you're scared, or get tongue-tied when the boss is chewing you out. The basal ganglia allow for a smooth integration of emotions, thoughts, and physical movement, and when there is too much input, they tend to lock up. A patient of mine was badly burned in a motorcycle accident in San Francisco. As he lay burning on the ground, people stood nearby, frozen with fear, unable

The Basal Ganglia System

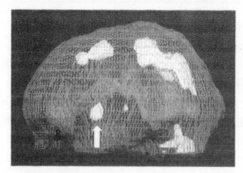

3-D side active view

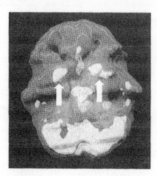

3–D underside active view

to move to help him. For years he was confounded by their actions, wondering why no one had moved to help him. "Didn't they care? Was I not worth trying to help?" he wondered. For years this man lived with both the physical pain from the accident and the emotional pain of feeling that others did not care enough to help him. He was relieved to learn a new interpretation of the situation: The intensity of emotion caused by the fiery accident had overwhelmed the onlookers' basal ganglia and they had become unable to move, even though most of them probably wanted to help.

When the basal ganglia are overactive (as we have seen in the case of people with anxiety tendencies or disorders), people are more likely to be overwhelmed by stressful situations and have a tendency to freeze or become immobile (in thoughts or actions). When their basal ganglia are underactive (as we have seen in people who have attention deficit hyperactivity disorder [ADHD]), often a stressful situation moves them to action. People with ADHD are frequently the first ones on the scene of an accident, and they respond to stressful situations without fear. I know, for example, that one of my friends who has ADHD is a lot quicker at responding to crises than I am (as mentioned in chapter 2, I have naturally overactive basal ganglia). I remember one situation where we were leaving a restaurant and paying the bill at the counter when the lady in front of us suddenly fell to the ground. My friend quickly went to her aid while I stood there frozen by the intensity of the situation. And I had medical training; my friend did not! I used to feel guilty about not moving quickly in those situations, but it has helped to learn that my brain just doesn't permit me to do so. The activity in my basal ganglia makes it harder to move quickly in anxiety-provoking situations.

Shifting and smoothing fine motor behavior is another basal ganglia function and is essential to handwriting and motor coordination. Again, let's use the example of attention deficit hyperactivity disorder. Many children and adults with ADHD have very poor handwriting. The act of handwriting is difficult and often stressful for them. Their writing may be choppy or sloppy. In fact, many teens and adults with ADHD print instead of writing in cursive. They find printing easier because it is not a smooth, continuous motor movement, but rather a start-and-stop motor activity. Many people with ADHD also complain that they have trouble getting their thoughts out of their head and onto paper, a term called finger agnosia (the fingers cannot tell what the brain is thinking). We know that the medications that help ADHD, such as the psychostimulants Ritalin, Dexedrine, or Adderall, work by enhancing the production of the neurotransmitter dopamine in the basal ganglia. These medications sometimes improve handwriting and enhance a person's ability to get his or her thoughts onto paper to an amazing extent. In addition, many people with ADHD say that their overall motor coordination is improved by these medications. Here is an example from one of my patients.

Tommy, age fourteen, handwriting, no medication

Hello, my name is Tommy.

Tommy's handwriting after ADHD diagnosis and treatment with stimulant medication

Another clue about the motor control functions of the basal ganglia comes from the understanding of two other illnesses, Parkinson's disease (PD) and Tourette's syndrome (TS). PD is caused by a deficiency of dopamine within the basal ganglia system. It is characterized by a "pill rolling" hand tremor, muscle rigidity, cogwheeling (jerking, stop-and-start movements when trying to rotate a joint), loss of agility, loss of facial expression, and slow movements. Often, giving persons dopamine-enhancing drugs, such as 1–dopa, significantly alleviates these symptoms, allowing smoother motor movements. The basal ganglia are also involved in suppressing unwanted motor activity. When there are abnormalities in this part of the brain, people are more at risk of Tourette's syndrome, which is a combination of motor and vocal tics (more on TS later in the chapter).

In our brain-imaging work, we have seen that the basal ganglia must also be involved in setting the body's "idle," or anxiety, level. Over-active basal ganglia are often associated with anxiety, tension, increased awareness, and heightened fear. Underactive basal ganglia can cause problems with motivation, energy, and get-up-and-go.

Interestingly, some of the most highly motivated individuals we have scanned, such as company CEOs, have significant increased activity in this part of the brain. We theorize that some people can use this increased activity in the form of motivation to become "movers" in society. My mother, for example, who like me has increased activity in this part of the brain, does tend to be a bit anxious, but she is a woman on the go. She plays golf four or five times a week, raised seven children without appearing stressed, and is always up "doing something" for other people. I believe that using the increased energy and drive from increased basal ganglia activity helps ward off anxiety.

Another interesting finding about this part of the brain is that the basal ganglia are likely involved in the pleasure control loops of the brain. One brain-imaging study performed by Nora Volkow's group at the Brookhaven National Laboratory in Upton, New York, looked at where cocaine and Ritalin work in the brain. Both were taken up mostly by the basal ganglia. Cocaine is an addictive substance; Ritalin, in doses prescribed for ADHD, is not. The study clearly showed why. Cocaine is a powerful enhancer of dopamine availability in the brain, and it has both very fast uptake and clearance from the brain. It comes on strong in a powerful wave, and then it's gone. The user gets a high high, and when it's gone, he or she wants more. In contrast, while Ritalin also increases the availability of dopamine to the basal ganglia, its effects are less powerful and it clears from the brain at a much slower rate. Dr. Volkow's group postulated that activation of the basal ganglia by cocaine perpetuates the compulsive desire for the drug. Ritalin, on the other hand, enhances motivation, focus, and follow-through, but does not give users a high or an intense desire to use more (unless at much higher doses than clinically prescribed). In fact, one the biggest clinical problems I have with teenagers who have ADHD is that they forget to take their medication.

Intense romantic love can also have a cocainelike effect on the brain, robustly releasing dopamine in the basal ganglia. Love has real physical effects. I had the opportunity to scan a close friend, Bill, shortly after he had met a new woman. He was head over heels for her. After their third date, when they spent the day at the beach in each other's arms, my friend came by my office to tell me about his newfound love. He was so happy he almost seemed to have a drug high. By coincidence,

Bill's Love-Affected Brain

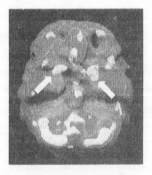

3-D underside active view

Note increased right and left basal ganglia activity (arrows).

while Bill was talking, my nuclear technician came into my office and told me we had an extra dose of the isotope and could do another scan if I had someone who needed one. Since I had an earlier scan of Bill's brain as part of our normal control group, I decided we'd scan him again and get a look at the brain of new love. To my amazement, his brain looked as if he had just taken a lot of cocaine. The activity in both the right and left basal ganglia was very intense, almost to the point of resembling seizure activity. Love has real effects on the brain, as powerful as addictive drugs.

PROBLEMS WITH THE BASAL GANGLIA SYSTEM

- *anxiety, nervousness*
- *panic attacks*
- *physical sensations of anxiety*
- *tendency to predict the worst*
- *conflict avoidance*
- *Tourette's syndrome/tics*
- *muscle tension, soreness*
- *tremors*
- *fine motor problems*
- *headaches*
- *low/excessive motivation*

Anxiety, Nervousness, and Panic Disorder

Excessive basal ganglia activity resets the body's idle to a revved-up level and can make people feel anxious, nervous, tense, and pessimistic. Almost all of the patients we have treated with panic disorder whom we've scanned had heightened basal ganglia activity.

Here's an example of panic disorder.

Gary

Gary came to see me about eight years ago. He had first gone to his doctor complaining of back pain. The doctor examined Gary's back and found a tender spot over his kidneys. He asked Gary to get a kidney X-ray. As soon as the doctor asked him to get this X-ray, Gary's thoughts took off: "The doctor is going to find out I have cancer." (Notice the leap in logic!) But his thoughts didn't stop there. "The doctor's going to find out I have cancer. I'm going to have to have chemotherapy." Ten seconds later, he'd already put himself into treatment. "I'm going to vomit my guts out, lose all my hair, be in a tremendous amount of pain, and then I'm going to die!" His mind did this all in a span of thirty seconds. Then Gary had a panic attack. His heart began to race. His hands became ice cold. He started to hyperventilate. And he broke out in a heavy sweat. He turned to the doctor and said, "I can't have that X-ray."

Bewildered, the doctor replied, "What do you mean? You came to see me to get help. I need this X-ray, so I can figure out ..."

Gary said, "No, you don't understand! I can't have the X-ray!"

The doctor found my number, called me, and said, "Daniel, please help me with this guy."

As Gary told me this story, I knew that he had a lifelong panic disorder. Gary was also an expert at predicting the worst, which was driving his panic symptoms.

In treating Gary, I taught him the Basal Ganglia Prescriptions given in chapter 6. I even went with him to have the kidney X-rays because it was important to have it done quickly. I hypnotized him, enabling him to be calm through the procedure. He did wonderfully. He breathed in a relaxed way, and he went through the procedure without any problems—until the X-ray technician came back into the room with a worried look on his face and asked Gary which side of his body was giving him pain. Gary grabbed his chest and looked at me like "You SOB! I knew you were lying to me about this! I'm going to die!" I patted him on the leg and said, "Look, Gary, before you die, let me take a look at the X-ray" (psychiatrists are also medical doctors). As I looked at his X-ray I could see that Gary had a big kidney stone, which can be terribly painful—but kidney stones don't usually kill anybody! Gary's basal ganglia, which were working too hard, put him through tremendous emotional pain by causing him to predict the worst possible outcome to situations.

Basal ganglia anxiety can make pain worse. As Gary became more anxious about his pain, the anxiety signals caused his muscles to contract; the smooth muscles in the ureter (the tube from the kidneys to the bladder) contracted, clamping down on the stone and intensifying the pain. A combination of psychotherapy, Nardil (phenelzine, a MAO-inhibitor antidepressant with antipanic qualities), and occasional use of Valium helped Gary live a more normal life.

Anxiety-provoking situations also cause many people with overactive basal ganglia to become frozen with fear and unable to leave their homes, a condition called agoraphobia (fear of being in public). I have treated many people who have been housebound for years (one woman for forty years) because of fear of having a panic attack.

Marsha

Marsha, a critical care nurse, was forced into treatment by her husband. She was thirty-six years old when she first began experiencing panic attacks. She was in a supermarket when all of a sudden she felt dizzy and short of breath, with a racing heart and a terrible sense of impending doom. She left her trolley in the shop and ran to her car, where she cried for over an hour. After her first episode, the panic

Marsha's Panic-Disorder-Affected Brain

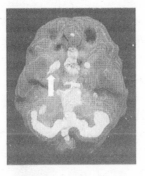

3-D underside active view

Note increased right basal ganglia activity (arrow).

attacks increased in frequency to the point where she stopped going out of her house, fearing that she'd have an attack and be unable to get help. She stopped working and made her husband take the children to and from school. She was opposed to any medication, because in the past her mother, in attempting to treat her own panic attacks, had become addicted to Valium and had often been quite mean to Marsha. Marsha did not want to see herself as being in any way like her mother. She believed that she "should" be able to control these attacks. Her husband, seeing her dysfunction only worsen, took her to see a family counselor. The counselor taught her relaxation and how to talk back to her negative thoughts, but it didn't help. Her condition worsened, and her husband brought her to see me. Given her resistance to medication, I decided to order a SPECT study to evaluate Marsha and then show her her own brain function.

Her SPECT study revealed marked increased focal activity in the right side of her basal ganglia. This is a very common finding in patients who have a panic disorder. Interestingly, patients who have active seizure activity also have focal areas of increased activity in their brains. Due to the intense level of emotions associated with panic attacks, my colleagues and I wonder if the basal ganglia findings are equivalent to behavioral seizures.

The findings on her scan convinced Marsha to try medication. I put her on Rivotril (clonazepam), an antianxiety medication that is also used for seizure control. In a short period of time she was able to leave her house, go back to work, and resume her life. In addition to the medication, I taught her the group of Basal Ganglia Prescriptions (given later), including sophisticated biofeedback and relaxation techniques, and worked with her to correct her negative "fortune-telling" thoughts. Several years later she was able to completely stop her medication and has remained panic free.

Post-Traumatic Stress Disorder

Mark

Mark, a fifty-year-old business executive, was admitted to the hospital shortly after he tried to kill himself. His wife had just started divorce proceedings, and he felt as though his life was falling apart. He was angry, hostile, frustrated, distrusting, and chronically anxious. His coworkers felt that he was "mad all the time." He also complained of a constant headache. Mark was a decorated Vietnam veteran, an infantry soldier with over one hundred kills. He told me that he had lost his humanity in Vietnam and that the experience had made him "numb."

In the hospital, he said that he was tormented by the memories of the past. Mark had post-traumatic stress disorder (PTSD). With his wife leaving him, he felt that he had no reason to live. Due to the severity of his symptoms, along with a history of a head injury in Vietnam, I ordered a brain SPECT study. It was abnormal, showing marked increased activity in the left side of his basal ganglia, the most intense activity in that part of the brain I had ever seen.

Left-sided basal ganglia findings are often seen in people who are chronically irritable or angry. Mood stabilizers, such as lithium, Tegretol, or Depakote, can be helpful in decreasing the irritability and calming down focal "hot" areas in the brain. I placed Mark on Depakote. Almost immediately, his headaches disappeared and he began to feel calmer. He stopped snapping at everyone, and he became more able to do the psychological work of healing from his divorce and the wounds from Vietnam.

In working with Mark, I often felt that his experiences in Vietnam had reset his basal ganglia to be constantly on the alert. Nearly every

Mark's PTSD- and Headache-Affected Brain

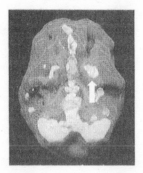

3-D underside active view
Note increased left basal ganglia activity (arrow).

day for thirteen months of the war, he had had to be "on alert" in order to avoid being shot. Through the years, he had never had the chance to learn how to reset his brain back to normal. The medication and therapy allowed him to relax and feel, for the first time in twenty-five years, that he had truly left the war zone.

Conflict Avoidance

Anxiety is, by definition, very uncomfortable. Thus, people who are anxious tend to avoid any situations that make them more uncomfortable, especially dealing with conflict. People who have basal ganglia problems tend to be frozen by conflict and consequently do what they can to avoid it. Unfortunately, conflict avoidance can have a serious negative impact on your life.

Loren

Loren, the owner of a neighborhood deli, hated conflict. He also had problems with chronic feelings of tension and anxiety. Out of fear of confrontation, these problems prevented him from firing employees who were not good for his business. They also caused him to be overly nice to people who were negative to him, so Loren grew to resent his own lack of assertiveness. His problems even caused marital difficulties. For years Loren wouldn't talk about the things in his marriage that made him unhappy. He would just hold them in until he finally exploded. Learning to deal with conflict was the centerpiece of his treatment.

Betsy

In a similar way, Betsy's conflict-avoidant tendencies were ruining her career. She worked at a local oil company. Being very bright, she advanced quickly until she got to a position in which she had to deal with high-powered men who were competitive and accustomed to conflict and confrontation. Betsy reacted to these men by becoming quiet and deferential. She looked for ways to please them, in order to avoid the anxiety that she perceived would overwhelm her if open conflict were to occur. Guess what happened? She stopped dead in her career. She was unable to be assertive and express her own ideas if they differed from those of others.

Betsy initially came to see me for a severe panic disorder that prevented her from driving. Her husband and friends had to drive her everywhere because she was afraid she'd have a panic attack.

In treatment, I taught her how to deal with conflict. I taught her how to face these men and not run away from them. Subsequently she began to speak up in meetings and stand up for her position in the company. Upper management began to pay attention to her in a positive way.

It's very important to learn ways to soothe your basal ganglia. Otherwise, the anxiety and programming from the past will rule your life.

Tourette's Syndrome (TS)

TS is a very interesting disorder that provides the bridge between the basal ganglia and two seemingly opposite disorders, attention deficit hyperactivity disorder (ADHD) and obsessive-compulsive disorder (OCD). TS is characterized by motor and vocal tics lasting more than a year. Motor tics are involuntary physical movements such as eye blinking, head jerking, shoulder shrugging, and arm or leg jerking. Vocal tics typically involve making involuntary noises such as coughing, puffing, blowing, barking, and sometimes swearing (coprolalia). TS runs in families and may be associated with several genetic abnormalities found in the dopamine family of genes. SPECT studies of TS patients, by my clinic and others, have found abnormalities in the basal ganglia of the brain. One of the most fascinating aspects of TS is its high association with both ADHD and OCD. It is estimated that 60 percent of people with TS have ADHD and 50 percent have OCD. On the surface it would appear that these are opposing disorders. People with ADHD have trouble paying attention, while people with OCD pay too much attention to their negative thoughts (obsessions) or behaviors (compulsions). In looking further at patients with both ADHD and OCD, I have found a high association of each disease in their family histories. So, for example, people with ADHD often have relatives with

OCD-like features and people with OCD have people in their families with ADHD. There is even a subtype of ADHD that has been termed overfocused ADHD; affected people have symptoms of both inattention and overfocus.

A crash course in the neurotransmitters (chemical messengers that help the brain to function) dopamine and serotonin is necessary here. In the brain there tends to be a balancing mechanism between dopamine and serotonin. This balance tends to be tipped in the basal ganglia. Dopamine is involved with motor movements, motivation, attention span, and setting the body's idle speed. Serotonin is more involved with mood control, shifting attention, and cognitive flexibility. When something happens in the brain to raise dopamine levels, serotonin becomes less effective; and when serotonin levels are raised, dopamine becomes less effective. For example, when I give someone a psychostimulant to treat ADHD, it works by effectively raising the availability of dopamine in the basal ganglia. This helps with focus, follow-through, and motivation. If I give him too much, he may become obsessive, moody, and inflexible (symptoms of too little serotonin). Likewise, if I give someone who has ADHD a medication that enhances serotonin availability in the brain, such as Prozac (a selective serotonin reuptake inhibitor), his ADHD symptoms are likely to become worse, but he won't care that they are worse and will also show lowered motivation.

Since the basal ganglia are involved with dopamine production (low in ADHD) and shifting and suppressing motor movements (lack of smoothness or cogwheeling may result in tics) and have been found to be overactive in OCD (in conjunction with the cingulate gyrus), the basal ganglia are likely to be significantly involved in all three of these disorders. Blocking dopamine with certain antipsychotic medications, such as Haldol (haloperidol) and Orap (pimozide), helps to suppress tics but makes ADHD symptoms worse. Psychostimulants, such as Ritalin (methylphenidate), Dexedrine (dexamfetamine sulphate), or Adderall (a combination of amphetamine salts), help ADHD symptoms but have a variable effect on tics (they may make them better or worse). In addition, as mentioned, psychostimulants tend to exacerbate OCD symptoms and cause people to focus more on the thoughts or behaviors that bother them. An interference mechanism in the basal ganglia is likely to be part of the picture, upsetting the dopamine-serotonin balance in the brain.

Fine Motor Problems

As discussed earlier, fine motor problems are often associated with basal ganglia abnormalities. We discussed handwriting problems earlier in this chapter. Another interesting connection probably related to basal ganglia activity is the development of fine motor tremors when we become anxious. When I lecture in front of an audience, I don't hold papers in my hands because the paper may start to rattle or shake in response to anxiety I feel. When the basal ganglia are overactive, we are more at risk of increased muscle tone or tremors. In my practice I have often prescribed the medication propranolol to calm the tremors musicians get during a performance.

Increased muscle tension related to overactive basal ganglia activity is often associated with headaches. I have noticed that a number of people with resistant headaches have intense focal areas of increased activity in the basal ganglia. This seems to occur with both muscle contraction headaches (often described as a pain in the back of the neck or as a tight band around the forehead) and migraines (usually one-sided throbbing headaches that may be preceded by a visual aura or other warning phenomena). Interestingly, often anticonvulsant medication such as Depakote or Tegretol, which decreases areas of overactivity in the brain, is helpful in decreasing some types of headaches.

Low and High Motivation

As mentioned, motivation tends to be low in dopamine-deficient states, such as ADHD. Interestingly, when serotonin levels are raised too high, decreased motivation also becomes a problem. Doctors know that when they overshoot the dose of serotonin-enhancing antidepressants (such as Prozac [fluoxetine], Lustral [sertraline], Seroxat [paroxetine], or Faverin [fluvoxamine]), lowered motivation is often the result. Many people have told me they stopped these medications because they stopped doing things that were important to their business or home life. One CEO told me he had stopped taking Lustral because he wasn't keeping up with his paperwork and he really didn't care. "That's not like me," he said.

Heightened dopamine or basal ganglia states may also cause increased or even excessive motivation. As I mentioned earlier, we found that many CEOs of corporations have enhanced basal ganglia activity. They also tend to work excessive hours. In fact, weekends tend to be the hardest time for these people. During the week, they charge through each day, getting things done. At the weekend, during unstructured time, they often complain of feeling restless, anxious, and out of sorts. Relaxation is foreign to them. In fact, it is downright uncomfortable. Workaholics may be made in the basal ganglia. Their internal idle speed, or energy level, doesn't allow them to rest. Of course, there is a positive correlate. Many of the people in society who make things happen are driven by basal ganglia that keep them working for long periods of time.

Basal Ganglia Checklist

Here is a basal ganglia system checklist. Please read this list of behaviors and rate yourself (or the person you are evaluating) on each behavior listed. Use the following scale and place the appropriate number next to the item. Five or more symptoms marked 3 or 4 indicate a high likelihood of basal ganglia problems.

0 = *never*
1 = *rarely*
2 = *occasionally*
3 = *frequently*
4 = *very frequently*

1........ Feelings of nervousness or anxiety
2........ Panic attacks
3........ Symptoms of heightened muscle tension (headaches, sore muscles, hand tremor)
4........ Periods of heart pounding, rapid heart rate, or chest pain
5........ Periods of trouble breathing or feeling smothered
6........ Periods of feeling dizzy, faint, or unsteady on your feet
7........ Periods of nausea or abdominal upset
8........ Periods of sweating, hot or cold flashes, cold hands
9........ Tendency to predict the worst
10........ Fear of dying or doing something crazy
11........ Avoidance of public places for fear of having an anxiety attack

12........ Conflict avoidance
13........ Excessive fear of being judged or scrutinized by others
14........ Persistent phobias
15........ Low motivation
16........ Excessive motivation
17........ Tics
18........ Poor handwriting
19........ Quick startle reaction
20........ Tendency to freeze in anxiety-provoking situations
21........ Excessive worry about what others think
22........ Shyness or timidity
23........ Low threshold of embarrassment

6

Mastering Fear:
Basal Ganglia Prescriptions

The following prescriptions will help you optimize and heal problems with the basal ganglia. They are based on what we have learned about the basal ganglia, as well as clinical experience with my patients. Remember, the basal ganglia are involved with integrating feelings and movement, shifting and smoothing motor behavior, setting the body's idle speed or anxiety level, modulating motivation, and driving feelings of pleasure and ecstasy.

BG PRESCRIPTION 1:
KILL THE FORTUNE-TELLING ANTS

People who have basal ganglia problems are often experts at predicting the worst. They have an abundance of fortune-telling ANTs (automatic negative thoughts). Learning to overcome the tendency toward pessimistic predictions is very helpful in healing this part of the brain. Through the years, I have met many people who tell me that they're pessimists. They say that if they expect the worst to happen in a situation, they will never be disappointed. Even though they may never be disappointed, they are likely to die earlier. The constant stress from negative predictions lowers immune system effectiveness and increases the risk of becoming ill. Your thoughts affect every cell in your body.

Learning how to kill the fortune-telling ANTs that go through your mind is essential to effectively dealing with the anxiety generated in this part of the brain. Whenever you feel anxious or tense, try the following steps.

Step 1

Write down the event that is causing you anxiety, for example, having to get up in front of people to give a speech.

Step 2

Notice and write down the automatic thoughts that come into your mind. Odds are, when you are anxious, your thoughts are predicting a negative outcome to a situation. Common anxiety-provoking thoughts include "They will think I'm stupid. Others will laugh at me. I will stumble on my words. I will shake and look nervous."

Step 3

Label or identify the thought as a fortune-telling ANT. Often, just naming the thought can help take away its power.

Step 4

Talk back to the automatic negative thought and "kill the ANT." Write down a response to defuse the negative thought. In this example, write something like "Odds are they won't laugh and I'll do a good job. If they do laugh, I'll laugh with them. I know that speaking in public is nerve-racking for many people, and probably some people will feel empathy for me if I'm nervous."

Do not accept every thought that comes into your mind. Thoughts are just thoughts, not facts. As such, when they are based on basal ganglia anxiety, they are often inaccurate. You do not have to believe every thought that comes into your mind. You can learn to change this pattern and help your basal ganglia cool down by predicting the best things.

BG PRESCRIPTION 2:
USE GUIDED IMAGERY

It is important to set (or reset) your basal ganglia to a relaxed, healthy level. This is best done by a regimen of daily relaxation. Taking twenty to thirty minutes a day to train relaxation into your body will have many beneficial effects, including decreasing anxiety, lowering blood pressure, lowering tension and pain in the muscles, and improving your temperament around others. Guided imagery is a wonderful technique to use on a daily basis.

Instructions: Find a quiet place where you can go and be alone for twenty to thirty minutes every day. Sit in a comfortable chair (you can lie down if you won't fall asleep) and train your mind to be quiet. In your mind's eye, choose your own special haven. I ask my patients, "If you could go anywhere in the world to feel relaxed and content, where would you go?" Imagine your special place with all of your senses. See what you want to see; hear the sounds you'd love to hear; smell and taste all the fragrances and tastes in the air; and feel what you would want to feel. The more vivid your imagination, the more you'll be able to let yourself go into the image. If negative thoughts intrude, notice them but don't dwell on them. Refocus on your safe haven. Breathe slowly, calmly, deeply. Enjoy your mini vacation.

BG PRESCRIPTION 3:
TRY DIAPHRAGMATIC BREATHING

Breathe slowly and deeply, mostly with your belly. This is one of the main exercises I teach my patients who have panic disorders. I actually write out a panic plan for them to carry with them. On the prescription it says: "Whenever you feel anxious or panicky, do the following:

- *breathe slowly and deeply with your belly,*
- *kill the fortune-telling ANTs,*
- *distract yourself from the anxiety,*
- *and if the above strategies are not completely effective, take the medication I prescribe for anxiety."*

Breathing is a very important part of the prescription. The purpose of breathing is to get oxygen from the air into your body and to blow off waste products such as carbon dioxide. Every cell in your body needs oxygen in order to function. Brain cells are particularly sensitive to oxygen, as they start to die within four minutes when they are deprived of it. Slight changes in oxygen content in the brain can alter the way a person feels and behaves. When a person gets angry, his or her breathing pattern changes almost immediately. Breathing becomes shallower and significantly faster. This breathing pattern is inefficient, and the oxygen content in the angry person's blood is lowered. Subsequently there is less oxygen available to a person's brain and he or she may become more irritable, impulsive, confused, and prone to negative behavior (such as yelling, threatening, or hitting another person).

Learn to breathe properly. Try this exercise:

Sit in a chair. Get comfortable. Close your eyes. Put one hand on your chest and one hand on your belly. Then, for several minutes, feel the rhythm of your breathing.

Do you breathe mostly with your chest? Mostly with your belly? Or with both your chest and belly?

The way you breathe has a huge impact on how you feel moment by moment. Have you ever watched a baby breathe? Or a puppy? They breathe almost exclusively with their bellies. They move their upper chest very little in breathing. Yet most adults breathe almost totally from the upper part of their chest.

To correct this negative breathing pattern, I teach my patients to become experts at breathing slowly and deeply, mostly with their bellies. In my office, I have some very sophisticated biofeedback equipment that uses strain gauges to measure breathing activity. I place one gauge around a person's chest and a second one around his or her belly. The biofeedback equipment measures the movement of the chest and belly as the person breathes in and out. If you expand your belly (using the diaphragm muscles there) when you breathe in, it allows room for your lungs to inflate downward, increasing the amount of air available to your body. I teach my patients to breathe with their bellies by watching their pattern on the computer screen. In about a half hour's time, most people can learn how to change their breathing patterns, which relaxes them and gives them better control over how they feel and behave.

If you do not have access to sophisticated biofeedback equipment, lie on your back and place a small book on your belly. When you breathe in, make the book go up, and when you breathe out, make the book go down. Shifting the center of breathing lower in your body will help you feel more relaxed and in better control of yourself. Practice this diaphragmatic breathing for five or ten minutes a day to settle down your basal ganglia.

This has been one of the most helpful exercises for me personally. When I first learned how to breathe diaphragmatically, I discovered that my baseline breathing rate was twenty-four breaths a minute and I breathed mostly with my upper chest. I had spent ten years in the military, being taught to stick my chest out and suck my gut in (the opposite of what is good for breathing). Quickly I learned how to quiet my breathing and help it be more efficient. Not only did it help my feelings of anxiety, it also helped me feel more settled overall. I still use it to calm my nerves before tough meetings, speaking engagements, and media appearances. I also use it, in conjunction with self-hypnosis, to help me sleep when I feel stressed. My current baseline breathing rate is less than ten times a minute.

BG PRESCRIPTION 4:
TRY MEDITATION/SELF-HYPNOSIS

There are many forms of meditation. They often involve diaphragmatic breathing and guided imagery. Herbert Benson, M.D., in his classic book, *The Relaxation Response*, describes how he had his patients focus on one word, and do nothing but that for a period of time each day. If other thoughts started to distract them, they were to train their mind to refocus on that one word. He reported startling results from this simple exercise: His patients had significant decreases in blood pressure and muscle tension.

Self-hypnosis taps into a natural "basal ganglia soothing" power source that most people do not even know exists. It is found within you, within your ability to focus your concentration. Many people do not understand that hypnosis is a natural phenomenon. It is an altered state we frequently go into and out of. Some natural examples of hypnosis include "highway hypnosis," in which our sense of time and consciousness becomes altered. Have you ever taken a long trip and not remembered a town you drove through? Or has a period of a couple of hours passed in what seemed like only twenty or thirty minutes? Time distortion is a common trait of hypnotic states. Have you ever become so engrossed in a good book or a good movie that two hours rushed by in what seemed like minutes? We become so focused that we enter a hypnotic state.

As you might imagine, because I have naturally overactive basal ganglia with a tendency toward anxiety, my medical internship year. produced only more anxiety. When I worked on the cardiac intensive care unit, I had a lot of trouble getting to sleep at night because I was so anxious over the condition of the patients under my care. Being tired the next day didn't help matters much. I had learned hypnosis as a medical student, and even used it with the nursing staff to help them stop smoking and lose weight. I hadn't thought of using it on myself. Besides, I rationalized, I wasn't really very hypnotizable. Late one evening, one of my patients had problems getting to sleep. He requested a sleeping pill. I thought it might be a better idea to use hypnosis to help him sleep. He was agreeable, and it worked quickly. When I made rounds the next morning, the patient asked me what he was going to do that night when I wasn't on call. I taught him self-hypnosis and came up with several sleep prescriptions. It then dawned on me to use self-hypnosis on myself. I learned that self-hypnosis, like most things, is a skill that gets better with practice. I got to the point where I could put myself to sleep in less than one minute through a simple self-hypnotic technique. Good sleep also helps calm anxiety. Sleep deprivation makes everything worse.

Here are the easy self-hypnotic steps I use personally. Set aside two to three ten-minute periods the first day and just go through the following six steps.

Relaxation

Step 1

Sit in a comfortable chair with your feet on the floor and your hands in your lap.

Step 2

Pick a spot on a wall that is a little bit above your eye level. Stare at the spot. As you do, count slowly to twenty. Notice that in a short while your eyelids begin to feel heavy. Let your eyes close. In fact, even if they don't feel as if they want to close, slowly close them anyway as you get to twenty.

Step 3

Next, take a deep breath, as deep as you can, and very slowly exhale. Repeat the deep breath and slowly exhale three times. With each breath in, feel your chest and belly rise and imagine breathing in peace and calmness. With each breath out, feel your chest and belly relax and blow out all the tension, all the things getting in the way of your relaxing. By this time, you'll notice a calm come over you.

Step 4

Next, tightly squeeze the muscles in your eyelids. Close your eyes as tightly as you can. Then slowly let the muscles in your eyelids relax. Notice how much more they have relaxed. Then imagine that relaxation spreading from the muscles in your eyelids to the muscles in your face—down your neck into your shoulders and arms—into your chest and throughout the rest of your body. The muscles will take the relaxation cue from your eyelids and relax progressively all the way down to the bottom of your feet.

Step 5

After your whole body feels relaxed, imagine yourself at the top of an escalator. Step on the escalator and ride down, slowly counting backwards from twenty. By the time you reach the bottom, you're likely to be very relaxed.

Step 6

Enjoy the tranquillity for several moments. Then get back on the escalator, riding up. Count to ten. When you get to ten, open your eyes, feel relaxed, refreshed, and wide awake.

To make these steps easy to remember, think of the following words:

FOCUS (focus on the spot)
BREATHE (slow, deep breaths)
RELAX (progressive muscle relaxation)
DOWN (ride down the escalator)
UP (ride up the escalator and open your eyes)

If you have trouble remembering these steps, you may want to record them and do the exercise as you listen to the tape.

When you do this the first few times, allow yourself plenty of time. Some people become so relaxed that they fall asleep for several minutes. If that happens, don't worry. It's actually a good sign— you're really relaxed!

When you've practiced this technique a few times, add visual imagery:

Visual Imagery

Choose a haven—a place where you feel comfortable, a place that you can imagine with all your senses. I usually "go" to the beach. I can relax there, and it calls up beautiful imagery for me. I can see the ocean, feel the sand between my toes, feel the warm sun and breeze on my skin, smell the salt air and taste it faintly on my tongue, hear the seagulls, the waves, children playing. Your haven can be a real or imagined place. It can be anywhere you'd like to spend time.

After you reach the bottom of the escalator, imagine yourself in your very special haven. Imagine it with all of your senses for several minutes.

This is where the fun starts. After you've gone through the relaxation steps and have imagined yourself in your haven, your mind is ripe for change.

Begin to experience yourself as you want to be—not as you currently are but as you *want* to be. Plan on spending at least twenty minutes a day on this refueling, life-changing exercise. You'll be amazed at the results.

During each session, choose an idea, ideal, or feeling state to focus on. Stay with the idea, ideal, or feeling state until you can imagine yourself engulfed in it. For example, if you want to be more relaxed, see yourself in a calm state, imagining it with all your senses. See yourself relaxed. Interact with others in a positive, relaxed way. Smell the environment around you. Feel your muscles relax. Taste a warm drink on your tongue, smell the aroma, feel the warm cup in your hands. Experience the relaxation. Make it real in your imagination, thereby beginning to make it real in your life.

If the relaxation does not come immediately, remember that self-hypnosis is not magic; it is a skill that needs attention and practice. It is well worth the effort.

Of note, I have a patient who tells me that whenever he comes out of a self-hypnotic state, his handwriting is better and he is much better coordinated overall. Sounds like basal ganglia soothing to me.

BG PRESCRIPTION 5:
THINK ABOUT THE "18/40/60 RULE"

People with basal ganglia problems often spend their days worrying about what other people think of them. To help them with this problem, I teach them the "18/40/60 Rule":

> When you're eighteen, you worry about what everybody is thinking of you;
>
> When you're forty, you don't give a damn about what anybody thinks of you;
>
> When you're sixty, you realize nobody's been thinking about you at all.

People spend their days worrying and thinking about themselves, not you. Think about your day. What have you thought about today—what others are doing or what you have to do or want to do? Odds are you've been thinking about yourself: what you have to do that day, who you're going to be with, what your bills are, the headaches your boss or children are giving you, whether your spouse will have any affection for you, and so on. People think about themselves, not you! You need to base your thoughts and the decisions you make on your goals—not your parents' goals, not your friends' goals, and not your coworkers' goals.

Worrying about what others think of them is the essence of people who have "social" phobias or those who are fearful or uncomfortable in social situations. The underlying problem is often that these people feel that others are judging them: their appearance, their clothes, their conversation, and so on.

My patients are amazed to learn that all of the energy they put into worrying about what others think of them is a total waste, energy they could more constructively put into meeting their own goals.

Did you know that one of the most common fears is the fear of public speaking? I have had a number of patients tell me that they failed a class in college because they refused to get up in front of the class and give a speech. That fear was based on how they felt others would judge them or their presentation. Those who have a fear of public speaking often tell themselves that people in the crowd will silently mock them or think bad things about them. The truth is, however, that probably some of the people in the audience aren't even listening to their presentation because they are thinking about their anxiety over their own presentation or about their own personal problems. The people in the audience who are listening are probably rooting for the speaker to do a good job, because they know from personal experience how hard it is to get up in front of a group of people to speak.

Stop worrying about what others think of you. Base your thoughts, your decisions, and your goals on what you want and what is important in your life. I am not advocating a self-centered life; most of us want to see ourselves in caring relationships with others and being able to be helpful to others. But you need to base your behavior on what you think, not on what you think others think.

BG PRESCRIPTION 6:
LEARN HOW TO DEAL WITH CONFLICT

As with relationships between countries, peace at any price is often devastating for relationships between people. Many people are so afraid of conflict with others that they do everything they can to avoid any turmoil. This "conflict phobia" actually sets up relationships for more turmoil rather than less.

Here are four typical scenarios of people who fear conflict:

1. In an attempt to be a "loving parent," Sara finds herself always giving in to her four-year-old son's temper tantrums. She is frustrated by how much the tantrums have increased in frequency over the past year. She now feels powerless and gives in just to keep the peace.

2. Billy, a ten-year-old boy, was bullied by a bigger ten-year-old named Ryan. Ryan threatened to hurt Billy if he didn't give him his lunch money. To avoid being hurt, Billy spent the year terrified by Ryan.

3. Kelly found herself feeling very distant from her husband, Carl. She felt that he always tried to control her and treated her like a child. He would complain about how much money she spent, what she wore, and who her friends were. Even though this really bothered Kelly, she said little because she didn't want to fight. However, she found that her interest in sex was nonexistent, she often felt tired and irritable, and she preferred to spend her free time with her friends rather than with Carl.

4. Bill worked as the foreman for Chet's company for six years. Over the past four years, Chet had become increasingly critical of Bill and belittled him in front of others. For fear of losing his job, Bill said nothing, but he became more depressed, started drinking more at home, and lost interest in his job.

Whenever we give in to the temper tantrums of a child or allow someone to bully or control us, we feel terrible about ourselves. Our self-esteem suffers, and the relationship with that other person is damaged. In many ways we teach other people how to treat us by what we tolerate and what we refuse to tolerate. "Conflict phobics" teach other people that it is okay to walk all over them, that there will be no consequences for misbehavior.

In order to have any personal power in a relationship, we must be willing to stand up for ourselves and for what we know is right. This does not mean we have to be mean or nasty; there are rational and kind ways to be firm. But firmness is essential.

Let's look at how the people in each of the four examples could handle their situations in more productive ways that would give them more power and more say in their lives.

1. Sara needs to make a rule that whenever her son throws a tantrum to get his way, he will not get what he wants, *period. No exceptions.* By giving in to his tantrums, Sara has taught her son to throw them, which not only hurts his relationship with his mother but will also teach him to be overdemanding with others and will damage his ability to relate socially to others. If Sara can be firm, kind, and consistent, she'll notice remarkable changes in a short time.

2. By giving in to the bully, Billy taught Ryan that his intimidating behavior was okay. Standing up to him early, even if it meant being beaten up, would have been better than spending a whole year in pain. Almost all bullies pick on people who won't fight back. They use intimidation and are rarely interested in real conflict.

3. Kelly made a strategic mistake by avoiding conflict early in her relationship with Carl. By giving in to his demands early on, she taught him that it was okay for him to control her. Standing up to him after years of giving in is very difficult but essential to saving the relationship. I see many, many people who even after years of giving in learn to stand up for themselves and change their relationship. Sometimes it takes a separation to convince the other person of your resolve, but the consequences of being controlled in a marriage are often depression and a lack of sexual desire. Standing up for oneself in a firm yet kind way is often marriage-saving.

4. Bill gave up his power when he allowed Chet to belittle him in front of others. No job is worth being tormented by your boss. Yet most people find that if they respectfully stand up to their boss, he or she is less likely to walk over them in the future. If, after standing up for yourself in a reasonable way, the boss continues to belittle you, it's time to look for a new job. Being in a job you hate will take years off your life.

Assertiveness means expressing your feelings in a firm, yet reasonable way. Assertiveness does not mean becoming mean or aggressive. Here are five rules to help you assert yourself in a healthy manner:

1. *Don't give in to the anger of others just because it makes you uncomfortable.*

2. *Don't allow the opinions of others to control how you feel about yourself. Your opinion, within reason, needs to be the one that counts.*
3. *Say what you mean and stick up for what you believe is right.*
4. *Maintain self-control.*
5. *Be kind, if possible, but above all be firm in your stance.*

Remember that we teach others how to treat us. When we give in to their temper tantrums, we teach them that that is how to control us. When we assert ourselves in a firm yet kind way, others have more respect for us and treat us accordingly. If you have allowed others to run over you emotionally for a long time, they'll be a little resistant to your newfound assertiveness. But stick to it, and you'll help them learn a new way of relating. You'll also help cool down your basal ganglia.

BG PRESCRIPTION 7:
CONSIDER BASAL GANGLIA MEDICATIONS

Antianxiety medications are often very helpful for severe basal ganglia problems. Nervousness, chronic stress, panic attacks, and muscle tension often respond to medications when the other techniques are ineffective. There are five classes of medication helpful in treating anxiety.

Benzodiazepines are common antianxiety medications that have been available for many years. Valium (diazepam), Xanax (alprazolam), Ativan (lorazepam) and oxazepam are examples of benzodiazepines. There are several advantages to these medications: They work quickly, they generally have few side effects, and they are very effective. On the negative side, long-term use can cause addiction. In the panic plan I discussed earlier, I often prescribe Xanax as a short-term anti-anxiety medication to use in conjunction with the other basal ganglia prescriptions.

BuSpar (buspirone) is often very effective in treating long-term anxiety. It also has the benefit of not being addictive. On the negative side, it takes a few weeks to be effective and it must be taken all of the time to work. It has been shown to have a calming effect on aggressive behavior.

Certain antidepressants, such as Tofranil (imipramine) and the MAO inhibitor Nardil (phenelzine), are especially helpful for people who have panic disorders. I have found these medications to be helpful in patients who have both limbic system and basal ganglia problems.

Focal basal ganglia abnormalities, like focal limbic system changes, are often helped with nerve-stabilizing medications, such as lithium, Tegretol, or Depakote.

The last class of medications I find helpful in severe cases of anxiety is antipsychotic medications, such as Risperdal (risperidone), Mellaril (thioridazine), and Haldol (haloperidol). Because of their side effects, I usually save these medications until I have tried other options. When psychotic symptoms are present, these medications are often lifesaving.

BG PRESCRIPTION 8:
WATCH YOUR BASAL GANGLIA NUTRITION

As mentioned in the Deep Limbic System Prescriptions chapter, what you eat has an important effect on how you feel. If your symptoms reflect heightened basal ganglia activity and anxiety, you'll do better with a balanced diet that does not allow you to get too hungry during the day. Hypoglycemic episodes make anxiety much worse. If you have low basal ganglia activity and low motivation, you will probably do better with a high-protein, low-carbohydrate diet to give yourself more energy during the day. It is also often helpful to eliminate caffeine, as it may worsen anxiety. Eliminating alcohol is often a good idea as well. Even though alcohol decreases anxiety in the short term, withdrawal from alcohol causes anxiety and places a person with anxiety at more risk of alcohol addiction.

Some herbal preparations such as valerian root have also been reported to help anxiety and are likely to have a calming effect on the basal ganglia. The B vitamins, especially vitamin B_6 in doses of 100 to 400 milligrams, are also helpful. If you take B_6 at these doses, it is important to take a B complex supplement as well. I also recommend GABA, an amino acid that has antianxiety qualities and is often used to help calm the brain. My patients have also found the scents from essential oils of chamomile and lavender to be calming.

7

Looking Into Inattention and Impulsivity:

The Prefrontal Cortex

FUNCTIONS OF THE PREFRONTAL CORTEX

- *attention span*
- *perseverance*
- *judgment*
- *impulse control*
- *organization*
- *self-monitoring and supervision*
- *problem solving*
- *critical thinking*
- *forward thinking*
- *learning from experience*
- *ability to feel and express emotions*
- *interaction with the limbic system*
- *empathy*

The prefrontal cortex (pfc) is the most evolved part of the brain. It occupies the front third of the brain, underneath the forehead. It is often divided into three sections: the dorsal lateral section (on the outside surface of the pfc), the inferior orbital section (on the front undersurface of the brain), and the cingulate gyrus (which runs through the middle of the frontal lobes). The cingulate gyrus, often considered to be part of the limbic system, will be covered in its own chapter. The dorsal lateral and inferior orbital gyrus are often termed the executive control center of the brain and will be discussed together in this chapter.

The Prefrontal Cortex

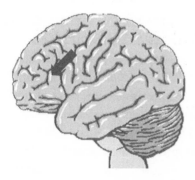

dorsal lateral prefrontal cortex
outside view

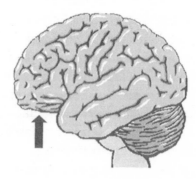

inferior orbital prefrontal cortex
outside view

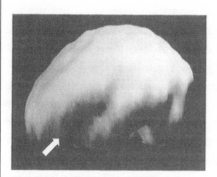

dorsal lateral prefrontal area
3-D side surface view

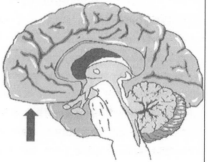

inferior orbital prefrontal area
inside view

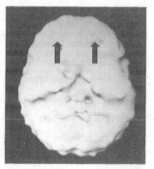

inferior orbital prefrontal area
3-D underside surface view

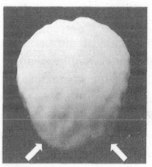

prefrontal area
3-D top-down surface view

When necessary, I'll distinguish what is known about their functions.

Overall, the pfc is the part of the brain that watches, supervises, guides, directs, and focuses your behavior. It supervises "executive functions," governing abilities such as time management, judgment, impulse control, planning, organization, and critical thinking. Our ability as a species to think, plan ahead, use time wisely, and communicate with others is heavily influenced by this part of the brain. The pfc is responsible for behaviors that are necessary for you to be goal-directed, socially responsible, and effective.

North Carolina neuropsychiatrist Thomas Gualtieri succinctly summarized the human functions of the pfc as "the capacity to formulate goals, to make plans for their execution, to carry them out in an effective way, and to change course and improvise in the face of obstacles or failure, *and to do so successfully, in the absence of external direction or structure.* The capacity of the individual to generate goals and to achieve them is considered to be an essential aspect of a mature and effective personality. It is not a social convention or an artifact of culture. It is hard wired in the construction of the prefrontal cortex and its connections."[*]

The pfc (especially the inferior orbital pfc) helps you think about what you say or do before you say or do it. For example, if you are having a disagreement with your spouse and you have good pfc function, you are more likely to give a thoughtful response that helps the situation. If you have poor pfc function, you are more likely to do or say something that will make the situation worse. The pfc helps you problem-solve, see ahead of a situation, and, through experience, choose among the most helpful alternatives. Playing a game such as chess effectively requires good pfc function.

This is also the part of the brain that helps you learn from mistakes. Good pfc function doesn't mean that you won't make mistakes. Rather, it generally means that you won't make the same mistake over and over. You are able to learn from the past and apply its lessons. For example, a student with good pfc function is likely to learn that if he or she starts a long-term project early, there is more time for research and less anxiety over getting it done. A student with decreased pfc function doesn't learn from past frustrations and may tend to put everything off until the last minute. Poor pfc function tends to appear in people who

[*] John Ratey, M.D., ed., *The Neuropsychiatry of Personality Disorders* (Cambridge, Mass.: Blackwell Science, 1995), p. 153.

have trouble learning from experience. They tend to make repetitive mistakes. Their actions are based not on experience, but rather on the moment, and on their immediate wants and needs.

The pfc (especially the dorsolateral pfc) is also involved with sustaining attention span. It helps you focus on important information while filtering out less significant thoughts and sensations. Attention span is required for short-term memory and learning. The pfc, through its many connections within the brain, helps you keep on task and allows you to stay with a project until it is finished. The pfc actually sends quieting signals to the limbic and sensory parts of the brain when you need to focus, and decreases the distracting input from other brain areas. When the pfc is underactive, you become more distractible (this will be discussed in detail under attention deficit hyperactivity disorder, below).

The pfc (especially the dorsolateral pfc) is also the part of the brain that allows you to feel and express emotions; to feel happiness, sadness, joy, and love. It is different from the more primitive limbic system. Even though the limbic system controls mood and libido, the prefrontal cortex is able to translate the workings of the limbic system into recognizable feelings, emotions, and words, such as love, passion, or hate. Underactivity or damage in this part of the brain often leads to a decreased ability to express thoughts and feelings.

Thoughtfulness and impulse control are heavily influenced by the pfc. The ability to think through the consequences of behavior—choosing a good mate, interacting with customers, dealing with difficult children, spending money, driving on the motorway—is essential to effective living, in nearly every aspect of human life. Without proper pfc function, it is difficult to act in consistent, thoughtful ways, and impulses can take over.

The pfc has many connections to the limbic system. It sends inhibitory messages that help keep it under control. It helps you "use your head along with your emotions." When there is damage or underactivity in this part of the brain, especially on the left side, the pfc cannot appropriately inhibit the limbic system, causing an increased vulnerability to depression if the limbic system becomes overactive. A classic example of this problem occurs in people who have had left frontal lobe strokes. Sixty percent of patients with these strokes develop a major depression within a year.

When scientists scan the prefrontal cortex with neuroimaging studies like SPECT, they often do two studies, one in a resting state

Left Frontal Lobe Stroke

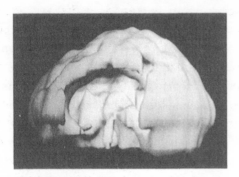 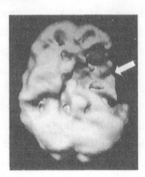

3-D side surface view *3-D underside surface view*
Notice large hole of activity in left frontal lobe.

and a second during a concentration task. In evaluating brain function, it is important to look at a working brain. When the normal brain is challenged by a concentration task, such as maths problems or sorting cards, the pfc activity increases. In certain brain conditions, such as attention deficit hyperactivity disorder and schizophrenia, prefrontal cortex activity decreases in response to an intellectual challenge.

PROBLEMS WITH THE PREFRONTAL CORTEX

- *short attention span*
- *distractibility*
- *lack of perseverance*
- *impulse control problems*
- *hyperactivity*
- *chronic lateness, poor time management*
- *disorganization*
- *procrastination*
- *unavailability of emotions*
- *misperceptions*
- *poor judgment*
- *trouble learning from experience*
- *short-term memory problems*
- *social and test anxiety*

Problems in the dorsal lateral prefrontal cortex often lead to decreased attention span, distractibility, impaired short-term memory, decreased mental speed, apathy, and decreased verbal expression. Problems in the inferior orbital cortex often lead to poor impulse control, mood control problems (due to its connections with the limbic system), decreased social skills, and decreased control over behavior.

People with pfc problems often do things they later regret, exhibiting problems with impulse control. They also experience problems with attention span, distractibility, procrastination, poor judgment, and problems expressing themselves. Situations that require concentration, impulse control, and quick reactions are often hampered by pfc problems. Test anxiety and social anxiety may be hallmarks of problems in the pfc. Tests require concentration and the retrieval of information. Many people with pfc problems experience difficulties in test situations because they have trouble activating this part of the brain under stress, even if they have adequately prepared for the test. In a similar way, social situations require concentration, impulse control, and dealing with uncertainty. Pfc deactivation often causes a person's mind to "go blank" in conversation, which naturally causes discomfort in social situations.

When men have problems in this part of the brain, their emotions are often unavailable to them and their partners complain that they do not share their feelings. This can cause serious problems in a relationship. Many women, for example, blame their male partners for being cold or unfeeling, when it is really a problem in the pfc that causes a lack of being "tuned in" to the feelings of the moment.

Attention Deficit Hyperactivity Disorder (ADHD)*

ADHD occurs as a result of neurological dysfunction in the prefrontal cortex. As I've mentioned, when people with ADHD try to concentrate, pfc activity decreases rather than increasing as it does in the normal brains of control group subjects. As such, people with ADHD show many of the symptoms discussed in this chapter, such as poor

---

* ADHD (attention deficit hyperactivity disorder) is also called ADD (attention deficit disorder). These are just names for the same disorder. Because half of the people who have ADHD are never hyperactive, many of us find the change frustrating. But, nonetheless, in this book I will refer to the disorder as ADHD.

internal supervision, short attention span, distractibility, disorganization, hyperactivity (although only half the people with ADHD are hyperactive), impulse control problems, difficulty learning from past errors, lack of forethought, and procrastination.

ADHD has been a particular interest of mine over the past fifteen years. Of note, two of my three children have this disorder. I tell people I know more about ADHD than I want to. Through the SPECT research done in my clinic, along with the brain-imaging and genetic work done by others, we have found that ADHD is basically a genetically inherited disorder of the pfc, due in part to a deficiency of the neurotransmitter dopamine.

Here are some of the common characteristics of ADHD that clearly relate this disorder to the pfc.

The Harder You Try, the Worse It Gets

Research has shown that the more people with ADHD try to concentrate, the worse things get for them. The activity in the pfc actually turns down, rather than turning up. When a parent, teacher, supervisor, or manager puts more pressure on a person with ADHD to perform, he or she often becomes less effective. Too frequently when this happens the parent, teacher, or boss interprets this decreased performance as willful misconduct, and serious problems arise. One man with ADHD whom I treat told me that whenever his boss puts intense pressure on him to do a better job, his performance becomes much worse, even though he really tries to do better. While it is true that almost all of us perform better with praise, I've found that it is essential for people with ADHD. When the boss encourages him to do better in a positive way, he becomes more productive. In parenting, teaching, supervising, or managing someone with ADHD, it is much more effective to use praise and encouragement, rather than pressure. People with ADHD do best in environments that are highly interesting or stimulating and relatively relaxed.

Short Attention Span

A short attention span is the hallmark of this disorder. People with ADHD have trouble sustaining attention and effort over prolonged periods of time. Their attention tends to wander and they are frequently off task, thinking about or doing things other than the task at hand. Yet one of the things that often fools inexperienced clinicians assessing this disorder is that people with ADHD do not have a short attention span for everything. Often, people with ADHD can pay attention just fine to things that are new, novel, highly stimulating, interesting, or frightening. These things provide enough intrinsic stimulation that they activate the pfc so the person can focus and concentrate. A child with ADHD might do very well in a one-on-one situation and completely fall apart in a classroom of thirty children. My son with ADHD, for example, used to take four hours to do half an hour's worth of homework, frequently getting off task. Yet if you gave him a car stereo magazine, he would quickly read it from cover to cover and remember every little detail in it. People with ADHD have long-standing problems paying attention to regular, routine, everyday matters such as homework, schoolwork, chores, or paperwork. The mundane is terrible for them, and it is *not* a choice. They need excitement and interest to kick in their pfc function.

Many adult couples tell me that in the beginning of their relationship, the partner with adult ADHD could pay attention to the other person for hours. The stimulation of new love helped him or her focus. But as the "newness" and excitement of the relationship began to fade (as it does in nearly all relationships), the person with ADHD had a much harder time paying attention, and his or her ability to listen faltered.

Distractibility

As mentioned above, the pfc sends inhibitory signals to other areas of the brain, quieting intake from the environment so that you can concentrate. When the pfc is underactive, it doesn't adequately dampen the sensory parts of the brain, and too many stimuli bombard the brain as a result. Distractibility is evident in many different settings for the person with ADHD. In class, during meetings, or while listening to a partner, the person with ADHD tends to notice other things going on and has trouble staying focused on the issue at hand. People with ADHD tend to look around the room, drift off, appear bored, forget where the conversation is going, and interrupt with extraneous information. Their distractibility and short attention span may also cause them to take much longer to complete their work.

Impulsivity

Lack of impulse control gets many ADHD people into hot water. They may say inappropriate things to parents, friends, teachers, supervisors, other employees, or customers. I once had a patient who had been fired from thirteen jobs because he had trouble controlling what he said. Even though he really wanted to keep several of the jobs, he would just blurt out what he was thinking before he had a chance to process the thought. Poorly thought-out decisions also relate to impulsivity. Rather than thinking a problem through, many ADHD people want an immediate solution and act without the necessary forethought. In a similar vein, impulsivity causes these people to have trouble going through the established channels at work. They often go right to the top to solve problems, rather than working through the system. This may cause resentment from coworkers and immediate supervisors. Impulsivity may also lead to such problem behaviors as lying (saying the first thing that comes into your mind), stealing, having affairs, and excessive spending. I have treated many ADHD people who have suffered with the shame and guilt of these behaviors.

In my lectures I often ask the audience, "How many people here are married?" A large percentage of the audience raises their hands. I then ask, "Is it helpful for you to say everything you think in your marriage?" The audience laughs, because they know the answer. "Of course not," I continue. "Relationships require tact. Yet because of impulsivity and a lack of forethought, many people with ADHD say the first thing that comes to mind. And instead of apologizing for saying something hurtful, many ADHD people will justify why they said the hurtful remark, only making the situation worse. An impulsive comment can ruin a nice evening, a weekend, even a whole marriage."

Conflict Seeking

Many people with ADHD unconsciously seek conflict as a way to stimulate their own pfc. They do not know they do it. They do not plan to do it. They deny that they do it. And yet they do it just the same. The relative lack of activity and stimulation to the pfc craves more activity. Hyperactivity, restlessness, and humming are common forms of self-stimulation. Another way I have seen people with ADHD "try to turn on their brains" is by causing turmoil. If they can get their parents or spouses to be emotionally intense or yell at them, that might increase activity in their frontal lobes and help them to feel more tuned in. Again, this is not a conscious phenomenon. But it seems that many ADHD people become addicted to the turmoil.

I once treated a man who would quietly stand behind a corner in his house and jump out and scare his wife when she walked by. He liked the charge he got out of her screams. Unfortunately for his wife, she developed an irregular heart rhythm because of the repetitive scares. I have also treated many adults and children with ADHD who seemed driven to get their pets upset by playing rough with or teasing them.

The parents of children with ADHD commonly report that the kids are experts at upsetting them. One mother told me that when she wakes up in the morning, she promises herself that she won't yell at or get upset with her eight-year-old son. Yet invariably by the time he is off to school, there have been at least three fights and both of them feel terrible. When I explained the child's unconscious need for stimulation to the mother, she stopped yelling at him. When parents stop providing the negative stimulation (yelling, spanking, lecturing, etc.), these children decrease the negative behaviors. Whenever you feel like screaming at one of these kids, stop yourself and instead talk as softly as you can. At least in that way you're helping to break their addiction to turmoil and lowering your own blood pressure.

Another self-stimulating behavior common in people with ADHD is worrying or focusing on problems. The emotional turmoil generated by worrying or being upset produces stress chemicals that keep the brain active. I once treated a women who had depression and ADHD. She started each session by telling me she was going to kill herself. She noted that this would make me anxious and seemed to enjoy telling me the gruesome details of how she would do it. After about a year of listening to her, I finally figured out that she wasn't really going to kill herself, she was using my reaction as a source of stimulation for her. After getting to know her well, I told her, "Stop talking about suicide. I do not believe you'll kill yourself. You love your four children, and I can't believe you would ever abandon them. I think you use this talk as a way to keep things stirred up. Without knowing, your ADHD causes you to play the game of 'Let's have a problem.' This ruins any joy you could have in your life." Initially, she was very upset with me (another source of conflict, I told her), but she trusted me enough to at least look at the behavior. Decreasing her need for turmoil became the major focus of psychotherapy.

A significant problem with using anger, emotional turmoil, and negative emotion for self-stimulation is damage to the immune system. The high levels of adrenaline produced by conflict-driven behavior decrease the immune system's effectiveness and increase vulnerability to illness. I have seen evidence of this deficiency over and over with the connection between ADHD and chronic infections, and in the increased incidence of fibromyalgia, chronic muscle pain thought to be associated with immune deficiency.

As noted, many people with ADHD tend to be in constant turmoil with one or more people, at home, work, or school. They seem to unconsciously choose people who are vulnerable and pick verbal battles with them. Many mothers of children with ADHD have told me that they feel like running away from home. They cannot stand the constant turmoil in their relationship with the child with ADHD. Many children and adults with ADHD have a tendency to embarrass others for little or no good reason, which consequently distances their "victims" from them and can result in social isolation. They may be the class clowns in school or the wisecrackers at work. *Witzelsucht* is a term in the neuropsychiatric literature that characterizes "an addiction to making bad jokes." It was first described in patients who had frontal lobe brain tumors, especially on the right side.

Disorganization

Disorganization is another hallmark of ADHD. It includes disorganization of physical space, such as rooms, desks, book bags, filing cabinets, and closets, as well as disorganization of time. Often when you look at work areas of people with ADHD, it is a wonder they can work there at all. They tend to have many piles of "stuff"; paperwork is often hard for them to keep straight; and they seem to have a filing system that only they can figure out (and then only on good days). Many people with ADHD are chronically late or put things off until the last possible minute. I've had several patients who have bought sirens from alarm companies to help them wake up. Imagine what their neighbors thought! They also tend to lose track of time, which contributes to lateness.

Start Many Projects, but Finish Few

The energy and enthusiasm of people with ADHD often push them to start many projects. Unfortunately, their distractibility and short attention span impair their ability to complete them. One radio station manager told me that he had started over thirty special projects the year before but completed only a handful. He told me, "I'm always going to get back to them, but I get new ideas that get in the way." I also treat a college professor who told me that the year before he saw me he had started three hundred different projects. His wife finished the thought by telling me he had completed only three.

Moodiness and Negative Thinking

Many people with ADHD tend to be moody, irritable, and negative. Since the pfc is underactive, it cannot fully temper the limbic system, which becomes overactive, leading to mood control issues. In another subtle way, as mentioned, many people with ADHD worry or become overfocused on negative thoughts as a form of self-stimulation. If they cannot seek turmoil from others in the environment, they seek it within themselves. They often have a "sky is falling" attitude that distances them from others.

ADHD used to be thought of as a disorder of hyperactive boys who outgrew it before puberty. We now know that most people with ADHD do not outgrow the symptoms of this disorder and that it frequently occurs in girls and women. It is estimated that ADHD affects seventeen million Americans and about 1.7 percent of the U.K. population, mostly children.

Kent

Kent was twenty-four years old when he first came to see me. He came for help because he had gone to junior college six straight semesters. He hadn't been able to finish one class! He wanted to go to medical school. Everybody told him he was nuts! How could he go to medical school if he couldn't even finish a junior college semester? Then his mother read my book *Windows into the ADD Mind*. She wondered if Kent didn't have attention deficit hyperactivity disorder.

After I took Kent's history, it was clear he had suffered from an undiagnosed lifelong case of ADHD. From the time he had been in kindergarten, he had had problems staying in his seat; he had been restless, distractible, disorganized, and labeled as an underachiever.

Kent's father requested that we do a brain SPECT study to look at his brain. He wanted to make sure Kent wasn't just looking for another excuse as to why he was failing in life. Kent's brain SPECT study at rest was normal. When Kent tried to concentrate, however, the prefrontal cortex of his brain turned off.

After the results of the clinical examination and brain SPECT studies, I put Kent on Adderall, a stimulant medication that is used to treat symptoms of ADHD. Kent had a remarkable response. He completed all of his classes at school the next semester. In eighteen months he got his associate of arts degree, and three years later he finished his bachelor's degree in biology. He has been accepted to medical school! I did a follow-up study of Kent's brain on Adderall several months after starting the medication. As you can see in the illustration, not only did he have a positive clinical response, he also had significant increased activity in the prefrontal cortex.

It's amazing how much his father's attitude has changed toward him. The father told me, "I thought he was just lazy. It makes me sad to think of all those years that he had a medical problem and I just hassled him for being lazy. I wish I could have those years back."

I have one man in my practice who has ten businesses because that's what he needs in order to keep himself turned on! When the brain is underactive, it's uncomfortable. Unconsciously, people learn how to turn it on, by conflict, coffee or cigarettes (both mild stimulants), anger, a fast-paced life, or highly stimulating physical activities, such as bungee jumping. (Bungee jumpers need to be screened for this problem!)

Kent's ADHD-Affected Brain, off and on Adderall

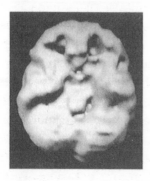 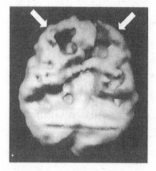

3-D underside surface view

At rest; note overall good activity.

During concentration; note markedly decreased pfc activity (arrows).

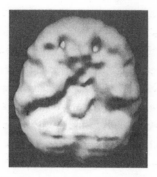

During concentration, with Adderall; note overall improved activity.

ADHD in the Family

Many psychiatric disorders are now thought to have significant genetic influences. ADHD is no exception. Here's a family case example.

Paul, age twenty, first came to see me because he was having trouble finishing his senior year at college. He was having difficulty completing term papers, he could not focus in class, and he had little motivation. He began to believe that he should drop out of school and go to work for his father. He hated the idea of quitting school so close to graduation. While I was writing up his history, Paul told me about bouts of depression that had been treated with Prozac in the past with little benefit.

Paul's brain SPECT study showed increased activity in his limbic system (consistent with depression) and deactivation of his prefrontal cortex during a concentration task (consistent with ADHD). He had a wonderful response to a combination of an antidepressant and a stimulant medication. He finished college and got the kind of job he wanted.

When Paul's mother, Pam, saw his good response to treatment, she came to see me for herself. As a child, she had had trouble learning. Even though she was very artistic, she had little motivation for school and her teachers labeled her as an underachiever. As an adult, Pam went back to school and earned a degree in elementary school teaching. In order to student teach, however, she had to pass the National Teacher's Exam. She had failed the test on four occasions. Pam was ready to give up and try a new avenue of study when she saw Paul get better. She thought maybe there was help for her. In fact, her brain SPECT studies were very similar to Paul's studies, and she responded well to the same combination of medications. Four months later, she passed the National Teacher's Exam.

With two successes in the family, the mother then sent her teenage daughter, Karen, to see me. Like her brother, Karen was a bright child who had underachieved in school. At the time she came to see me, she lived in Los Angeles and was enrolled in a broadcast journalism course. She complained that learning the material was hard for her. She was also moody, restless, easily distracted, and impulsive, and had a quick temper. Several years earlier she had been treated for alcohol and amphetamine abuse. She said that the alcohol settled her restlessness and the amphetamines helped her to concentrate. Karen's brain SPECT studies were very similar to her brother's and mother's. Once on medication, she was amazed at the difference. She could concentrate in class and finished her work in half the time it had taken before. Karen's level of confidence increased to the point where she could look for work as a broadcaster, something she had been unable to do previously.

The most reluctant member of the family to see me was the father, Tim—even though Pam, Paul, and Karen told him that he should. He said, "There's nothing wrong with me; look at how successful I am." But his family knew different. Even though Tim owned a successful grocery store, he was reclusive and distant. He got tired early in the day, was easily distracted, and had a scattered approach to work. His success at work was due in part to his good employees, who made his ideas happen. He also had trouble learning new games, such as cards, which caused him to avoid certain social situations. Tim enjoyed high-stimulation activities, such as riding motorcycles, even at the age of fifty-five. Looking back, Tim had done poorly in high school. He had barely got through college even though he had a very high IQ. He had tended to drift from job to job until he was able to buy the grocery store. Tim's wife finally convinced him to see me. She was getting ready to divorce him because she felt that he didn't care about her. He later told me that he was too physically and emotionally drained to share much of his life with her.

During our first session, Tim told me that he couldn't possibly have ADHD because he was a success in business. But the more questions I asked him about his past, the more lights went on in his mind. His childhood nickname had been "Speedy." He often hadn't done his homework. He had often been distracted or bored in school. His energy was gone by the end of the morning. When I asked about his organization at work, he replied that her name was Elsa, his assistant. At the end of the interview, I commented, "If you really do have ADHD, I wonder how successful you could be given what you've already accomplished." Tim's brain SPECT studies showed the classic pattern for ADHD. When he tried to concentrate, the prefrontal cortex of his brain turned off, rather than on. When I told him this, it really sank in. "Maybe that's why it is hard for me to learn games. When I'm in a social situation and I'm pressed to learn or respond, I just freeze up. So I avoid these situations."

Tim had a remarkable response to Ritalin. He was more awake during the day, he accomplished more in less time, and his relationship with his wife dramatically improved. In fact, they both said they couldn't believe that their relationship could be so good, after all the years of distance and hurt.

Psychotic Disorders

Psychotic disorders, such as schizophrenia, affect a person's ability to distinguish reality from fantasy. These disorders are complex and involve several brain areas, but at least in part, the neurotransmitter abnormalities cause decreased prefrontal cortex activity.

Schizophrenia is a chronic, long-standing disorder characterized by delusions, hallucinations, and distorted thinking. When I first started ordering SPECT studies on schizophrenic patients, I began to understand why they distorted incoming information. The following case is a good example.

Julie

Julie was forty-eight years old when we met. She had a history of hospitalizations for paranoid thinking, hearing voices, and delusional thinking. Her main delusion centered around being assaulted by someone who put an electrical probe inside her head that "blasted her with electricity." She had been on multiple medication trials without success. Due to her lack of responsiveness to standard treatments, I ordered a brain SPECT study.

In a sense, Julie was right. She *was* being blasted with electricity (note the multiple hot spots across her brain), but because she had such poor prefrontal cortex activity, she was unable to process the physiological nature of her illness and developed delusions to explain the pain she experienced. With the information from the SPECT study, Julie was placed on a high therapeutic dose of Depakote, which lessened her pain and anxiety. For the first time, she was willing to entertain the possibility that her symptoms were the result of abnormal brain activity rather than an outside attack. A repeat SPECT study eight months later showed a marked decrease in the hot spots in her brain along with subsequent increased activity in her prefrontal cortex.

Julie's Schizophrenia-Affected Brain

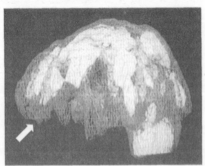

front

3-D left-side surface view

Note markedly decreased prefrontal activity (arrow) and multiple hot spots across the cortex.

Derrick

Derrick, a thirteen-year-old boy, was brought to see me because he was severely anxious. He was displaying psychotic symptoms, feeling that other children were talking about him behind his back and that they were out to embarrass him in front of his whole school. He started to avoid all contact with his peer group. He would hide in the middle of clothes racks at the mall if he saw people he knew, for fear that they might laugh at him or talk about him to others. He was petrified by his thoughts and stopped going to school. He even seriously entertained the idea of suicide. He had crying spells, sleeplessness, and intense anxiety. He wasn't able to rationally discuss any of these feelings. I saw him for months in psychotherapy and tried him on several antidepressant and antipsychotic medications without a therapeutic response. A SPECT scan was done when he was off all medication to help us understand what was going on.

Derrick's SPECT study showed marked decreased activity in his prefrontal cortex at rest, a common finding in psychotic disorders. It is also a finding in some psychotic depressions. The study led me to try alternative medications that were more effective. Within two months there was a dramatic clinical improvement in his condition. His mood was better, he had no suicidal thoughts, he was less sensitive to others, and he was more able to entertain alternatives to his distorted thoughts. Seven months later, he was much more like a normal teenager. A repeated SPECT study performed six months later showed normalization of his prefrontal cortex activity. Six years later, I see Derrick every six months. He is an honors student at a highly prestigious university.

The SPECT study was very important in the treatment process. It clearly showed Derrick's parents that his problems were based on brain abnormalities and that he couldn't help what he thought or felt. They were able to respond in a more understanding and helpful manner, lowering the level of stress at home.

Head Injuries

Due to its location, the pfc is especially susceptible to head injury. Many people do not fully understand how head injuries, sometimes even "minor" ones in which no loss of consciousness occurs, can alter a person's character and ability to learn. This is particularly true when the head injury occurs in the brain's executive director, or pfc. Your brain is very soft. Your skull is very hard. Your brain sits in a closed space that has many sharp edges. Unfortunately for the pfc, the inferior orbital cortex sits on top of several sharp, bony ridges, and the dorsal lateral prefrontal cortex lies just beneath the place where many blows to the head occur.

It is important to note that many people forget they've had a significant head injury in their lifetime. In our clinic we ask patients several times whether or not they have had a significant head injury. Our intake paperwork asks the question "Have you ever had a head injury?" The historian, who gathers patients' histories before they see the doctor, asks them again about head injuries. The computer testing we have patients complete asks a third time about head injuries. If I see no, no, no to the question of head injuries, I'll ask again. If I get a fourth no, I will then say, "Are you sure? Have you ever fallen out of a tree, fallen off a fence, or dived into a shallow pool?" I am constantly amazed at how many people remember head injuries that they'd long forgotten or felt were too insignificant to remember. One patient, when asked the question for the fifth time, put his hand on his forehead and said, "Oh yeah! When I was five years old, I fell out of a second-story window." Likewise, I have had other patients forget they went through windshields, fell out of moving vehicles, or were knocked unconscious when they fell off their bicycles. Head injuries are very important. I often tell my patients that their brain is more sophisticated than any computer we can think of designing. You can't drop a computer without the potential of causing serious damage. In the same way, the brain is fragile, and if trauma occurs in sensitive parts of the brain, it has the potential to alter one's ability to function.

Phineas P. Gage provided scientists with an extreme example of pfc dysfunction secondary to a head injury. This was one of the first cases in the medical literature about the outcome of prefrontal cortex damage. In 1848, at the age of twenty-five, Gage was an up-and-coming railroad construction foreman in Vermont working for the Rutland and Burlington Railroad. His job involved using a long tamping iron to ignite explosives to forge a path for the railroad. One day a horrible accident occurred; the explosion sent the tamping iron, which was 1.25 inches in diameter, 3.5 feet long, and weighed 13.5 pounds, through the front part of Gage's skull. It went through his left eye, through the left prefrontal cortex, and out the top front part of his skull, leaving a circular 3.5-inch opening, destroying his left prefrontal cortex and surrounding areas of the brain. Initially the interest in the case was due to Gage's survival, which was called "unprecedented in surgical history." Later, in 1868, his doctor turned his attention to the personality changes in Gage. Before the accident, Gage had been an honest, reliable, deliberate person and a good worker. After the accident, even though he did not appear to suffer any intellectual impairment, he was described as childish, capricious, and obstinate, showed poor judgment, used profane language, and was inconsiderate of others. In short, his doctor concluded that "Gage was no longer Gage." In many ways, the pfc contains our ability to be ourselves.

Zachary

The two following cases provide modern-day examples similar to that of Gage.

Zachary, age ten, was a fun-loving, active boy who was affectionate, sweet, and eager to please. He did well in kindergarten and was liked by the other children. One summer, between kindergarten and first grade, Zachary was riding in the front seat of a car with his mother on a trip to his grandparents' house. All of a sudden a drunk driver swerved into their lane, causing Zachary's mother to quickly jerk the car to the side

Zachary's Trauma-Affected Brain

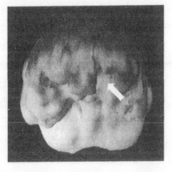

3-D front-on surface view
Note markedly decreased activity in the left prefrontal cortex.

of the road. She lost control, and the car hit a tree. Zachary's mother's leg was broken in the accident, and Zachary, thankfully restrained by a seat belt, hit his head against the side window. He was unconscious, but only for about ten minutes.

About six weeks later, Zachary began to change. He exhibited aggressive behavior, breaking his own toys and hurting his younger brother. He began swearing, blurted out statements at inappropriate times, and interrupted frequently. He became rude, contrary, argumentative, and conflict-seeking. He lost his friends at school the next year because he said things that hurt their feelings. He started to tease the two cats at home, so much so that they started to avoid him whenever he came into the house. Six months after the accident, his mother knew that something was seriously wrong. She took him to a counselor, who thought the problem was psychological, a result of the accident. The counselor thought that Zachary and his mother were too close and developed strategies to help Zachary become more independent. That only seemed to make things worse. After two years of counseling, which didn't seem to help much, the mother consulted Zachary's pediatrician. He diagnosed Zachary with ADHD and put him on Ritalin. But that didn't help very much either. In fact, it only seemed to make him more aggressive. When Zachary was brought to see me at age nine, I thought he might have a chronic post-concussive syndrome, secondary to the accident. His brain SPECT study revealed marked decreased activity in the left pfc and decreased activity in the left occipital cortex, indicating both a front and back injury (common in head injuries). In addition, there was decreased activity in his left temporal lobe. Given this constellation of findings, I put Zachary on a combination of medication (an anticonvulsant, to stabilize his aggressiveness and help his temporal lobe function, and Symmetrel (amantadine) to help with focus, concentration, and impulse control). He was also placed in a special class at school and given cognitive retraining exercises. Over the next several months, his behavior began to improve.

Tim

Tim, age fifteen, was a high school sophomore. From his early youth he had exhibited severe behavior problems. He was hyperactive, impulsive, moody, and frequently angry, especially whenever someone would tell him no. His temper flared quickly, often over minor or trivial incidents. He had already been arrested for shoplifting, he frequently skipped school, and he was defiant and abusive toward his parents. He did not get along with other teens at school and seemed to "never fit in." He smoked a pack of cigarettes a day and frequently used marijuana and cocaine. He had already been in one treatment program and was on his way to a second when his parents brought him to our clinic. He had tried numerous medications without success.

His brain SPECT study showed one of the most severe cases of damage to the left prefrontal cortex that I have ever seen. When he was eighteen months old, he had fallen down a flight of stairs. His mother said he had never been quite the same since then. She knew there was a difference in his personality. Given the level of functional damage to Tim's brain, I decided to put him on a combination of an anticonvulsant medication and a stimulant. It helped lessen the rage and improve his impulse control. Given the level of damage, Tim's chances to gain full executive function are not very promising. The goal of treatment is to utilize every prescription available to help him develop auxiliary internal supervision mechanisms. Otherwise, legal authorities may have to impose external supervision in some form of a contained setting, basically through no fault of Tim's. He doesn't have the capacity for internal supervision that is housed in the prefrontal cortex.

Tim's Trauma-Affected Brain

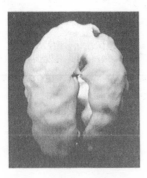 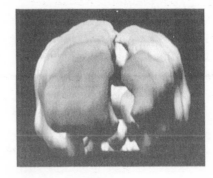

D top-down surface view   *3-D front-on surface view*

Notice the large defect in the left mid-frontal region.

Understanding the functions and problems of this part of the brain is often essential to the healing process of people who suffer.

Prefrontal Cortex Checklist

Here is the prefrontal cortex checklist. Please read this list of behaviors and rate yourself (or the person you are evaluating) on each behavior listed. Use the following scale and place the appropriate number next to the item. Five or more symptoms marked 3 or 4 indicate a high likelihood of prefrontal cortex problems.

0 = *never*
1 = *rarely*
2 = *occasionally*
3 = *frequently*
4 = *very frequently*

1........ Inability to give close attention to details or avoid careless mistakes
2........ Trouble sustaining attention in routine situations (homework, chores, paperwork, etc.)
3........ Trouble listening
4........ Inability to finish things, poor follow-through
5........ Poor organization of time or space
6........ Distractibility
7........ Poor planning skills
8........ Lack of clear goals or forward thinking
9........ Difficulty expressing feelings
10........ Difficulty expressing empathy for others
11........ Excessive daydreaming
12........ Boredom
13........ Apathy or lack of motivation
14........ Lethargy
15........ A feeling of spaciness or being "in a fog"
16........ Restlessness or trouble sitting still
17........ Difficulty remaining seated in situations where remaining seated is expected
18........ Conflict seeking

19........ Talking too much or too little

20........ Blurting out of answers before questions have been completed

21........ Difficulty awaiting turn

22........ Interruption of or intrusion on others (e.g., butting into conversations or games)

23........ Impulsivity (saying or doing things without thinking first)

24........ Trouble learning from experience; tendency to make repetitive mistakes

8

Becoming Focused:
Prefrontal Cortex Prescriptions

The prefrontal cortex is the most evolved part of the brain. As such, it is essential in helping you reach your goals. To review, the prefrontal cortex is involved with concentration, attention span, judgment, impulse control, and critical thinking. It controls your ability to look at situations, organize your thoughts, plan what you want to do, and carry out your plans. Healing this part of the brain requires the development of a concept I call "total focus."

PFC PRESCRIPTION 1:
DEVELOP AND MAINTAIN CLEAR FOCUS
(THE ONE-PAGE MIRACLE)

Developing an ability to stay totally focused will help guide your thoughts and behavior and give you an "auxiliary prefrontal cortex." It will help strengthen the conscious part of your mind.

In order to be successful in the world, we need to have clearly defined goals. Specifically, we need to know who we are and what we want to accomplish in our relationships, at work, and within ourselves. When we know what we want, we are more likely to change our behavior to get it. Being goal-directed helps keep our behavior on track.

When I first mention goal setting to my patients, they generally look at me with blank stares or mutter something vague about a career or money. Goal setting is not for some far-off dream. It is for now, and it is very specific. Making goals that you can focus on daily will make a big difference in your life.

I have my patients, whether they are six or seventy-five years old, do a goal-setting exercise I developed called the One-Page Miracle (OPM). In studying successful children and adults, I have found that the one thing they have in common is a sense of personal responsibility and clear goals. The One-Page Miracle will help guide nearly all of your thoughts, words, and actions. I've seen this exercise quickly focus and change many people.

Here's how to develop your own OPM. Take one sheet of paper and clearly write out your major goals. Use the following main headings: Relationships, Work, Money, and Myself. Under "Relationships," write the subheadings spouse/lover, children, extended family, and friends. Under "Work," write current and future work goals, and include a section on how you want to get along with your employer. Under "Money," write your current and future financial goals. Under "Myself," write out body, mind, spirit, and interests.

Next to each subheading, clearly write out what's important to you in that area; write what you want, not what you don't want. Be positive and write in the first person. Keep a copy with you for several days so you can work on it over time. After you finish the initial draft (you'll want to update it frequently), place this piece of paper where you can see it every day, such as in your briefcase, on your refrigerator, by your bed, or on the bathroom mirror. In that way, every day you can focus your eyes on what's important to you. This makes it easier for you to supervise yourself and to match your behavior to get what you want. Your life will become more conscious, and you will spend your energy on goals that are important to you.

I separate the areas of relationships, work, money, and self in order to encourage a more balanced approach to life. We burn out when our lives become unbalanced and overextended in one area at the expense of others.

Here is an actual example of an OPM I did with one of my patients who had a prefrontal cortex injury. Jarred was married with three children, and he was an attorney in private practice. Since the injury he had had significant impulse control problems and spent excessive time at work, which were the reasons he came to see me.

After you look at the example, fill out an OPM for yourself. After you complete this exercise, put it up where you can see and read it every day. It is a great idea to start the day off by reading the OPM to get focused for the day.

Jarred's
One-Page Miracle
What Do I Want for My Life?

RELATIONSHIPS
Spouse: A close, kind, caring, loving partnership with my wife.
Children: To be a firm, kind, positive force in my children's lives. To be continually present in their lives in a way that enhances their development as responsible, happy people.
Extended Family: To continue to keep close contact with my parents and siblings, to provide support and love.
Friends: To take time to maintain and nurture my friendships.

WORK (To be the best attorney I can be)
To have the best business possible, while maintaining a balanced life. Specifically, my work activities focus on spending time taking care of my current clients, doing activities to obtain new clients, and giving back by doing some voluntary work each month. I will focus on my goals at work and not get distracted by things not directly related to my goals.

MONEY (Money is for needs, wants, and security)
Short term: To be thoughtful of how our money is spent, to ensure it is directly related to my family's and my needs and goals.
Long term: To save 10 percent of everything I earn. I pay myself and my family before other things. I'll put away $2,500 each month in pension plan, giving me the desired result of $5,000 per month after the age of sixty-five.

MYSELF (To be the healthiest person I can be)
Body: To take care of my body on a daily basis.
Mind: To feel stable, positive, and grateful, to live in a way that makes me feel proud.
Spirit: To live close to God and be the kind of person He would want me to be.

Your Name:

One-Page Miracle
What Do I Want for My Life?

RELATIONSHIPS

Spouse/Lover:

_____

Children:

_____

Extended Family:

_____

Friends:

_____

WORK (To be the best   I can be)

_____

_____

_____

MONEY (Money is for needs, wants, and security)
Short term:

_____

Long term:

_____

MYSELF (To be the healthiest person I can be)

Body:

_____

Mind:

_____

Spirit:

_____

Teach yourself to be focused on what's important to you. This auxiliary prefrontal cortex will help you keep your life on track.

PFC PRESCRIPTION 2:
FOCUS ON WHAT YOU LIKE A LOT
MORE THAN WHAT YOU DON'T LIKE

The prefrontal cortex is intimately involved with focus, concentration, and attention span. What we attend to and focus on has a very significant impact on how we feel and act day to day. As I mentioned, many people with pfc challenges, especially people with ADHD, tend to be conflict-driven as a way to "turn on" prefrontal cortex activity. Unfortunately, this behavior has many negative side effects, especially on relationships and immune system functioning. Focusing on what you like about your life and on what you like about others is a powerful way to keep your prefrontal cortex healthy.

To that end, I collect penguins. I have six hundred of them in my office, everything that you could imagine in penguin, including a penguin weather vane, penguin clocks, pens, pencils, puppets, dolls, watches, ties, a penguin sewing kit, a penguin vacuum cleaner, and even a pair of penguin boxer shorts given to me by a nine-year-old patient. I know this might sound a bit odd, but I tell people that given that I'm a psychiatrist I'm allowed to be a bit odd. My friends and family have an easy time buying for me at Christmas. Let me tell you why I collect penguins and how they relate to the prefrontal cortex.

While I was doing my fellowship in child and adolescent psychiatry, my family and I lived in Hawaii. When my son was seven years old, I took him to a marine life educational and entertainment park for the day. We went to the killer whale show, the dolphin show, and finally the penguin show. The penguin's name was Fat Freddie. He did amazing things: He jumped off a twenty-foot diving board; he bowled with his nose; he counted with his flippers; he even jumped through a hoop of fire. I had my arm around my son, enjoying the show, when the trainer asked Freddie to get something. Freddie went and got it, and he brought it right back. I thought, "Whoa, I ask this kid to get something for me, and he wants to have a discussion with me for twenty minutes, and then he doesn't want to do it!" I knew my son was smarter than this penguin.

I went up to the trainer afterward and asked, "How did you get Freddie to do all these really neat things?" The trainer looked at my son, and then she looked at me and said, "Unlike parents, whenever

Freddie does anything like what I want him to do, I notice him! I give him a hug, and I give him a fish." The light went on in my head.

Whenever my son *did* what I wanted him to do, I paid little attention to him, because I was a busy guy, like my own father. However, when he *didn't* do what I wanted him to do, I gave him a lot of attention because I didn't want to raise a bad kid! I was inadvertently teaching him to be a little monster in order to get my attention. Since that day, I have tried hard to notice my son's good acts and fair attempts (although I don't toss him a fish, since he doesn't care for them) and to downplay his mistakes. We're both better people for it.

I collect penguins as a way to remind myself to notice the *good* things about the people in my life a lot more than the bad things. This has been so helpful for me as well as for many of my patients. It is often necessary to have something that reminds us of this prescription. It's not natural for most of us to notice what we like about our life or what we like about others, especially if we unconsciously use turmoil to stimulate our prefrontal cortex.

Focusing on the negative aspects of others or of your own life makes you more vulnerable to depression and can damage your relationships.

Jamie

Let me give you a clear example of how powerfully this prescription can work. Seven years ago I met Jamie, a fourteen-year-old teenager who was admitted to the hospital after a suicide attempt. She had tried to kill herself because she was doing so poorly in school and couldn't keep up academically with her friends. On the night of her suicide attempt, she had a terrible fight with her mother, who berated her poor performance in school. Jamie had a family history of depression on her father's side, and her mother had many ADHD symptoms (although her mother refused to be evaluated and treated for it). Jamie felt sad and had a tendency to look at the negative side of things. She was also disorganized, had lifelong trouble focusing on her schoolwork, and was impulsive. She was diagnosed with depression and ADHD. Jamie's SPECT study showed decreased pfc activity and increased limbic activity. I started her on medication (which over time became a combination of Prozac and Ritalin) and began seeing her in psychotherapy. Over several months, Jamie's condition significantly improved. Her mood was better. School was easier for her. She had better frustration tolerance and impulse control. Our initial weekly visits after leaving the hospital turned into every two weeks and then monthly by the end of the first year. She maintained good stability, except for one area of her life: She continued to fight with her mother.

Two years after I began seeing Jamie, she came into my office and burst into tears. "I just can't stand my mother," she started the session. "All she does is pick on me and try to get me upset. I know you've told me not to react to her, but I can't help it. She knows every button on my body." As she finished telling me about her latest fight with her mother, she looked around my office and asked, "Dr. Amen, how come a grown man collects penguins?" A bit amazed, I asked, "You've just noticed the penguins? After two years?" I then told her the story about Fat Freddie. Then I taught her about the concept of *behavioral shaping,* what the trainer had done to get Fat Freddie to be a star performer. I told her, "Let me teach you how to shape the behavior of your mother. Every time your mother is inappropriate with you, conflict-seeking toward you, rude, or mean to you, I want you to keep quiet and not react."

"Oh, Dr. Amen," she said, "I don't know if I can do that. I've tried."

I replied, "I know, but I want you to try with this new understanding. And every time your mother is appropriate with you, listens to you, and is helpful to you, I want you to put your arms around her and tell her how much you love and appreciate her." Jamie said she would try her best.

When she came back a month later, she told me that she had had the best month she had ever had with her mother. Her mother had yelled at her only once, and she hadn't reacted. And she had given her mother a lot of hugs. "I think I get what you're teaching me, Dr. Amen," she said with a smile. "I have power to help things or make things worse. Even though I'm not responsible for how my mother acts, I have a big influence on the situation." I was proud of Jamie. She had learned that by focusing on what she liked about her mother a lot more than on what she didn't like, she could have a positive impact on a negative situation. I taught her not to be a victim of her mother, but to use her own positive power in the situation.

PFC PRESCRIPTION 3:
HAVE MEANING, PURPOSE, STIMULATION, AND EXCITEMENT IN YOUR LIFE

Meaning, purpose, stimulation, and excitement in your life help prevent shutdown and encourage you to focus by activating your prefrontal cortex. As I mentioned, in my clinical practice I treat many patients with ADHD. One of the most interesting parts of the disorder is that there is often an inconsistency of symptoms. People with ADHD often struggle with routine, mundane activities. However, when they are engaged in interesting, exciting, stimulating tasks, they often excel. A very important prescription I give my patients is to ensure that they have positive meaning and stimulation in their lives, whether it is in their work, their relationships, or their spirituality. It can make all the difference between success and chronic failure. A man with ADHD in a boring job he dislikes is likely to need more medication to be effective. If he is in a job that excites and motivates him, he is likely to need less medication. The situation will provide the stimulation. Let me give you an example.

Seth

Seth, a very successful owner of several video outlets, came into my office feeling very frustrated. He had had a nice response to treatment for his ADHD, so I wondered what had gone wrong. "Doc," he started, "I just feel like I have a bad character. I must be a bad person. I try and try to get my paperwork done, but I just can't bring myself to do it. It bores me literally to tears. Even with the medication and therapy, I still can't get it done." I asked for more information. "I sit down to do it," he continued, "when the meds are fully effective, and I just stare at the paperwork. I don't know what holds me back." "Seth," I replied, "it may have nothing to do with your character. You are a loving husband and father, you have a successful business that gives jobs to lots of people, and you care about others. Maybe what you have is a paperwork disability. Many people with ADHD excel at things they like to do and are terrible at things that provide little motivation, like paperwork. Maybe you need to hire someone to do the paperwork. That will leave you more time to grow the business further."

What Seth said next hit the mark. "That makes perfect sense to me. When I was a teenager, I loved to sail. But I never wanted to go out when the water was calm. I waited for the storm warnings to come up before I went out. During the storm I would be scared to death and wondered why I would do such a crazy thing. But when the storm was over and I got back to shore, I couldn't wait to go out again. It was the excitement and stimulation that motivated me."

Seth hired someone to do his paperwork. His business grew as he spent more time on the things he did best.

PFC PRESCRIPTION 4:
GET ORGANIZED; GET HELP
WHEN YOU NEED IT

People who have pfc difficulties often have problems with organization. Learning organizational skills can be very helpful. Day planners and computer organizational programs can be lifesaving. It is also important to know your limitations and, when possible, surround yourself with people who can help organize you. These people can be intimately involved with your life, such as a spouse or friend, or they can be people who work for you. The most successful people I have seen who have ADHD or other prefrontal cortex problems are those people who have others help them with organization. Don't be embarrassed to ask for help.

Here are some tips to help with organization:

- *Set clear goals for your life (as mentioned in pfc Prescription 1) in the following areas: relationships (spouse/lover, children, family, and friends), work, money, physical health, emotional health, and spirituality. Then ask yourself every day, "Is my behavior getting me what I want?" This critical exercise will help you stay on track in your life. Manage your time in a way that is consistent with the goals you have for your life.*
- *Take the extra time to organize your work area on a regularly scheduled basis. Devote some time each week to organization. Otherwise procrastination will take over.*
- *Keep up with the paperwork or have someone do it for you.*
- *Prioritize your projects.*

- *Make deadlines for yourself.*
- *Keep TO DO lists, and revise them on a regular basis.*
- *Keep an appointment and planning book with you at all times.*
- *Use a portable cassette recorder to help you remember ideas throughout the day or make notes on your mobile or BlackBerry.*
- *Break down overwhelming tasks into small tasks. This happens on assembly lines every day. Remember, "A journey of a thousand miles begins with one step."*
- *Do unpleasant tasks first. That way, you'll have the more pleasurable ones to look forward to. If you save the unpleasant tasks for last, you'll have little incentive to get to them.*
- *Use file folders, desk organizers, and labeled storage boxes to organize your paperwork*
- *Hire a professional organizer to help you get and stay organized. When my son with ADHD was sixteen years old, I hired a professional organizer to help him. He didn't want to listen to me (what did I know—I was only his dad). She was a gifted woman who helped him immensely. She organized his room with him, as well as his book bag for school, his assignment book, and his study schedule. She helped him set up systems, and then she came back once a month to work with him and help him maintain what he learned. Today he is good with organization. Like many people with ADHD, it's not natural for him, but he has the basics down and he is not a victim of his tendencies toward disorganization.*

PFC PRESCRIPTION 6:
CONSIDER BRAIN-WAVE
BIOFEEDBACK TRAINING

I've discussed ADHD as primarily a problem in the prefrontal cortex. Medication is the cornerstone of the "biological" treatments for ADHD, but it is not the only biological treatment. Over the past fifteen years, researchers including Joel Lubar, Ph.D., of the University of Tennessee, have demonstrated the effectiveness of a powerful adjunctive tool in the treatment of ADHD and other prefrontal cortex problems: brain-wave or EEG biofeedback.

Biofeedback in general is a treatment technique that utilizes instruments to measure physiological responses in a person's body (such as hand temperature, sweat gland activity, breathing rates, heart rates, blood pressure, and brain-wave patterns). The instruments feed the information on these body systems to the patient, who can then learn how to change them. In brain-wave biofeedback, we measure the level of brain-wave activity throughout the brain.

There are five types of brain-wave patterns:

- delta brain waves (1–4 cycles per second): very slow brain waves, occurring mostly during sleep;
- theta brain waves (5–7 cycles per second): slow brain waves, occurring during daydreaming, relaxation, and twilight states;
- alpha brain waves (8–12 cycles per second): brain waves occurring during relaxed states;
- SMR (sensorimotor rhythm) brain waves (12–15 cycles per second): brain waves occurring during states of focused relaxation;
- beta brain waves (13–24 cycles per second): fast brain waves occurring during concentration or mental work states.

In evaluating more than six thousand children with ADHD, Dr. Lubar found that the basic problem with these children is that they lack the ability to maintain "beta" concentration states for sustained periods of time. He also found that these children have excessive "theta" day-dreaming brain-wave activity. Dr. Lubar found that through the use of EEG biofeedback, children could be taught to increase the amount of "beta" brain waves and decrease the amount of "theta," or daydreaming, brain waves.

The basic biofeedback technique teaches children to play games with their minds. The more they can concentrate and produce "beta" states, the more rewards they can accrue. With my clinic's EEG bio-feedback equipment, for example, a child sits in front of a computer monitor and watches a game screen. If he increases the "beta" activity or decreases the "theta" activity, the game continues. The game stops, however, when the player is unable to maintain the desired brain-wave state. Children find the screens fun, and we gradually shape their brain-wave pattern to a more normal one. From the research, we know that this treatment technique is not an overnight cure. Children often have to practice this form of biofeedback for between one and two years.

In my experience with EEG biofeedback and ADHD, many people are able to improve their reading skills and decrease their need for medication. Also, EEG biofeedback has helped to decrease impulsivity and aggressiveness. It is a powerful tool, in part because the patient becomes part of the treatment process by taking more control over his own physiological processes.

The use of brain-wave biofeedback is considered controversial by some clinicians and researchers. More research needs to be done and published in order to demonstrate its effectiveness. Also, in some circles, EEG biofeedback has been oversold. Some clinics have advertised the ability to cure ADHD with biofeedback, without the use of medication. Unfortunately, overselling this treatment technique has hurt its credibility. Still, in my clinical experience, I find EEG biofeedback to be a powerful and exciting treatment with a developing future.

PFC PRESCRIPTION 7:
TRY AUDIOVISUAL STIMULATION

A treatment similar to EEG biofeedback is called audiovisual stimulation. This technique was developed by psychologists Harold Russell, Ph.D., and John Carter, Ph.D., at the University of Texas in Galveston. Both Dr. Russell and Dr. Carter were involved in the development of treatment of ADHD children with EEG biofeedback. They wanted to develop a treatment technique that could become widely available to children who needed it.

Based on a concept termed *entrainment*, in which brain waves tend to pick up the rhythm in the environment, they developed special glasses and headphones that flash lights and sounds at a person at specific frequencies to help the brain "tune in" and become more focused. Patients wear these glasses for twenty to thirty minutes a day.

I have tried this treatment on a number of patients with some encouraging results. One patient who developed tics on both Ritalin and Dexedrine tried the glasses for a month. His ADHD symptoms significantly improved. When he went off the audiovisual stimulator, his symptoms returned. The symptoms again subsided when he retried the treatment.

I believe that audiovisual stimulation techniques show promise for the future, but more research is needed.

PFC PRESCRIPTION 8:
DON'T BE ANOTHER PERSON'S STIMULANT

As mentioned, many people with prefrontal cortex problems tend to be conflict-seeking to stimulate their brain. It is critical for you to not feed the turmoil, but rather to starve it. The more someone with this pattern unknowingly tries to upset or anger you, the more you need to be quiet, calm, and steady. I teach parents of ADHD children to stop yelling. The more they yell and increase the emotional intensity in the family, the more the children seek turmoil. I also teach siblings and spouses to maintain a low voice and a calm demeanor. The harder the person with ADHD tries to escalate the situation, the less intense the respondent should be.

It is fascinating how this prescription works. In general, the conflict-seeking people are used to being able to get you upset. They have mastered all your emotional buttons, and they push them with regularity. When you begin to deny them the drama and adrenaline rush (by being less reactive and calmer in stressful situations), they initially react very negatively, almost as if they are going through a drug withdrawal. In fact, when you first become calmer they may even get worse in the short term. Stick with it, and they'll improve in the long term.

Here are some strategies for dealing with a person who has a tendency toward conflict-seeking behavior:

- *Don't yell.*
- *The more their voice goes up, the more your voice should go down.*
- *If you feel the situation starting to get out of control, take a break. Saying you have to go to the bathroom may be a good prescription. The person probably won't try to stop you. It may be a good idea to have a thick book ready if he or she is really upset and you need to stay away for a long time.*
- *Use humor (but not sarcasm or angry humor) to defuse the situation.*
- *Be a good listener.*
- *Say you want to understand and work on the situation, but you can do this only when things are calm.*

PFC PRESCRIPTION 9:
CONSIDER PREFRONTAL CORTEX MEDICATION

Medications that aid prefrontal cortex performance need to be specifically tailored to the problem. Those people who have ADHD often respond very well to stimulant medications such as Ritalin (methylphenidate). This medication works by stimulating the neurotransmitter dopamine, which in turn helps to prevent the prefrontal cortex shutdown that happens in ADHD. Contrary to popular belief, this medication is very safe and well tolerated, and it makes a difference almost immediately.

I have seen this medication change people's lives. I did SPECT studies of one ten-year-old boy with ADHD on and off his medication. With 10 milligrams of Ritalin three times a day, he clearly has more access to the activity in the prefrontal cortex, so he's better able to focus, set goals, organize, plan, and control his impulses.

For a year, I kept a log of what my ADHD adult patients told me about the effectiveness of their medication. The following are some of their comments.

> "I experienced an increased awareness of the world around me. I saw the hills for the first time when driving to work. I saw the bay when I crossed over the bridge. I actually noticed the color of the sky!"
>
> "I experienced a 180-degree difference in my attitude."
>
> "I look at my children and say, 'Aren't they cute?' rather than complaining about them."
>
> "I could sit and watch a movie for the first time in my life."
>
> "I am able to handle situations where I used to be hysterical. I am able to see when I'm starting to overreact."
>
> "The lens on my life is much clearer."
>
> "It amazes me that a little yellow pill [5 mg of Ritalin] can take me from wanting to jump off the bridge to loving my husband and enjoying my children."
>
> "I'm not running at train wreck speed."
>
> "For the first time I felt in charge of my life."
>
> "I used to think I was stupid. It seemed everyone else could do more things than me. I'm starting to believe that there may be intelligent life in my body."
>
> "I sleep much better. Can you believe I'm taking a stimulant and it calms me down?"

Before and After Stimulant Medication

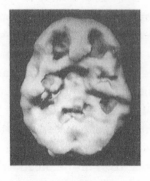 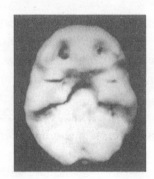

3-D underside surface view

ADHD, concentration, no medication; note markedly decreased prefrontal and temporal lobe activity.

ADHD, concentration, with Ritalin 15 mg; note marked overall improvement.

"I used to be the kind of person who would go walking by myself in downtown Detroit at 2 am. Now on the medication I would never do something so stupid. Before, I just wouldn't think about the consequences."

"Now I can give talks in front of groups. Before, my mind would always go blank. I organized my life around not speaking in public. Now my brain feels calmer, clearer."

"I'm not as intimidated by others as I used to be."

"My husband may not be as happy as before I was on medication. Now I can think, and he doesn't win all of the arguments. I'm going to have to retrain him to not always expect to get his way."

"I feel in control of my life."

"I can't stand useless confrontation, when I used to thrive on it!"

Certainly not everyone with ADHD experiences a dramatically positive response to stimulant medication, but many do. When they gain access to their prefrontal cortex, it is often amazing how much more effective they can be.

Several "stimulating" antidepressants are also helpful in ADHD. Norpramin (desipramine) and Tofranil (imipramine) increase the neurotransmitter noradrenaline and are especially helpful for people with ADHD and anxiety or depressive symptoms. Zyban (bupropion) increases the neurotransmitter dopamine and is often helpful for people with ADHD and depression or low energy. Efexor (venlafaxine) increases the neurotransmitters serotonin, noradrenaline, and, in higher doses, dopamine, and is most helpful for people with ADHD who overfocus or are obsessive.

PFC PRESCRIPTION 10:
WATCH YOUR PREFRONTAL CORTEX NUTRITION

Nutritional intervention can be especially helpful in this part of the brain. For years I have recommended a high-protein, low-carbohydrate diet that is relatively low in fat to my patients with ADHD. This diet has a stabilizing effect on blood sugar levels and helps both with energy level and concentration. Unfortunately, most Western diets are filled with refined carbohydrates, which have a negative impact on dopamine levels in the brain and concentration. With both parents working outside the home, there is less time to prepare healthy meals, and fast-food meals have become more the norm. The breakfast of today typically consists of foods that are high in simple carbohydrates, such as frozen waffles or pancakes, Pop Tarts, muffins, pastry, cereal. Sausage and eggs have gone by the wayside in many homes because of the lack of time and the perception that fat is bad for us. Even though it is important to be careful with fat intake, the breakfast of old is not such a bad idea for people with ADHD or other dopamine-deficient states.

The major sources of protein I recommend include lean meats, eggs, low-fat cheeses, nuts, and pulses. These are best mixed with a healthy portion of vegetables. An ideal breakfast is an omelet with low-fat cheese and lean meat, such as chicken. An ideal lunch is a tuna, chicken, or fresh fish salad, with mixed vegetables. An ideal dinner contains more carbohydrates for balance with lean meat and vegetables. Eliminating simple sugars (such as cakes, sweets, ice cream, pastries) and simple carbohydrates that are readily broken down to sugar (such as bread, pasta, rice, potatoes) will have a positive impact on energy level and cognition. This diet is helpful in raising dopamine levels in the brain. It is important to note, however, that this diet is not ideal for people with cingulate or overfocus issues, which usually stem from a relative deficiency of serotonin. Serotonin and dopamine levels tend to counterbalance each other; whenever serotonin is raised, dopamine tends to be lowered and vice versa.

Nutritional supplements can also have a positive effect on brain dopamine levels and help with focus and energy. I often have my patients take a combination of tyrosine (500–1,500 milligrams two to three times a day); OPC (oligomeric procyanidius) grape seed or pine bark, found in health food stores (1 milligram per pound of body weight); and gingko biloba (60–120 milligrams twice a day). These supplements help increase dopamine and blood flow in the brain, and many of my patients report that they help with energy, focus, and impulse control. If you want to try these supplements, check with your doctor.

PFC PRESCRIPTION 11:
TRY MOZART FOR FOCUS

One controlled study found that listening to Mozart was helpful for children with ADHD. Rosalie Rebollo Pratt and colleagues studied nineteen children, ages seven to seventeen, with ADHD. They played recordings of Mozart for them three times a week during brain-wave biofeedback sessions. They used 100 Masterpieces, vol. 3, which included Piano Concerto no. 21 in C, The Marriage of Figaro, Flute Concerto no. 2 in D, Don Giovanni, and other concertos and sonatas. The group that listened to Mozart reduced their theta brain-wave activity (slow brain waves that are often excessive in ADHD) in exact rhythm to the underlying beat of the music, and displayed better focus and mood control, diminished impulsivity, and improved social skill. Among the subjects who improved, 70 percent maintained that improvement six months after the end of the study without further training. (Findings reprinted in the International Journal of Arts Medicine, 1995.)

9

Looking Into Worry and Obsessiveness:
The Cingulate System

FUNCTIONS OF THE CINGULATE SYSTEM

- *ability to shift attention*
- *cognitive flexibility*
- *adaptability*
- *movement from idea to idea*
- *ability to see options*
- *ability to "go with the flow"*
- *ability to cooperate*

Traversing longitudinally through the central deep aspects of the frontal lobes is the cingulate gyrus. It's the part of the brain that allows you to shift your attention from one thing to another, to move from idea to idea, to see the options in life. Feelings of safety and security have also been attributed to this part of the brain. In my experience, the term that best relates to this part of the brain is *cognitive flexibility*.

Cognitive flexibility defines a person's ability to go with the flow, adapt to change, deal successfully with new problems. Many situations in life demand cognitive flexibility. For example, when you start a new job, you need to learn a new system of doing things. Even if you did something another way at a previous job, learning how to shift to please a new boss or adapt to a new system is critical to job success. Pupils need cognitive flexibility in order to be successful in school. Once children begin having various teachers throughout the day, it

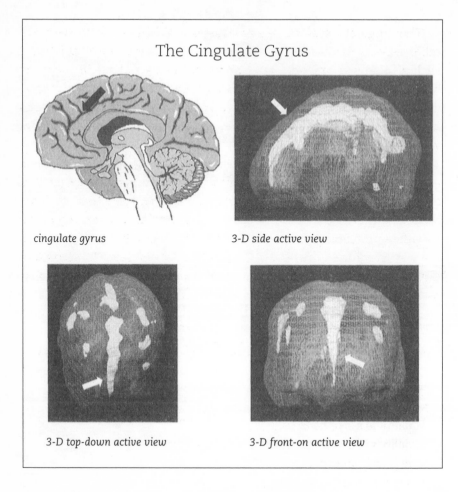

The Cingulate Gyrus

cingulate gyrus

3-D side active view

3-D top-down active view

3-D front-on active view

is necessary to shift learning styles in order to adapt to the different styles of the teachers. Flexibility is also important in friendships. What works in a friendship with one person may not be at all effective with someone else.

Effectively managing change and transitions is an essential ingredient in personal, interpersonal, and professional growth. The cingulate system can be of great help or hindrance to this process. When it is working properly, we are more able to roll with the circumstances of the day. When it is impaired or overactive, cognitive flexibility is diminished.

Along with shifting attention, we have seen that cooperation is also influenced by this part of the brain. When the cingulate works effectively, it's easy to shift into cooperative modes of behavior. People with cingulate problems have difficulty shifting attention and get stuck in ineffective behavior patterns.

The cingulate system has also been implicated (along with the other aspects of the prefrontal cortex) in "future-oriented thinking," such as planning and goal setting. When this part of the brain works well, it is easier to plan and set reasonable goals. On the negative side, difficulties in this part of the brain can cause a person to perceive fearful situations where there are none, predict negative events, and feel very unsafe in the world.

Seeing options is crucial to adaptable behavior. In my profession, adaptable doctors readily utilize new ideas and technology (after a scientific basis is developed), and they are open to give their patients the latest information on what is new and exciting. Doctors who have cingulate problems (I have scanned many) tend to be rigid, do things the way they have always been done, and be autocratic ("Do it my way if you want me to treat you"). Being able to see options and new ideas protects against stagnation, depression, and hostile behavior.

PROBLEMS WITH THE CINGULATE SYSTEM

- *worrying*
- *holding on to hurts from the past*
- *getting stuck on thoughts (obsessions)*
- *getting stuck on behaviors (compulsions)*
- *oppositional behavior*
- *argumentativeness*
- *uncooperativeness; tendency to say no automatically*
- *addictive behaviors (alcohol or drug abuse, eating disorders)*
- *chronic pain*
- *cognitive inflexibility*
- *obsessive-compulsive disorder (OCD)*
- *OCD spectrum disorders*
- *eating disorders*
- *road rage*

When the cingulate system is abnormal, people have a tendency to get stuck on things, locked into things, to rethink the same thought over and over and over. They may become worriers and continually obsess on the same thought. They may hold on to hurts or grudges from the past, unable to let them go. They may also get stuck on negative behaviors or develop compulsions such as hand washing or excessively checking locks.

One patient who had difficulties in this part of the brain described this phenomenon as "like being on a rat's exercise wheel, where the thoughts just go over and over and over." Another patient told me, "It's like having a reset button that is always on. Even though I don't want to have the thought anymore, it just keeps coming back."

The clinical problems associated with the cingulate will be discussed shortly. There are also a number of what I call "subclinical patterns" associated with abnormalities in this part of the brain. Subclinical problems are those that don't reach the intensity or cause the dysfunction of a fully-fledged disorder, but can nonetheless erode our quality of life. Worrying, holding on to hurts from the past, cognitive inflexibility, and rigidity may not send you to the therapist, but they can make your life unnecessarily gloomy.

Worrying

Even though we all worry at times (and some worry is necessary to keep us working or studying in school), people who have an overactive cingulate may have integrated chronic worrying into their personality. They may worry to the point of causing emotional and physical harm to themselves. Whenever repetitive negative concerns circle through the mind, it can cause tension, stress, stomachaches, headaches, and irritability. Chronically expressing worries often irritates others and makes a person seem less powerful and perhaps even less mature.

At a dinner party, an old friend of mine who is also a doctor complained that his wife worried "all the time." "She worries for the whole family," he told me. "It upsets me and the children. Her constant worry seems to be associated with her chronic headaches and irritability. How do I help her relax so that she won't get so upset about the little things in life?" he queried. I had known my friend's wife for many years. Even though she had never been clinically depressed and wouldn't fit the diagnostic criteria for panic disorder or OCD (obsessive-compulsive disorder), I knew that it was in her personality to worry. Members of her family, which she had discussed with me on several occasions, did have clinical problems (such as alcoholism, drug abuse, and compulsive behaviors) associated with the cingulate system.

Holding on to Hurts

Holding tightly on to hurts from the past can cause serious problems in a person's life. I once treated a woman who was very angry with her husband. On a trip to Hawaii, her husband had allowed his eyes to wander toward some of the scantily dressed women on the beach at Waikiki. The wife had become irate. She felt he had been unfaithful to her with his eyes. Her anger had ruined the whole trip, and she continued to bring up the incident years later.

Another cingulate example occurred in a newly blended family. Don married Laura, who had a three-year-old son, Aaron. Laura and Aaron had been living with her parents. Shortly after the wedding Don, Laura, and Aaron went to visit Laura's parents. During the visit Aaron asked for a second bowl of ice cream. Don told him no because it might ruin his dinner. Laura's parents undermined Don's new authority in front of the little boy by saying he could have the second helping of ice cream. Frustrated, Don tried to discuss the issue. The grandparents told him he was being silly. What did he know, they thought, he was new to fatherhood. When Don tried further to talk to them, they just dismissed him. The grandparents, unable to let go of the incident, refused to even speak to Don or Laura for the next eighteen months. Many family cutoffs are due to excessive cingulate activity.

Cognitive Inflexibility

Cognitive inflexibility, the inability to roll with the ups and downs of everyday life, is at the root of most cingulate problems. A friend's six-year-old daughter, Kimmy, provides a perfect example of cognitive inflexibility. Her older sister was instructed by her mother to get Kimmy ready to go out for the day. The older sister picked out a shirt and pair of trousers for Kimmy. Kimmy complained that the shirt and trousers looked stupid. She had the same complaint for the next three outfits that her sister chose for her. Kimmy wanted to wear a sundress (it was February and cold outside). She cried and cried to get her way. Nothing else would do. Once she got the idea of the sundress in her head, she couldn't shift away from it.

In couples counseling through the years, I have frequently heard another example of cognitive inflexibility: the need to do something

now. Not five minutes from now, but *now*! Here's a fairly common scenario: A wife asks her husband to get some clothes out of the dryer
and put the clothes from the washer into the dryer. He asks her to wait
a few minutes because he's watching the end of a basketball game.
She becomes irate and says that it needs to be done now. They get
into a fight. She doesn't feel comfortable until the chore is finished. He
feels intruded upon, pushed around, and generally degraded. The need
to do it *now* can cause some serious relational problems. Of course, if
the husband said he would help, then didn't, we could understand her
need to have it done now.

There are many more everyday examples of trouble shifting attention or cognitive inflexibility. Here's a short list:

- *Only eating specific foods, being unwilling to try new tastes*
- *Having to keep a room a certain way*
- *Having to make love the same way every time (or avoiding
  lovemaking because of feeling uncomfortable about the messiness
  that is involved with it)*
- *Becoming upset if the plans for the evening change at the last minute*
- *Having to do things a certain way at work, even if it's not in the
  business's best interest (e.g., not being flexible enough to meet an
  important customer's needs)*
- *Making other family members do chores such as the dishes in a
  certain way (this often alienates others and they become less willing
  to help)*

Cognitive inflexibility can insidiously destroy happiness, joy, and
intimacy.

∧ ⁊

The Automatic No

Because they have problems shifting attention, many people with cingulate overactivity become stuck on the word *no. No* seems to be the
first word they say, without ever really thinking about whether or not
no is even in their best interest. One of my patients told me about his
father. Whenever my patient would ask his father for something, such
as permission to borrow the car, the father would automatically say
no. The children in the family all knew that if they wanted something

from their father, he would first say no to them, and then a week or two later he would think about the request and sometimes change his mind. "No" was always his first response.

I have had several employees who clearly had cingulate problems. Frequently they would be uncooperative and find ways not to do what was asked of them. They seemed to frequently argue with requests and tell me why things couldn't be done, rather than constructively try to solve problems.

When partners have cingulate problems, they often get the opposite of what they want. One man told me that whenever he wanted to make love with his wife, he had to act as if he really didn't want to make love. He said, "If I would ask her directly, she would say no ninety-nine out of one hundred times. If I would lock our bedroom door at night [a sign that he wanted to be intimate with her], she would automatically become tense and say she wasn't interested. If I acted uninterested, just rubbed her back for a long time, then maybe I would have a chance. The amount of work and planning it took to make it happen often wasn't worth the effort." The "automatic no" puts a great strain on many different types of relationships.

Road Rage

Something happens to many people when they get behind the wheel of a car; a territorial animal comes growling to the surface. Cingulate people tend to be the worst. The problem again is trouble shifting attention. For example, if you are driving on a motorway and someone accidentally cuts you off, most people would think to themselves, "You bastard," and then leave the situation alone. People with cingulate problems say to themselves, "You bastard, you bastard, you bastard, you bastard ..." and they cannot get the thought out of their head. I have known many cingulate people who have acted out their frustrations by doing crazy things on the road, such as swearing, gesturing, chasing, or harassing the other driver. I have one patient, a very bright, successful professional, who on several occasions chased other drivers who had cut him off and on two occasions got out of the car and bashed their windows in with a baseball bat he kept in the car. After the second incident, he came to see me. He said, "If I don't get help for this, I'm sure I'll end up in jail." His cingulate gyrus was markedly

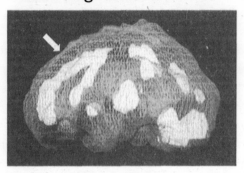

Road-Rage-Affected Brain

3-D side active view

Notice markedly increased cingulate activity (arrow).

overactive, causing him to get locked into the negative thoughts and subsequently be less able to control his frustration.

Obsessive-Compulsive Disorder

Gail

On the outside, Gail was normal. She went to work every day, she was married to her childhood sweetheart, and she had two small children. On the inside, she felt like a mess. Her husband was ready to leave her, and her children were often withdrawn and upset. She was distant from her family and locked into the private hell of obsessive-compulsive disorder. She cleaned her house for hours every night after work. She screamed at her husband and children when anything was out of place. She would become especially hysterical if she saw a piece of hair on the floor, and she was often at the sink washing her hands. She also made her husband and children wash their hands more than ten times a day. She stopped making love to her husband because she couldn't stand the feeling of being messy.

On the verge of divorce, Gail and her husband came to see me. At first, her husband was very skeptical about the biological nature of her illness. Gail's brain SPECT study showed marked increased activity in the cingulate system, demonstrating that she really did have trouble shifting her attention.

Gail's OCD-Affected Brain

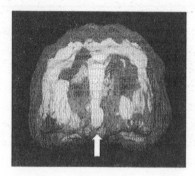

3-D front-on active view
Note heavily increased cingulate activity (arrow).

With this information, I placed Gail on Lustral. Within six weeks, she had significantly relaxed, her ritualistic behavior had diminished, and she stopped making her kids wash their hands every time they turned around. Her husband couldn't believe the change. Gail was more like the woman he had married.

Obsessive-compulsive disorder (OCD) affects somewhere between two and four million people in the United States and between two to three percent of the U.K. population. This disorder, almost without exception, dramatically impairs a person's functioning and often affects the whole family. OCD is often unnoticed by people in the outside world, but not by those who live with the obsessive-compulsive person.

The hallmarks of this disorder are obsessions (recurrent disgusting or frightening thoughts) or compulsions (behaviors that a person knows make no sense but feels compelled to do anyway). The obsessive thoughts are usually senseless and repugnant. They may involve repetitive thoughts of violence (such as killing one's child), contamination (such as becoming infected by shaking hands), or doubt (such as having hurt someone in a traffic accident, even though no such accident occurred). The more a person tries to control them, the more powerful they become.

The most common compulsions involve hand washing, counting, checking, and touching. These behaviors are often performed according to certain rules in a very strict or rigid manner. For example, a person with a counting compulsion may feel the need to count every crack on the pavement on the way to work or school. What would be a five-minute walk for most people could turn into a three- or four-hour trip for a person with obsessive-compulsive disorder. A part of the individual generally recognizes the senselessness of the behavior and doesn't get pleasure from carrying it out, although doing it often provides a release of tension.

The intensity of OCD varies widely. Some people have mild versions, where, for example, they have to make the house perfect before they go on vacation or they spend the vacation worrying about the condition of the house. The more serious forms can cause a person to be housebound for years. I once treated an eighty-three-year-old woman who had obsessive sexual thoughts that made her feel dirty inside. It got to the point where she would lock all her doors, draw the curtains, turn off the lights, take the phone off the hook, and sit in the middle of a dark room, trying to stop the abhorrent sexual thoughts as they came into her mind. Her life became paralyzed by this behavior, and she needed to be hospitalized.

Exciting research in the past few years has shown a biological pattern associated with OCD. Brain SPECT studies have shown increased blood flow in the cingulate system, along with increased activity in the basal ganglia (often the anxiety component of the problem).

Like most forms of psychiatric illness, part of effective treatment for OCD often involves medication. Currently, there are eight "anti-obsessive medications" and more on the way. The current medications that have shown effectiveness with OCD are Anafranil (clomipramine), Prozac (fluoxetine), Lustral (sertraline), Seroxat (paroxetine), Efexor (venlafaxine), Zispin (mirtazapine), and Faverin (fluvoxamine). These medications have provided many patients with profound relief from OCD symptoms.

In addition, behavior therapy is often helpful. The patient is gradually exposed to the situations most likely to bring out the rituals and habits. The therapist teaches the patient thought-stopping techniques and strongly encourages him or her to face his or her worst fear (for example, by persuading a patient with a fear of dirt or contamination to play in the mud).

OCD Spectrum Disorders

There is a group of disorders that have been recently labeled obsessive-compulsive spectrum disorders. People with these disorders get stuck on unwanted, repetitive thoughts and cannot get them out of their minds unless they act in a specific manner. According to psychiatrist Ronald Pies, postulated OCD spectrum disorders include: trichotillomania (pulling out one's own hair), onychophagia (nail biting), Tourette's syndrome (involuntary motor and vocal tics), kleptomania, body dysmorphic disorder (feeling that a part of the body is excessively ugly), hypochondria, autism, compulsive shopping, pathological gambling, chronic pain, addictive disorders, and eating disorders. I would also add oppositional defiant disorder.

A sample of repetitive thoughts that significantly interfere with behavior might include:

- *Chronic pain:* "I hurt! I hurt! I hurt!"
- *Eating disorders, such as anorexia and bulimia:* "I'm too fat! I'm too fat! I'm too fat!" despite rational evidence to the contrary.
- *Addictive disorders:* "I need a drink! I need a drink!"
- *Pathological gambling:* "Next time I'll win! Next time I'll win! Next time I'll win!"
- *Compulsive shopping:* "I need to buy this one thing! I need to buy this one thing! I need to buy this one thing!"
- *Oppositional defiant disorder:* "No I won't! No I won't! You can't make me!"

In 1991, Susan Swedo, M.D., at the National Institutes of Mental Health in Bethesda, Maryland, hypothesized that patients with trichotillomania would exhibit the same brain imaging as those with OCD. At rest, these patients exhibited a different brain pattern. Yet when these patients were treated with the antiobsessive antidepressant Anafranil, there was decreased activity in the cingulate aspect of the frontal lobes, which has also been found with successful treatment of OCD with antiobsessive antidepressants.

Here are several case examples from my own practice to illustrate OCD spectrum disorders.

Chronic Pain

Stewart

Stewart, a forty-year-old roofer, had hurt his back ten years earlier when he fell off a roof. He had undergone six back operations but remained in constant pain. He was essentially bedridden and about to lose his family because all he could think about was the pain. The threat of losing his family catalyzed him to get a psychiatric evaluation. His SPECT revealed marked overactivity in the cingulate system. He was placed on 200 milligrams of Anafranil per day. After five weeks, he reported that his back still hurt, but he was much less focused on the pain. He was able to get out of bed and go back into education. Other researchers have also reported several cases of intractable pain that were responsive to treatment with antiobsessive medications.

Eating Disorders

Leslie

Twenty-year-old Leslie suffered from bulimia for three years. She got to the point where she was using laxatives several times a day in increasing doses, along with exercising for two to three hours a day. Her binges were also becoming more frequent. When she sought treatment, she felt totally out of control. During her initial evaluation, she said she knew her behavior was abnormal and she hated it. However, when she got the urge to eat, she felt she had to give in to it, and afterward she could not get the thoughts of being overweight out of her head. She had a maternal aunt who had been diagnosed with obsessive-compulsive disorder. Leslie's brain SPECT study revealed increased activity in the cingulate system along with increased activity in her right basal ganglia. With this information, she was placed in an eating disorders group and given Prozac (an antiobsessive antidepressant). Over the next three months, she improved markedly, to the point where she was eating normally, not taking any laxatives at all, and exercising less than an hour a day.

In 1992, the Prozac Bulimia Nervosa Collaborative Study Group reported that daily therapy with 60 milligrams of Prozac significantly decreased the frequency of binge eating and self-induced vomiting. In the medical literature Prozac has been reported to decrease activity in the cingulate in obsessive-compulsive patients.

Drug or Alcohol Addiction

Joshua

Joshua began using drugs and alcohol at the age of twelve. When his parents finally caught on to his drug abuse at the age of sixteen, Joshua reported that he had used LSD more than a hundred times and he was drinking a pint of whiskey a day. He said that he was unable to stop, even though he had wanted to many times. When his parents brought him in for evaluation, it was revealed that there was a strong history of drug and alcohol abuse on both sides of his family, even though neither of his parents drank alcohol or abused drugs. After his SPECT study revealed significant overactivity in the cingulate system, Joshua was placed on Lustral in addition to his individual and support group therapy. He reported that he still had periodic cravings for the substances, but that he could avoid them more easily with the behavioral techniques he learned. He was able to get the thoughts about drugs and alcohol out of his head.

Pathological Gambling

Many people enjoy gambling. They feel happy when they win, discouraged when they lose. And they realize that gambling is a game of chance, like many things in life. Some people, however, become addicted to gambling and it can ruin every aspect of their lives. Pathological gambling is defined by the American Psychiatric Association as persistent and recurrent maladaptive gambling behavior that disrupts personal, family, or vocational pursuits. Pathological gambling usually starts with an important "big win." The high from the win gets "stuck" in a gambler's head, and he or she begins to chase it, even to the point of self-destruction.

Adam

Adam came to our office out of desperation. His wife had just left him, and he had seen an attorney to discuss filing for bankruptcy. His gambling had got out of control. He was a successful entrepreneur who had worked hard at starting his own business, but in the few years before he came to see me he had begun neglecting his business to spend more of his time at the racetrack and drive back and forth to Reno and Lake Tahoe. In our first session he told me, "I feel compelled to gamble. I know it is ruining my life, but it seems I have to place a bet or the tension just builds and builds. Before I started losing everything, I knew I could win. It was all I thought about!" Adam came from an alcoholic home; both his father and paternal grandfather were alcoholics. Even though Adam himself had never had a problem with alcohol, he clearly had an addiction. Explaining the cingulate system to Adam was helpful. He could identify many people in his family who had problems shifting attention. "You should see our family gatherings," he told me. "Someone is always mad at someone else. People in my family can hold grudges for years and years." In addition to going to Gamblers Anonymous and psychotherapy, Adam took a small daily dose of Prozac to help him shift away from the obsessive thoughts about gambling. Eventually he was able to reconnect with his wife and rebuild his business.

Compulsive Spending

Compulsive shopping is another manifestation of problems in the cingulate system. Compulsive shoppers get high from the pursuit and purchase of goods. They spend inordinate amounts of time thinking about shopping activities. This addiction can ruin their financial status and their relationships and have a negative impact on their work.

Jill

Jill worked as the office manager for a big law firm in San Francisco. Before work, during her lunch hours, and after work she found herself drawn to the stores at Union Square, near her office. She felt a rush of internal excitement as she picked out clothes for herself and her family members. She also enjoyed buying presents for others, even if they were just acquaintances. It was the act of shopping that was important. Even though she knew she shouldn't be spending the money, it felt too good to stop. She and her husband had many fights over the money she spent during her shopping sprees. She began embezzling money from work. She took care of the company chequebook and began to write and cash cheques to fictitious vendors in order to cover her personal debt. When a business audit almost found her out, she stopped. But her addiction didn't. Her husband finally divorced her when he uncovered credit card debt in the amount of thirty thousand dollars. Ashamed, scared, and depressed, Jill entered treatment. All her life she had been a worrier. In her teens she had had an eating disorder, and she had a cousin who had obsessive-compulsive disorder. Her SPECT study revealed a markedly overactive cingulate system. When she got locked into a train of thought or behavior (spending) she had real problems shifting away from it. Lustral (an antiobsessive antidepressant) was helpful for her as part of the healing process.

Oppositional Defiant Disorder

Oppositional defiant disorder (ODD) is considered a behavioral disorder of children and teenagers who are negativistic, hostile, defiant, and contrary. They tend to be argumentative, are easily annoyed, and lose their temper often, especially when they do not get their way. These children are chronically uncooperative. They tend to say no even when saying yes is clearly in their own best interest. The question I ask parents to help me diagnose this disorder is "How many times out of ten when you ask this child to do something will he (or she) do it the first time without arguing or fighting?" Most children will comply seven to eight times out of ten without a problem. For most ODD children the answer is usually three or fewer; for many of them it is zero.

David

I first met David when he was seven years old. He came into my office with his mother. He was wearing typically dirty shoes, and the minute he sat down, he put his feet up on my navy-blue leather couch. His mother, embarrassed by his rudeness, took his feet off the couch. He put them back on the couch. She took them off. He put them back on again. Looking angry, she took them off again. Right away, he put them back on and she took them off. I was watching the cingulate of the mother/son pair in action. David had to have his feet on the couch, mostly because his mother didn't want them on the couch (he also probably wanted to see what would happen if he irritated me). His mother couldn't stand the fact that he wouldn't listen to her, and she had to have his feet off the couch. Seeing the mother/son cingulate in action, I knew that many of their problems probably stemmed from an inability to shift attention and to hold their own positions. To confirm my suspicions about David, I said ten innocuous things, such as "The weather is good today ... Don't you think California is nice? [he was from out of state] ... I like your outfit" and so on. David argued with eight of the ten things I said. "The weather is awful ... I hate California ... My mother made me wear this stupid outfit ..." With an incredulous look on her face, David's mother argued with him: "This is beautiful weather ... Yesterday you said you wanted to live in California ... This is your favorite outfit ..." Further conversation with his mother suggested we had a generational cingulate problem.

When I first suggested a connection between cingulate overactivity and oppositional defiant-disorder, many of my colleagues did not take me seriously. How could ODD, which is an externalizing behavior disorder, be related to OCD, an internal anxiety disorder? After seeing this pattern over years it makes perfect sense to me. These children cannot shift their attention. They get stuck on No, No way, Never, You can't make me do it. They often have "cingulate parents," and many of them have a family history of OCD and other cingulate problems.

One of the most interesting findings among the patients we studied was that mothers or fathers who had obsessive thoughts, compulsive behaviors, or inflexible personality styles tended to have children with ODD. We studied eleven cases that exhibited this parent-child pattern and obtained brain SPECT studies on both the parent and the child. In nine out of the eleven, both the parent's and the child's brain SPECT study revealed increased cingulate activity. Both a biological explanation for this finding and behavioral etiology can be entertained. One can postulate that the finding of increased cingulate activity (biological component) can cause parents to have problems shifting attention and become stuck on thoughts or behaviors and cause them to be inflexible, while the child's inability to shift attention causes his behavior to appear oppositional. It is also possible that the parent's rigid style causes the child to react in an oppositional way (the behavioral part) as a way to gain independence and autonomy, which induces the subsequent SPECT finding.

As mentioned above, it has been observed that the brain SPECT abnormalities in the cingulate normalize with effective treatment. This does not appear to be merely variability from test to test, as researchers have shown that without intervening in some way, the brain SPECT patterns change very little. In the following case of ODD, follow-up data were obtained.

Jeremy

Jeremy, age nine, was evaluated for significant oppositional behavior. He had been suspended from school five times for refusing to do what he was told and being openly defiant with his teacher. His parents were told not to bring him back to school until they sought professional help. His clinical evaluation was consistent with a diagnosis of oppositional defiant disorder. His brain SPECT study revealed marked increased cingulate activity. When he improved only minimally with behavioral interventions, he was placed on Anafranil. Within two weeks, he showed marked clinical improvement. After two months, his brain SPECT study was repeated and revealed essentially normal cingulate activity. The following year, Jeremy did well in school; in fact, his teacher that year could not understand why his former teachers had warned her about him.

Stress Often Increases Activity in the Cingulate System

In many children and teenagers with ODD, I obtain both rest and concentration SPECT studies. Interestingly, in about half of the cases, I see a further increase in cingulate activity when these patients try to concentrate. Clinically, I find that this correlates with those oppositional children and teens who get worse ("more stuck") under pressure or when they are pushed to comply with certain requests. I have seen this occur frequently on an adolescent treatment unit. Some of these teens would become so "stuck" that they refused to comply with the staff requests and ended up on restriction or even, in some cases, in restraints because they could not shift their attention in order to behave more appropriately. It can be particularly bad if a cingulate teen meets up with a cingulate nurse who cannot back off a little to let the situation defuse.

Ken and Katie

Ken's family illustrates the problems an overactive cingulate can cause. His wife and two daughters came to his office to pick him up and go out to dinner. His youngest daughter, Katie, smiled when she saw him and gave him a big hug. As they were going to drive in two separate cars, Ken said to her, "Come on, Katie, ride with me in my car." Katie had been diagnosed with attention deficit hyperactivity disorder, and she was often oppositional with Ken. He wanted to spend some extra time with her on the way to the restaurant. As soon as he said, "Come with me," she said, "No. I don't want to." Ken's feelings were a little hurt. He replied, "Come on, Katie, I want to be with you." She said, "No! I'm going with Mummy." Not one to give up easily, Ken physically picked her up and put her in the car. She yelled, screamed, and cried halfway to the restaurant (real quality time). All of a sudden she stopped crying, dried her eyes, and said, "I'm sorry, Daddy. I really wanted to go with you." When he had pushed Katie to go with him, her brain locked. She got stuck on her first reaction and became unable to think about what she actually wanted to do.

Katie's SPECT study showed increased activity in the cingulate system. All of Ken's children are grandchildren of alcoholics. I have seen a significant connection between a family history of alcoholism and increased activity in the cingulate system.

Given that children and teens with ODD tend to "lock up" cognitively when they are pushed to comply, I have found behavioral techniques, such as giving options and distraction, more effective in obtaining compliance. When you give oppositional children or teens an option as to *when* they might do something, they tend to be less likely to get stuck on "No, I won't do it." When they are stuck on a negative thought or behavior, I have found it helpful to distract them for a bit and then come back to the issue at hand later. Ken would have been better at

getting Katie to go with him in the car if he had given her a choice
rather than just telling her she was going to go with him.

Therapy for a Family with Similar Brain SPECT Findings

The following family case study demonstrates how the same brain
finding can present itself clinically in different ways. Brain SPECT studies were obtained on a mother and two of her children.

Celina, Samuel, and Laura

Celina is a thirty-six-year-old woman who had experienced depressive
feelings after the birth of her first child ten years prior to her evaluation. She suffered from significant irritability, crying spells, sleeplessness, lack of appetite and weight loss, problems concentrating, and
difficulty in managing her children. Her condition was brought to a
crisis with suicidal behavior when she separated from her husband.
She was initially seen by another psychiatrist and started on an antidepressant, which had little effect. I started to see her in psychotherapy
and placed her on a different antidepressant. It had a positive effect,
and she did well. After several months, she decided that she "should
be stronger than the depression" and took herself off the medication.
Within several weeks her depression worsened, but she was resistant
to restarting the antidepressant.

In an effort to demonstrate to her that her depression existed on a
biological level as well as on a psychological level, a brain SPECT study
was performed. Celina's SPECT study revealed increased activity in her
limbic system (consistent with the underlying depressive disorder)
and markedly increased cingulate activity.

I asked her more pointed questions to see if she had obsessive-
compulsive disorder. Although she denied it at the initial evaluation,
in fact she was perfectionistic at home and had repetitive negative
thoughts. She tearfully remarked, "You mean my husband was right
when he thought it was strange that I had to have all the shirts in the
drawer buttoned a certain way and put just so in the drawer or I would
become very upset?"

Celina then reported rituals that her eight-year-old daughter, Laura, would perform before entering a new room, such as running a finger under her nose and licking her lips. Laura also had a locking compulsion. Every time someone left the house, she would be right behind, locking the door. Imagine how irritated her brother and sister were because they could never go out of the house to play without being locked out!

I was also seeing Celina's ten-year-old son, Samuel, for attention deficit hyperactivity disorder and oppositional defiant disorder. Samuel's ADHD symptoms did not respond to Ritalin or Dexedrine (stimulants used to treat ADHD). Celina reported that once Samuel got a thought in his mind, he was unable to let it go. He would follow her around the house for two and a half hours asking her the same questions she had already answered. Samuel was also one of the most negative, hostile children I had ever met. Even though his mother was depressed, he defied her, yelled at his sisters, and seemed to do whatever he could to make the turmoil in the home worse.

Brain SPECT studies were done on both children to see if there might be a genetic component to their problems and/or a similar response to treatment. Interestingly, both of them also showed increased cingulate activity. Neither of the children had limbic system findings or showed evidence of clinical depression.

Based on the SPECT and clinical information, Celina was placed on Prozac (which has been shown to normalize or calm cingulate hyperactivity) to decrease her depression and help lessen her obsessive thinking and compulsive behaviors. She had a dramatically positive response and reported that she was no longer bothered when things weren't "just so." The scan also convinced her that her condition was at least, in part, biological and not her fault or the result of a weak will, which encouraged her to take her medication for a longer period of time.

Additionally, Samuel was started on Prozac and had a similarly positive response. His behavior became much less oppositional, and his school performance dramatically improved. He made the honor roll for the first time in his life and was placed in the gifted-and-talented program the following year.

Initially Laura refused to take medication, and her ritualistic behaviors continued. Approximately eight months later, she agreed to start Prozac, and her compulsive behaviors diminished. The family dynamics improved significantly after the mother, Samuel, and Laura were treated with medication and psychotherapy.

It was clear that the family dynamics in this family operated and interacted on many levels. The mother's depression and obsessive thinking contributed to the anxiety and behavior problems in her children, and the cerebral blood flow abnormalities in the children probably added to their difficult behavior, which further stressed the mother.

Cingulate System Checklist

Here is the cingulate system checklist. Please read this list of behaviors and rate yourself (or the person you are evaluating) on each behavior listed. Use the following scale and place the appropriate number next to the item. Five or more symptoms marked 3 or 4 indicate a high likelihood of cingulate problems.

0 = *never*
1 = *rarely*
2 = *occasionally*
3 = *frequently*
4 = *very frequently*

1........ Excessive or senseless worrying
2........ Being upset when things do not go your way
3........ Being upset when things are out of place
4........ Tendency to be oppositional or argumentative
5........ Tendency to have repetitive negative thoughts
6........ Tendency toward compulsive behaviors
7........ Intense dislike of change
8........ Tendency to hold grudges
9........ Trouble shifting attention from subject to subject
10........ Trouble shifting behavior from task to task
11........ Difficulties seeing options in situations
12........ Tendency to hold on to own opinion and not listen to others
13........ Tendency to get locked into a course of action, whether or not it is good
14........ Being very upset unless things are done a certain way
15........ Perception by others that you worry too much
16........ Tendency to say no without first thinking about question
17........ Tendency to predict negative outcomes

10

Getting Unstuck:
Cingulate System Prescriptions

The cingulate system of the brain allows us to shift our attention from thing to thing, idea to idea, issue to issue. When it is dysfunctional, we have a tendency to get locked into negative thoughts or behaviors; we have trouble seeing the options in situations. Healing this part of the mind involves training the mind to see options and new ideas.

Throughout this book I have written about the use of medications in healing the brain. I will do so in this chapter as well. It is important to remember, however, that your day-to-day thoughts and behaviors also have a powerful effect on your brain chemistry. UCLA psychiatrist Jeffrey Schwartz demonstrated, through award-winning research, a powerful mind-body lesson. He and other researchers at UCLA studied people who had obsessive-compulsive disorder with PET scans, reporting findings similar to those presented in this book. Interestingly, when these patients were treated with antiobsessive medication, the overactive parts of their brains slowed toward normal activity. This was a revolutionary finding: Medications help heal the dysfunctional patterns of the brain. What was more striking, however, was that those patients who were treated without medication, through the use of behavior therapy alone, also showed normalization of the abnormal activity in their brain when the treatment was effective. Changing behavior can also change brain patterns.

CG PRESCRIPTION 1:
NOTICE WHEN YOU'RE STUCK, DISTRACT YOURSELF, AND COME BACK TO THE PROBLEM LATER

The first step to overcoming cingulate dysfunction is to notice when you're stuck and distract yourself. Becoming aware of circular or looping thoughts is essential to gaining control over them. Whenever you find your thoughts cycling (going over and over), distract yourself from them. Get up and do something else. Distraction is often a very helpful technique. Here's an example.

Maurie

Maurie, age thirty-two, came to see me for chronic tension. He incessantly worried about his job. Despite getting good performance reviews, he felt that his boss didn't like him. The constant worry frequently upset him. He couldn't get these thoughts out of his head. Over and over they went. He complained of headaches, tension, and irritability at home. No amount of rational discussion helped. I gave him the task of writing down the times he was stuck on these negative thoughts about work. They occurred every several hours. The ANT-killing exercise (see pages 66–68) was helpful for him, but it didn't completely prevent these thoughts from circling in his head. His homework became distraction. Every time one of these thoughts came into his mind, I told him he had to sing a song. He picked out several songs he liked and rotated through them whenever the thoughts started to bother him. This worked for him. He liked the music, and he felt that it gave him a measure of control over his troubling thoughts.

Some of my cingulate patients find it helpful to make a list of all the things they can do to distract themselves when they get harassing thoughts. Here are some examples:

- Sing a favorite song.
- Listen to music that makes you feel positive.
- Take a walk.
- Do a chore.
- Play with a pet.
- Do structured meditation.

■ *Focus on a word and do not allow any other thoughts to enter your mind (imagine a broom that sweeps out all other thoughts).*

If you actively distract yourself from repetitive thoughts or block them, over time they will lose their control over you.

CG PRESCRIPTION 2:
THINK THROUGH ANSWERS BEFORE
AUTOMATICALLY SAYING NO

As mentioned, many cingulate people have an automatic tendency to say no. Fight the tendency. Before answering questions or responding to requests in a negative way, take a breath and think first whether or not it is best to say no. Often it is helpful to take a deep breath, hold it for three seconds, and then take five seconds to exhale, just to get extra time before responding. For example, if your spouse asks you to come to bed and make love, take a deep breath before responding that you're tired, too busy, or not in the mood. Use the time during the deep breath to ask yourself whether you really want to deny your partner. Is it in your best interest to say no and continue doing what you're doing, or is it in your best interest to get close to your partner? The automatic no has ruined many relationships. Take enough time to ask yourself if saying no is really what you want to say.

CG PRESCRIPTION 3:
WRITE OUT OPTIONS AND SOLUTIONS WHEN YOU
FEEL STUCK

When you are stuck on a thought, it is often helpful to write it down. Writing it down helps to get it out of your head. Seeing a thought on paper makes it easier to deal with in a rational way. When repetitive thoughts cause sleeping problems, keep a pen and paper near your bed to write them out. After you write out a thought that has "got stuck," generate a list of things you can do about it and things you can't do about it. For example, if you are worried about a situation at work, such as whether you'll get a promotion, do the following:

1. Write out the thought: *"I'm worried about whether or not I'll get the promotion at work."*
2. Make a list of the things you can do about the worry: *"I can do the best job I can at work." "I will continue to be reliable, hardworking, and creative." "I will make sure the boss knows I desire the promotion." "In a confident (not bragging) way, I will make sure the boss knows about my contributions to the company."*
3. Make a list of the things you cannot do about the worry: *"I cannot make the decision for the boss." "I cannot want the promotion any more than I do." "I cannot will the promotion to happen. Worrying will not help." "I cannot make the promotion happen (although I do have lots of influence on the process by my attitude and performance)."*

Use this simple exercise to unlock the thoughts that keep you awake at night feeling tense.

CG PRESCRIPTION 4:
SEEK THE COUNSEL OF OTHERS WHEN YOU FEEL STUCK

When all of your efforts to get rid of repetitive thoughts are unsuccessful, it is often helpful to seek the counsel of others. Finding someone to discuss the worries, fears, or repetitive behaviors with can be very helpful. Often just talking about feeling stuck will open new options. Through the years, I have used mentors to help me through some of the problems I've had to face. Others can be a "sounding board," helping you to see options and offering reality checks.

Several years after I started performing SPECT studies on my patients, I was professionally attacked by some of the researchers in the field. I had sent a letter to several of them, asking for their help and collaboration. No response. I was very excited about the clinical usefulness of SPECT in day-to-day clinical practice, and I wanted to share my excitement and newfound knowledge with others. The attack on my work caused me a lot of anxiety and sleepless nights. (Remember, I have right basal ganglia overactivity, and I have a strong tendency to avoid conflict and confrontation.)

I sought the advice of a close friend who had seen the development

of my work and who had referred to me many patients who had benefited from this technology. When I told him about the attack on my
work, he smiled. He wondered why I had expected anything different.
He said, "People who say things that differ from the norm used to get
burned at the stake. The more controversial, the more of a nerve you're
striking in the established community." When he said, "What else would
you expect?" it suggested a new way to interpret what had happened. I
could look differently at the behavior of these other researchers. (In fact,
one of the most vocal detractors of my work himself published research
findings a year later confirming what I had seen clinically.) When you're
stuck, allow others to help you with the unsticking process.

CG PRESCRIPTION 5:
MEMORIZE AND RECITE THE SERENITY PRAYER
WHEN BOTHERED BY REPETITIVE THOUGHTS

The Serenity Prayer is repeated daily by millions of people around
the world, especially those in twelve-step programs. It is a beautiful
reminder that there are limits to what we can do in life and we need
to respect that. Many people find it helpful to repeat this prayer every
time they are bothered by repetitive negative thoughts. I recommend
that you memorize at least the first four lines of the prayer (change it
as needed to fit your own beliefs).

> God, grant me the serenity
> to accept the things I cannot change,
> the courage to change the things I can,
> and the wisdom to know the difference.
> Living one day at a time,
> enjoying one moment at a time;
> accepting hardship as a pathway to peace,
> taking as Jesus did this sinful world as it is,
> not as I would have it, trusting that you will make
> all things right if I surrender to your will;
> so that I may be reasonably happy in this life
> and supremely happy with you in the next.
> —Attributed to Reinhold Niebuhr

CG PRESCRIPTION 6:
DON'T TRY TO CONVINCE SOMEONE ELSE WHO IS STUCK; TAKE A BREAK AND COME BACK LATER

If you're locked in the middle of an argument with someone who's stuck, take a break! Take ten minutes, take ten hours, take ten days! If you distract yourself from a lose-lose situation, you're often able to come back later and work it out.

I learned long ago not to try to argue with people who have cingulate system problems. When another person is "stuck" on a thought or behavior, logical reasoning usually won't work. One of the best techniques I've found to deal with those who get stuck is as follows: I will briefly make the point I want to make. If I can tell the other person is getting locked into his or her position, I try to change the subject and distract him or her from the topic. Distraction allows time for the other person's subconscious mind to process what I said without having to lock in on it or fight it. Often, when we come back to the issue, the other person has a more open mind to the situation. Here's an example.

Jackie came to see me about marital problems. Her husband traveled and was unable to attend many of the sessions. In the individual sessions, I saw that Jackie frequently became locked into her position and left little room for alternative explanations of behavior. Her husband said that she would go on and on for hours and not listen to anything he said. As I realized this was her pattern, I used the brief "attack and retreat" model I described. When she complained about her husband not paying attention to her, I wondered aloud if it wasn't because he felt she didn't listen to his opinion. Immediately she said I was wrong. She said that she was a very good listener. I didn't argue with her, but went on to something else for a while. The next session, Jackie talked about listening more to her husband. Her subconscious was able to hear what I said, as long as I didn't activate her getting locked into opposing me.

This is often a very helpful technique to use with teenagers. Many teens argue and oppose their parents as part of the natural individuation and separation process. I teach parents to get out of struggles with their teenagers by briefly making their points and moving on to other topics. For important issues, come back to them at later times.

One of the best marital suggestions I give couples, which I also mentioned in chapter 8, is "Go to the bathroom." When you can see that your partner is beginning to get into cingulate territory and is starting to go over the same point again and again, excuse yourself and say you have to go to the bathroom. Few people will argue with you when nature calls, and it is often helpful just to take a break. If the cingulate problem in the other person seems particularly strong, take a big book with you and settle in for a lengthier stay.

CG PRESCRIPTION 7:
TRY MAKING PARADOXICAL REQUESTS

Remember "reverse psychology"? It works with cingulate people. But you need to be sly about it. In "reverse psychology," you basically ask for the opposite of what you want. When you want a kiss from a naturally oppositional two-year-old, say, "I don't want a kiss." The next moment the child is begging to give you a kiss. When you want someone to help you with a chore, say, "You probably wouldn't want to help me with this chore." Family therapists have developed whole paradoxical treatment prescriptions to deal with resistant couples. The therapists bet on the couple's resistance to suggestions. For example, if the couple is having problems spending time together and finding time for sex, the therapist would tell them not to spend any time together and definitely not to have sex. Many couples find that after the paradoxical suggestions they start to spend more time together and make love more regularly and passionately than they have in years.

Paradoxical suggestions and interventions have been used as therapeutic prescriptions by psychotherapists for many years. These interventions have gone under many names, such as *antisuggestion, negative practice, paradoxical intention, confusion technique, declaring hopelessness, restraining change, prescribing a relapse,* and *therapeutic double blind.* Basically, they all involve suggesting the opposite of the desired response. A common paradoxical suggestion is given to people who have trouble sleeping: "Stay awake as long as possible when going to bed." In treating male patients who could not urinate in public lavatories because of anxiety, psychologists L. M. Ascher and R. M. Turner told them they should go to public lavatories and go through the entire procedure of urinating (stand in front of the urinal, unzip their pants, and take out their penis), but refrain from urinating. With repeated trials, the men were able to overcome their fear of urinating in public. It is my contention that these tactics probably work best on cingulate clients.

Whenever you want a cingulate person to do something for you, it is best to make it look as if it is his or her idea. If you ask for many things directly, you are likely to be disappointed. Ask for the person's input. Get his or her feedback. Here are some examples:

- *If you want someone to meet you for dinner, it is often best to ask what time is good for him or her as opposed to telling him or her to meet you at a certain time.*
- *If you want a hug, it is often best to say something like "You probably wouldn't want to give me a hug."*
- *If you want him or her to go to the store with you, say something like "You probably wouldn't want to go with me."*
- *If you want someone to finish a report by next Thursday, say, "You probably can't finish the report by next Thursday."*
- *If you want a child to comply with a request without giving you a problem, say, "You probably wouldn't be able to do this without getting upset, would you?"*

CG PRESCRIPTION 8: LEARN HOW TO DEAL WITH OPPOSITIONAL CHILDREN

There are two prescriptions I find essential in dealing with oppositional children. Remember, oppositional children often become rigid or stuck in negative behavior patterns. Effectively intervening with them can make a significant difference in their lives. The first prescription is to know when to distract their attention in order to break the loops of thoughts or behaviors that cause them to be oppositional. Distraction, as mentioned above, is a very powerful technique in helping cingulate thinkers get unstuck. Distract the child away from the pattern by changing the subject, getting him or her to do something physical (such as taking a walk or playing a game), or working with a predetermined distraction prescription.

Josh

One prescription I use is having the parent read from a favorite book when the child begins to get stuck or locked into a negative thought or behavior. For example, eight-year-old Josh got stuck on being afraid of going to school. Before school he would complain of headaches, stomachaches, and anything else he thought his mother would accept to keep him home from school. When she caught on to his ploy, she would try to make him go to school anyway. When that happened, the little boy would scream, cry, throw tantrums, and threaten to run away from home. As the problem escalated, she brought Josh to see me. Not only was he anxious about school, his behavior was typically oppositional. The first intervention was to tell Josh in no uncertain terms that he was going to school! It was the law. It was good for him. And if we allowed him to stay home from school, he would become more afraid of it and would actually become "frozen by his fears." To help him, on mornings when he felt as if he couldn't go to school or he was worried about school, his mum or dad would distract him from his bad thoughts. Josh was very interested in insects. He had many beloved books about insects. When Josh became upset, his parents would read to him about a new insect and try to make it as interesting as possible. If Josh still gave his parents a problem about going to school, then he had to spend the day sitting on his bed without watching television or being able to go out to play. If he was too sick to go to school, then he was too sick to do anything else. Before this intervention Josh had problems eight mornings out of ten. After the first month, Josh's problems in the morning diminished to two mornings out of ten. By the third month, the problem was eliminated. Both parts of the intervention were crucial to its success. His parents had to let Josh know clearly that his fearful, oppositional behavior would not get him anything positive. The parents would not be bullied. He was going to school, or he would have to sit on his bed all day long (no secondary gain by being sick). Second, the parents used distraction to help Josh shift his attention away from his fears that got stuck.

It is essential that parents assert their ultimate authority over cingulate children. Parents cannot allow oppositional behavior to prevail. If they do, it only reinforces the oppositional behavior, which could ruin a child's life. Permissive parents don't teach their children to deal with authority, and those kids have trouble socially and in school. Authoritative, firm parents tend to raise the most effective children. Just as when people who have OCD give in to their obsessive thoughts or compulsive behaviors those behaviors become stronger and harder to fight, when you give in to oppositional children and allow them to oppose you and disobey their oppositional behavior only becomes worse. The earlier you train oppositional children out of this behavior, the better off everyone will be. To that end, I have developed a set of parenting rules that is the first step in dealing with these children. It is important to clearly spell out the rules and make sure the child knows you are going to back them up. Here are two of the rules that deal with oppositional behavior:

Do what Mum and Dad say the first time.

No arguing with parents.

These rules spell out that you have authority as parents and will not allow your child to argue with you. If you make it a rule for children to comply the first time, then they know that is what is expected of them. You must also quickly intervene if they do not comply the first time. Do not tell a child to do something eight times. Your chance of abusing the child verbally or physically goes up dramatically if you repetitively tell him or her to do things and don't intervene early. For example, if you tell a child to do something and he or she refuses to do it or doesn't do it within a reasonable period of time, very quickly say, "You have a choice. You can do it now, or you can take a time-out and then you can do it. I don't care, it's up to you." If the child doesn't move quickly to do what you asked, then put him or her in time-out. Repeat as necessary. Deal with misbehavior quickly, firmly, and unemotionally. The more emotional you get, the more these children tend to misbehave. Consistency is essential here.

The second rule, "No arguing with parents," is very important for oppositional children. If you allow the child to argue with you, then you are only reinforcing and strengthening his or her cingulate resistance. Of course, you want to hear your child's opinion. But draw the line between stating one's opinion and arguing. You might want to tell your child, "As your parents, we want to hear your opinion, but arguing means you have made your point more than twice."

These parenting interventions are always more effective when you do them in the context of a good relationship with your child. Parents who become "limbically bonded" to their children by spending time and listening to them have fewer problems with oppositional behavior.

In summary, use distraction when necessary but also be firm and authoritative with oppositional children. Pick your battles with them, and do not fight over every issue. Unfortunately, oppositional children often have one or two cingulate parents, which only feeds the negative family dynamics. Flexibility on the parents' part is often very helpful.

CG PRESCRIPTION 9:
CONSIDER CINGULATE MEDICATIONS

Medications are often very helpful in the cingulate part of the brain, especially those medications that modulate the neurotransmitter serotonin.

Medications that increase serotonin in the brain are termed serotonergic. These include Prozac, Lustral, Seroxat, Anafranil, Efexor, Zispin and Faverin. Several research studies have shown that when these medications are effective, they normalize activity in the cingulate system. Clinically, I have seen these medications decrease patients' repetitive thoughts and compulsive behaviors, calm overfocus or worry, and relax people who have a tendency to be frozen by their inability to see options. When these medications work, they often have a dramatic effect on thoughts and behaviors.

Rob

Rob, a forty-eight-year-old married systems analyst, came to see me because he had problems with holding grudges, "getting stuck" in loops of negative thinking, obsessive thoughts, moodiness, irritability, periodic intense suicidal thoughts, and problems with anger control. "I am the anger broker of the Valley," he reported during the initial session. His wife also reported frequent episodes when Rob would become upset about something, be unable to shift away from the thoughts that were upsetting him, lose control, and exhibit aggressive behavior such as breaking furniture or punching holes in the walls. Rob had a childhood history of oppositional behavior. As part of his evaluation, a brain SPECT study was done that showed markedly increased uptake in his cingulate gyrus. I started him on Anafranil (clomipramine), which has been used in patients with obsessive thinking. Over two months of treatment, his dose of Anafranil was increased to 225 milligrams a day. Rob and his family noted a positive response. He was less irritable, markedly less aggressive, more flexible, and happier. He reported that he was more effective in interpersonal relationships, especially with his children.

After three years of continued clinical improvement on the same dose of Anafranil (two brief trials at lowering the dosage caused a resumption of symptoms) a follow-up brain SPECT study revealed a marked normalization of Rob's brain activity.

Rob's SPECT Studies

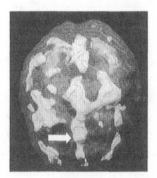 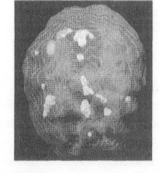

3-D top-down active view

Before treatment; note markedly increased cingulate activity.

After treatment with Anafranil; note normal cingulate activity.

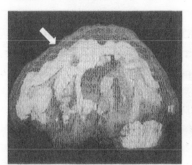 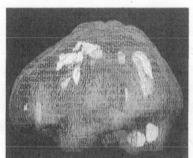

3-D side active view

Before treatment; note markedly increased cingulate activity (arrow).

After treatment with Anafranil; note normal cingulate activity.

Medications don't work all of the time, and sometimes they have side effects that can be annoying and even disturbing. Yet serotonergic medications are some of the newest and most effective weapons in the arsenal against human emotional pain and suffering. They have helped millions of people live more normal lives.

In addition, St John's wort, a natural herbal treatment, in my experience can also be very helpful in raising serotonin levels and calming the cingulate part of the brain. St John's wort has been studied head to head with several antidepressants and found to be just as effective with fewer side effects. It has been used for many years in Germany, where it is prescribed seven times more often than Prozac. The usual dose of St John's wort is 300 milligrams (containing 0.3% hypericin) three times a day. I have used St John's wort in my clinic for several years and find it a very helpful treatment. Here's an example.

Linda

Linda was twenty-six years old when she first came to see me. She had been raped violently twice, had been in a physically abusive love relationship, and had experienced the deaths of a great many friends while still a teenager. Her symptoms were depression, anxiety, worrying, and drug use. Her baseline SPECT study showed marked over-activity in the cingulate (problems shifting attention), basal ganglia (anxiety), and limbic areas (depression and mood dyscontrol). After four psychotherapy sessions with EMDR (eye movement desensitization and reprocessing, a specific treatment technique for traumatic events) and one month of St John's wort (900 milligrams a day), Linda felt significantly better. When we repeated her SPECT study, there was marked normalization of activity in all three areas.

Even though St John's wort can be effective, it is not completely without side effects. One of my patients experienced a seriously slowed heart rate. Another patient who had got worse on Prozac found that St John's wort made her worse as well. If you have significant struggles with mood or behavior, I recommend you work closely with a psychiatrist and discuss any herbal treatments with him or her.

CG PRESCRIPTION 10:
TRY NUTRITIONAL INTERVENTIONS

Low serotonin levels and increased cingulate activity are often associated with worrying, moodiness, emotional rigidity, and irritability. There are two ways that food can increase serotonin levels. Foods high in carbohydrate, such as pasta, potatoes, bread, pastries, crisps, and

Linda's SPECT Studies

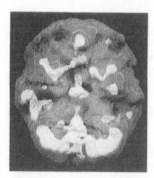 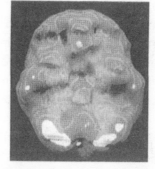

3-D underside active view

Before treatment; note markedly increased cingulate, basal ganglia, and limbic activity.

After treatment with St John's wort; note normal cingulate, basal ganglia, and limbic activity.

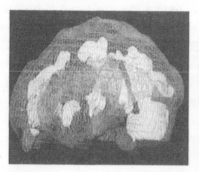 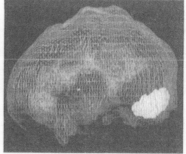

3-D side active view

Before treatment; note markedly increased cingulate, basal ganglia, and limbic activity.

After treatment with St John's wort; note normal cingulate, basal ganglia, and limbic activity.

popcorn, increase l–tryptophan levels (the natural amino acid build-ing block for serotonin) in the blood, resulting in more l–tryptophan being available to enter the brain, where it is converted to serotonin. The calming effect of serotonin can often be felt in thirty minutes or less by eating these foods. Cerebral serotonin levels can also be raised by eating foods rich in tryptophan, such as chicken, turkey, salmon, beef, peanut butter, eggs, green peas, potatoes, and milk. Many people unknowingly trigger cognitive inflexibility or mood problems by eating diets that are low in l–tryptophan. For example, the high-protein, low-carbohydrate diets that I recommend for low-dopamine states (related to prefrontal cortex underactivity) often make cingulate problems worse. L-tryptophan is a relatively small amino acid. When you eat a high-protein diet, the larger amino acids compete more successfully to get into the brain, causing lower levels of brain serotonin and more negative emotional reactiveness.

Nutritional supplementation with l-tryptophan can also be very helpful. L-tryptophan was taken off the market a number of years ago because one contaminated batch, from one manufacturer, caused a rare muscle disease and a number of deaths. The l-tryptophan actually had nothing to do with the deaths. L-tryptophan is a naturally occur-ring amino acid found in milk, meat, and eggs. Many of my patients have found it very helpful for improving sleep, decreasing aggressive-ness, and improving mood control. In addition, it does not have side effects for most people, which is a real advantage over antidepressants. L-tryptophan was recently reapproved by the Food and Drug Admin-istration and is now available. I recommend l-tryptophan in doses of 1,000–3,000 milligrams taken at bedtime. There have also been some recent studies with inositol, from the B vitamin family, which you can get from a health food store. In doses of 12–20 milligrams a day it has been shown to decrease moodiness, depression, and problems of over-focus. Check with your doctor if you want to try these supplements.

CG PRESCRIPTION 11:
EXERCISE

Exercise can also be very helpful in calming worries and increas-ing cognitive flexibility. Exercise works by increasing brain levels of l-tryptophan. As mentioned above, l-tryptophan is a relatively small amino acid and has trouble competing against the larger amino acids to enter the brain. During exercise, more of the large amino acids are utilized to replenish muscle strength, which causes a decrease in the availability of these larger amino acids in the bloodstream. As such, l-tryptophan can compete more effectively to enter the brain and raise brain serotonin levels. In addition, exercise increases your energy levels and may distract you from the bad thoughts that tend to loop. I often recommend exercise for oppositional children as a way to improve their l-tryptophan levels and increase cooperation.

11

Looking Into Memory and Temper:
The Temporal Lobes

Ninety-four-year-old father to his sixty-eight-year-old son: "One day you wake up and realize that you're not eighty-one anymore. You begin to count the minutes, not the days, and you realize that you're not going to be around. All you have left is the experiences. That's all there is."

—from Grumpy Old Men

FUNCTIONS OF THE TEMPORAL LOBES

Dominant Side (usually the left)

- *understanding and processing language*
- *intermediate-term memory*
- *long-term memory*
- *auditory learning*
- *retrieval of words*
- *complex memories*
- *visual and auditory processing*
- *emotional stability*

Nondominant Side (usually the right)

- *recognizing facial expressions*
- *decoding vocal intonation*

- *rhythm*
- *music*
- *visual learning*

For too many years the temporal lobes have largely gone unnoticed in human psychology. They are rarely discussed in psychiatric circles, and few neurologists have been concerned with the rich contribution they make to who we are and how we experience life. Until we were able to map activity in the temporal lobes, their function remained mysterious. Many professionals basically thought of them as armrests for the brain. The brain-imaging work we have done at our clinic clearly shows that the temporal lobes play an integral part in memory, emotional stability, learning, and socialization.

The most precious treasures we have in life are the images we store in the memory banks of our brains. The sum of these stored experiences is responsible for our sense of personal identity and our sense

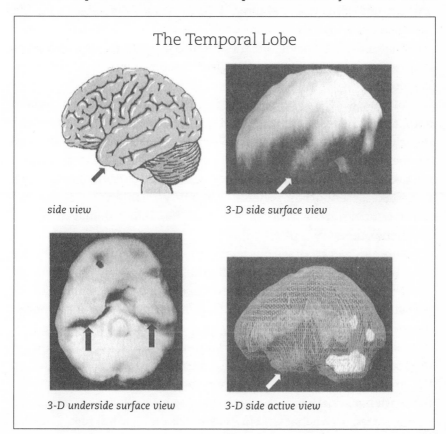

The Temporal Lobe

side view

3-D side surface view

3-D underside surface view

3-D side active view

of connectedness to those around us. Our experiences are enormously significant in making us who we are. The temporal lobes, on either side of the brain behind the eyes and underneath the temples, store the memories and images and help us define our sense of ourselves.

On the dominant side of the brain (the left side for most people), the temporal lobes are intimately involved with understanding and processing language, intermediate- and long-term memory, complex memories, the retrieval of language or words, emotional stability, and visual and auditory processing.

Language is one of the keys to being human. It allows us to communicate with other human beings and to leave a legacy of our thoughts and actions for future generations. Receptive language, being able to receive and understand speech and written words, requires temporal lobe stability. The ability to accurately hear your child say, "I love you," or to listen and be frightened by a scary story is housed in this part of the brain. The dominant temporal lobe helps to process sounds and written words into meaningful information. Being able to read in an efficient manner, remember what you read, and integrate the new information relies heavily on the dominant temporal lobe. Problems here contribute to language struggles, miscommunication, and reading disabilities.

I often tell my patients that it is their memories that give them both their greatest joys and their greatest sorrows. Memories can make us strong and self-confident (remember the times you felt most competent), or they can bring us to our knees (remember your biggest mistakes). Memories influence every action and pattern of action you undertake. Essential components of memory are integrated and stored in the temporal lobes. When this part of the brain is damaged or dysfunctional, memory is often impaired.

Memories can sabotage our chances for success and effectiveness. I once treated a couple with severe marital problems. The husband had problems with depression and attention deficit hyperactivity disorder. His wife tended to be rigid and unforgiving. Ultimately her memories destroyed the relationship. Shortly after they began therapy, the husband's problems were diagnosed and treated with medication. He got significant relief from his symptoms. Everyone except his wife noticed the improvement. Because his more positive behavior was inconsistent with her experience, she could not see his progress and remained in old patterns of behavior. She was stuck on blaming him. She was unwilling to get help for herself, and ultimately the marriage died. It was her memories, rather than the new reality, that killed it.

Through our research we have also found that emotional stability is heavily influenced by the dominant temporal lobe. The ability to consistently feel stable and positive, despite the ups and downs of everyday life, is important for the development and maintenance of consistent character and personality. Optimum activity in the temporal lobes enhances mood stability, while increased or decreased activity in this part of the brain leads to fluctuating, inconsistent, or unpredictable moods and behaviors.

The nondominant temporal lobe (usually the right) is involved with reading facial expressions, processing verbal tones and intonations from others, hearing rhythms, appreciating music, and visual learning.

Recognizing familiar faces and facial expressions and being able to accurately perceive voice tones and intonations and give them appropriate meaning are critical social skills. Being able to tell when someone is happy to see you, scared of you, bored, or in a hurry is essential for effectively interacting with others. Quaglino, an Italian ophthalmologist, reported on a patient in 1867 who, after a stroke, was unable to recognize familiar faces despite being able to read very small type. Since the 1940s, more than one hundred cases of prosopagnosia (the inability to recognize familiar faces) have been reported in the medical literature. Patients who have this disorder are often unaware of it (right-hemisphere problems are often associated with neglect or denial of illnesses), or they may be ashamed at being unable to recognize close family members or friends. Most commonly, these problems were associated with deficits of the right temporal lobe. Results of current research suggest that knowledge of emotional facial expressions is inborn, not learned (infants can recognize their mother's emotional faces). Yet when there are problems in this part of the brain, social skills can be impaired.

The temporal lobes help us process the world of sight and sound, and give us the language of life. This part of the brain allows us to be stimulated, relaxed, or brought to ecstasy by the experience of great music. The temporal lobes have been called the "interpretive cortex," as they interpret what we hear and integrate it with stored memories to give meaning to the incoming information. Strong feelings of conviction, great insight, and knowing the truth have also been attributed to the temporal lobes.

PROBLEMS WITH THE DOMINANT (USUALLY LEFT) TEMPORAL LOBE

- *aggression, internally or externally directed*
- *dark or violent thoughts*
- *sensitivity to slights; mild paranoia*
- *word-finding problems*
- *auditory processing problems*
- *reading difficulties*
- *emotional instability*

PROBLEMS WITH THE NONDOMINANT (USUALLY RIGHT) TEMPORAL LOBE

- *difficulty recognizing facial expression*
- *difficulty decoding vocal intonation*
- *implicated in social-skill struggles*

PROBLEMS WITH EITHER OR BOTH TEMPORAL LOBES

- *memory problems, amnesia*
- *headaches or abdominal pain without a clear explanation*
- *anxiety or fear for no particular reason*
- *abnormal sensory perceptions, visual or auditory distortions*
- *feelings of déjà vu or jamais vu*
- *periods of spaciness or confusion*
- *religious or moral preoccupation*
- *hypergraphia, excessive writing*
- *seizures*

Temporal lobe abnormalities occur much more frequently than previously recognized. You'll note that many of the above symptoms are often thought of as psychological when, in reality, for many they are biological. The temporal lobes sit in a vulnerable area of the brain in the temporal fossa (or cavity), behind the eye sockets and underneath the temples. The front wall of the cavity includes a sharp bony ridge

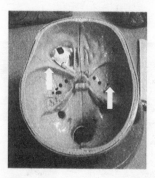

Model showing the base of the skull (thick arrow points to temporal fossa where the temporal lobe sits; thin arrow points to sharp wing of lesser sphenoid bone).

(the lesser wing of the sphenoid bone), which frequently damages the front part of the temporal lobes in even minor head injuries. (God would have done better to put bumper guards on that ridge.) Since the temporal lobes sit in a cavity surrounded by bone on five sides (front, back, right side, left side, and underside) they can be damaged by a blow to the head from almost any angle.

Temporal lobe problems can come from many different sources, the most common being genetics, head injuries, and toxic or infectious exposure. The temporal lobes, prefrontal cortex, and cingulate gyrus are the parts of the brain most vulnerable to damage by virtue of their placement within the skull. They are also the most heavily involved in thinking and behavior.

Blaine

Blaine, age sixty, came to see me because his wife heard me speak at a conference and she was sure he had a temporal lobe problem. He had memory lapses. He was moody and he was often aggressive. He also frequently saw shadows out of the corner of his eyes and heard an annoying "buzzing" sound, for which his doctor could not find a cause. His temper flare-ups just seemed to come out of the blue. "The littlest things set me off. Then I feel terribly guilty," he said. When Blaine was five years old, he had fallen off a porch headfirst into a pile of bricks. As a schoolboy, he had had a terrible time learning to read and had

Blaine's Brain

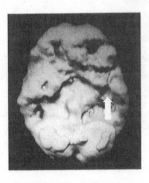

3-D underside surface view

Notice decreased left temporal lobe activity (arrow).

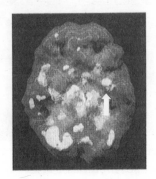

3-D underside active view

Notice increased deep left temporal lobe activity (arrow).

frequently got into fights. His brain SPECT study showed significant abnormalities in his left temporal lobe: a decrease in activity in both the front and back and an area of increased activity deep within. Seeing these abnormalities, it was clear to me that many of Blaine's problems came from the instability of his left temporal lobe, probably a result of his childhood accident. I placed him on Depakote, an antiseizure medication known to stabilize activity in the temporal lobes. When I spoke to him three weeks later, he was elated. The buzzing and shadows had gone away, and he had not lost his temper since he had started the medication. He said, "That was the first time in my life I can remember going three weeks and not screaming at someone." Four years later his temper remains under control.

Common problems associated with left temporal lobe abnormalities include aggression (internally or externally directed), dark or violent thoughts, sensitivity to slights, mild paranoia, word-finding problems, auditory processing problems, reading difficulties, and emotional instability. Let's look at each of these in detail.

The aggressiveness often seen with left temporal lobe abnormalities can be expressed either externally toward others or internally in aggressive thoughts about oneself. Aggressive behavior is complex, but in a large study performed in my clinic on people who had assaulted another person or damaged property, more than 70 percent had left temporal lobe abnormalities. It seems that temporal lobe damage or dysfunction makes a person more prone to irritable, angry, or violent thoughts (much more on this will be discussed in the chapter on violence). One patient of mine with temporal lobe dysfunction (probably inherited, as his father was a "rageaholic") complains of frequent, intense violent thoughts. He feels shame over having these thoughts. "I can be walking down the street," he told me, "and someone accidentally brushes against me, and I get the thought of wanting to shoot him or club him to death. These thoughts frighten me." Thankfully, even though his SPECT study confirmed left temporal lobe dysfunction, he had good prefrontal cortex function, so he is able to supervise his behavior and maintain impulse control over his terrible thoughts. In a similar case, Misty, a forty-five-year-old woman, came to see me about her angry outbursts. One day, someone had accidentally bumped into her in the supermarket and she had started screaming at the woman. "I just don't understand where my anger comes from," she said. "I've had sixteen years of therapy, and it is still there. Out of the blue, I'll go off. I get the most horrid thoughts. You'd hate me if you knew." She had fallen off the top of a bunk bed when she was four years old and had been unconscious for only a minute or two. The front and back parts of her left temporal lobe were clearly damaged. A small daily dose of Depakote was very helpful in calming the "monster" within.

I often see internal aggressiveness with left temporal lobe abnormalities, expressed in suicidal behavior. In a study from our clinic we saw left temporal lobe abnormalities in 62 percent of our patients who had serious suicidal thoughts or actions. After I gave a lecture about the brain in Oakland, a woman came up to me in tears. "Oh, Dr. Amen," she said, "I know my whole family has temporal lobe problems. My paternal great-grandfather killed himself. My father's mother and father killed themselves. My father and two of my three uncles killed themselves, and last year my son tried to kill himself. Is there help for us?" I had the opportunity to evaluate and scan three members of her family. Two had left temporal lobe abnormalities, and Depakote was helpful in their treatment.

In terms of suicidal behavior, one very sad case highlights the involvement of the left temporal lobes. For years I wrote a column in my local newspaper about the brain and behavior. One column was about temporal lobe dysfunction and suicidal behavior. A week or so after it appeared a mother came to see me. She told me that her twenty-year-old daughter had killed herself several months earlier and she was grief stricken over the unbelievable turn of events in her life. "She was the most ideal child a mother could have," she said. "She did well in school. She was polite, cooperative, and a joy to have around. Then it all changed. Two years ago she had a bicycle accident. She accidentally hit a branch in the street and was flipped over the handlebars, landing on the left side of her face. She was unconscious when an onlooker got to her, but shortly thereafter she came to. Nothing was the same after that. She was moody, angry, easily set off. She started to complain of 'bad thoughts' in her head. I took her to see a therapist, but it didn't seem to help. One evening, I heard a loud noise out front. She had shot and killed herself on our front lawn."

Her tears made me cry. I knew that her daughter might well have been helped if someone had recognized her "minor head injury," which had likely caused temporal lobe damage; anticonvulsant medication might well have prevented her suicide. Of interest, in the past twenty years psychiatrists have been using anticonvulsants to treat many psychiatric problems. My suspicion is that we are frequently treating underlying physiological brain problems that we label as psychiatric.

People with left temporal lobe abnormalities are often more sensitive to slights and even appear mildly paranoid. Unlike people with schizophrenia, who can become frankly paranoid, people with temporal lobe dysfunction often think others are talking or laughing about them when there is no evidence for it. This sensitivity can cause serious relational and work problems.

Reading and language-processing problems are also common when there is dysfunction in the left temporal lobe. Being able to read in an efficient manner, remember what you read, and integrate the new information relies heavily on the dominant temporal lobe. It is currently estimated that nearly 20 percent of the U.S. and U.K. population have difficulty reading. Our studies of people with dyslexia (underachievement in reading) often show underactivity in the back half of the left temporal lobe. Dyslexia can be inherited, or it can be brought about after a head injury damaging this part of the brain. Here are two illustrative cases.

Denise

Thirteen-year-old Denise came to see me because she was having problems with her temper. She had pulled a knife on her mother, which had precipitated the referral. She also had school problems, especially in the area of reading, for which she was in special classes. Due to the seriousness of her aggression and learning problems I decided to order a SPECT study at rest and during concentration. At rest her brain showed mild decreased activity in the back half of her left temporal lobe. When she tried to concentrate, the activity in her left temporal lobe completely shut down. As I showed Denise and her mother the scans, I told Denise that it was clear that the more she tried to read, the harder reading would become. As I said this Denise burst into tears. She cried, "When I read I am so mean to myself. I tell myself, 'Try harder. If you try harder then you won't be so stupid.' But trying harder doesn't seem to help." I told her it was essential for her to talk nicely to herself and that she would do better reading in an interesting, fun, and relaxed setting. I sent Denise to see the educational therapist who works in my office. She taught her a specialized reading program that showed her how to visualize words and use a different part of the brain to process reading.

Carrie

Carrie, a forty-year-old psychologist, came to see me two years after she sustained a head injury in a car accident. Before the accident she had had a remarkable memory and had been a fast, efficient reader. She said reading had been one of her academic strengths. After the accident, she had memory problems and struggled with irritability, and reading became difficult. She said that she had to read passages over and over to retain any information and that she had trouble remembering what she read for more than a few moments. Again, her SPECT study showed damage to the front and back of her left temporal lobe (the pattern typically seen in trauma). I had her see my biofeedback technician to enhance activity in her left temporal lobe. Over the course of four months she was able to regain her reading skills and improve her memory and her control over her temper.

In our experience, left temporal lobe abnormalities are more frequently associated with externally directed discomfort (such as anger, irritability, aggressiveness), while right temporal lobe abnormalities are more often associated with internal discomfort (anxiety and fearfulness). The left-right dichotomy has been particularly striking in our clinical population. One possible explanation is that the left hemisphere of the brain is involved with understanding and expressing language, and perhaps when the left hemisphere is dysfunctional, people express their discomfort inappropriately. When the nondominant hemisphere is involved, the discomfort is more likely to be expressed nonverbally.

Mike

Nondominant (usually right) temporal lobe problems more often involve social skills problems, especially in the area of recognizing facial expressions and voice intonations. Mike, age thirty, illustrates the difficulties we have seen when there is dysfunction in this part of the brain. Mike came to see me because he wanted a date. He had never had a date in his life and was very frustrated by his inability to successfully ask a woman out on a date. During the evaluation Mike said he was at a loss as to what his problem was. His mother, who accompanied him to the session, had her own ideas. "Mike," she said, "misreads situations. He has always done that. Sometimes he comes on too strong, sometimes he is withdrawn when another person is interested. He doesn't read the sound of my voice right either. I can be really mad at him, and he doesn't take me seriously. Or he can think I'm mad, when I'm nowhere near mad. When he was a little boy Mike tried to play with other children, but he could never hold on to friends. It was so painful to see him get discouraged." Mike's SPECT study showed marked decreased activity in his right temporal lobe. His left temporal lobe was fine. The intervention that was most effective for Mike was intensive social skills training. He worked with a psychologist who coached him on facial expressions, voice tones, and proper social etiquette. He had his first date six months after coming to the clinic.

Abnormal activity in either or both temporal lobes can cause a wide variety of other symptoms, including abnormal perceptions (sensory illusions), memory problems, feelings of déjà vu (that you have previously experienced something even though you haven't), jamais vu (not recognizing familiar places or people), periods of panic or fear for no particular reason, periods of spaciness or confusion, and preoccupation with religious or moral issues. Illusions are very common temporal lobe symptoms. Common illusions include:

- *seeing shadows or bugs out of the corner of the eyes*
- *seeing objects change size or shape (one patient would see lampposts turn into animals and run away; another would see figures in a painting move)*
- *hearing bees buzzing or static from a radio not there*
- *smelling odors or getting odd tastes in the mouth*
- *feeling bugs crawling on the skin or other skin sensations*

Unexplained headaches and stomachaches are also common in temporal lobe dysfunction. Recently, the anticonvulsant Depakote received a clinical indication for migraine headaches. Often when headaches or stomachaches are due to temporal lobe problems, anticonvulsants seem to be helpful. Many of the patients who experience sudden feelings of anxiety, nervousness, or panic make secondary associations to the panic and develop fears or phobias. For example, if you are in a park the first time you experience a feeling of panic or dread, you may then develop anxiety every time you go into a park.

Moral or religious preoccupation is a common symptom with temporal lobe dysfunction. I have a little boy in my practice who, at age six, made himself physically sick by worrying about all of the people who were going to hell. Another patient spent seven days a week in church, praying for the souls of his family. He came to see me because of his temper problems, frequently directed at his family, which were often seen in response to some perceived moral misgiving or outrage. Another patient came to see me because he spent so many hours focused on the "mysteries of life" that he could not get any work done and was about to lose his job.

Hypergraphia, a tendency toward compulsive and extensive writing, has also been reported in temporal lobe disorders. One wonders whether Ted Kaczynski, the Unabomber, didn't have temporal lobe problems, given the lengthy, rambling manifesto he wrote, his proclivity toward violent behavior, and his social withdrawal. (His loathing of high technology would make submitting to a SPECT scan out of the question for him.) Some of my temporal lobe patients spend hours and hours writing. One patient used to write me twenty- and thirty-page letters, detailing all the aspects of her life. As I learned about temporal lobe hypergraphia and had her treated with anticonvulsant medication, her letters became more coherent and were shortened to two or three pages giving the same information. Of note, many people with temporal lobe problems have the opposite of hypergraphia; they are unable to get words out of their heads and onto the page. I know a therapist who's a wonderful public speaker but cannot get the thoughts out of his head to write his book. On his scan there was decreased activity in both temporal lobes. On a very small daily dose of Depakote, his ideas were unlocked and he could write for hours at a time.

Harriet

Memory problems have long been one of the hallmarks of temporal lobe dysfunction. Amnesia after a head injury is frequently due to damage to the inside aspect of the temporal lobes. Brain infections can also cause severe memory problems. Harriet was a very gracious eighty-three-year-old woman who had lost her memory fifteen years earlier during a bout of encephalitis. Even though she remembered events before the infection, she could remember only small bits and pieces afterward. An hour after she ate, she would feel full but couldn't remember what she had eaten. Harriet said, "I left my brain to the local medical school, hoping my problems would help someone else, but I don't think they'll do anything with my brain except give it to medical students to cut up. Plus I want to know what the problem is. And write it down. I won't remember what you tell me!" Harriet's brain showed marked damage in both temporal lobes, especially on the left side, as if the virus had gone to that part of her brain and chewed it away.

Alzheimer's disease, a devastating progressive form of senile dementia, is the cause of one of the most common memory problems in the elderly. Unfortunately, it robs many people of their retirement years and can leave families physically, emotionally, and financially exhausted. SPECT is an important tool in diagnosing this disorder. Before functional studies were available, the only way to diagnose Alzheimer's was

Harriet's Encephalitis-Affected Brain

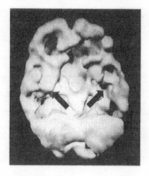

3-D underside surface view
Note markedly decreased activity in both temporal lobes (arrows).

through autopsy. SPECT studies show a typical Alzheimer's pattern of decreased perfusion in both temporal lobes and decreased activity in the parietal lobes. Sometimes this pattern is seen three to six years before the onset of symptoms. Some of the new anti-Alzheimer's drugs are showing promise in arresting the progression of this disorder and have been shown on SPECT to actually improve perfusion in the parts of the brain mostly involved in memory and thinking, such as the temporal lobes. On page 206 is a scan of a man with Alzheimer's disease who had become forgetful, got frequently lost away from home, forgot how to do simple things such as dress himself, and was increasingly aggressive toward his wife.

Fyodor Dostoyevsky was reported to have had bouts of "temporal lobe seizures." He felt his affliction was a "holy experience." One of his biographers, Rene Fueloep-Miller, quotes Dostoyevsky as saying that his epilepsy "rouses in me hitherto unsuspected emotions, gives me feelings of magnificence, abundance and eternity." In *The Idiot*, Dostoyevsky writes:

There was always one instant just before the epileptic fit ... when suddenly in the midst of sadness, spiritual darkness and oppression, his brain seemed momentarily to catch fire, and in an extraordinary rush, all his vital forces were at their highest tension. The sense of life, the consciousness of self, were

Alzheimer's Disease-Affected Brain

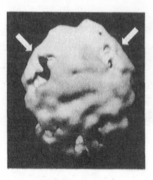

3-D top-down surface view

Note markedly decreased parietal lobe activity (arrows).

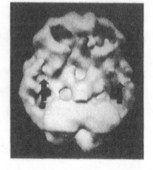

3-D underside surface view

Note markedly decreased temporal lobe activity (arrows).

multiplied almost ten times at these moments which lasted no longer than a flash of lightning. His mind and his heart were flooded with extraordinary light; all his uneasiness, all his doubts, all his anxieties were relieved at once; they were all resolved in a lofty calm, full of serene, harmonious joy and hope, full of reason and ultimate meaning. But these moments, these flashes, were only a premonition of that final second (it was never more than a second) with which the fit began. That second was, of course, unendurable. Thinking of that moment later, when he was well again, he often said to himself that all these gleams and flashes of supreme sensation and consciousness of self, and therefore, also of the highest form of being, were nothing but disease, the violation of the normal state; and if so, it was not at all the highest form of being, but on the contrary must be reckoned the lowest. Yet he came at last to an extreme paradoxical conclusion. "What if it is disease?" he decided at last. "What does it matter that it is an abnormal intensity, if the result, if the sensation, remembered and analyzed afterwards in health, turns out to be the acme of harmony and beauty, and gives a feeling, unknown and undivined till then, of completeness, of proportion, of reconciliation, and of startled prayerful merging with the highest synthesis of life?

Bryce

Lewis Carroll is reported to have had "temporal lobe experiences," which were described in the visual distortions of Alice in *Alice's Adventures in Wonderland*. Seven-year-old Bryce became very upset when his mother read *Alice's Adventures in Wonderland* to him. He said that he felt like Alice. "I have weird things happen to me," he told her. "I see things." During the day he saw objects change shapes, often getting smaller. He also saw green, shadowy ghosts at night. Bryce also had a lot of anxiety symptoms. Frightened that Bryce was losing his mind (a cousin had been diagnosed with a "schizophrenic-like" illness), his mother brought him to see me. On hearing of these symptoms, I suspected that one or both of his temporal lobes were acting up. His brain SPECT study confirmed abnormalities in his right temporal lobe and increased basal ganglia activity. I prescribed Depakote (an antiseizure medication effective in the temporal lobes), and he was also placed in psychotherapy to decrease his anxiety. Within two weeks, Bryce's strange experiences disappeared, and over the next six months his anxiety lessened.

Bryce's Brain, Affected by Temporal Lobe Epilepsy

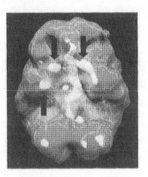

3-D underside active view

Notice area of increased activity in deep right temporal lobe (up arrow) and in basal ganglia (down arrows).

Ellen and Jack

Ellen and Jack had similar histories: both had been somewhat reclusive; both had periods of spaciness; and both had periods of panic for no particular reason. Both had religious experiences that occupied a good deal of their lives. Ellen, age thirty-two, was nearly paralyzed by her deep religious feelings, unable to work and socially isolated. Jack took great interest in her periods of "deep spiritual awakening," but was never able to make out what they meant. Ellen was brought to my office by her parents, who were concerned about her social isolation. Jack wanted an evaluation for the panic attacks. The couple's SPECT studies revealed marked increased activity in the deep aspects of their temporal lobes. The majority of their symptoms went away on Depakote. Even taking Depakote, both remained deeply religious people, but they were no longer constantly preoccupied with their thoughts.

Jim

Like Ellen and Jack, Jim was bothered by periods of spaciness and panic. He also had periods of "religious thoughts," in which he felt the "presence of the devil" and was unsure and afraid. His fear of the devil haunted him, made him reclusive, and made him seem paranoid to his family. There was an interesting difference between Jim's SPECT study and Ellen's and Jack's studies: Jim's study revealed abnormal activity in the left temporal lobe, not the right. In my experience, left temporal lobe problems are often associated with very negative or "dark" thoughts. After Jim was placed on Depakote, the "presence of the devil" was gone.

Temporal Lobe Checklist

Here is the temporal lobe checklist. Please read this list of behaviors and rate yourself (or the person you are evaluating) on each behavior listed. Use the following scale and place the appropriate number next to the item. Five or more symptoms marked 3 or 4 indicate a high likelihood of temporal lobe problems.

0 = never
1 = rarely
2 = occasionally
3 = frequently
4 = very frequently

1.......... Short fuse or periods of extreme irritability
2.......... Periods of rage with little provocation
3.......... Frequent misinterpretation of comments as negative when they are not
4.......... Irritability that tends to build, then explodes, then recedes; person often feels tired after a rage
5.......... Periods of spaciness or confusion
6.......... Periods of panic and/or fear for no specific reason
7.......... Visual or auditory changes, such as seeing shadows or hearing muffled sounds
8.......... Frequent periods of déjà vu (feelings of being somewhere you have never been) or jamais vu (not recalling a familiar place or person)
9.......... Sensitivity or mild paranoia
10........ Headaches or abdominal pain of uncertain origin
11........ History of a head injury or family history of violence or explosiveness
12........ Dark thoughts, such as suicidal or homicidal thoughts
13........ Periods of forgetfulness
14........ Memory problems
15........ Reading comprehension problems
16........ Preoccupation with moral or religious ideas

Enhancing Experience:
Temporal Lobe Prescriptions

The following prescriptions are geared toward optimizing and healing the temporal lobes. They are based on what we have learned about the temporal lobes, as well as clinical experience with my patients. Remember that the temporal lobes are involved with mood stability, understanding and processing language, memory, reading social cues (facial expression and voice intonation), rhythm, and music.

TL PRESCRIPTION 1:
CREATE A LIBRARY OF WONDERFUL EXPERIENCES

Strive for a series of experiences that keep you motivated, healthy, and excited about your life. As the temporal lobes store the experiences of your life, keeping them stimulated with positive ones will help keep you healthy. Celebrate your life on a regular basis; make your experiences count.

Record the memorable experiences of your life with pictures, videos, diary entries, and so on. Develop a library of wonderful experiences. Reexperience them whenever you can. Experiences are your link to life itself. Can it be possible that home movies really are therapeutic? Perhaps not for family and friends, but they certainly are for you.

TL PRESCRIPTION 2:
SING WHENEVER/WHEREVER YOU CAN

Singing in the shower may be healing to your temporal lobes. Song has long been known to have healing qualities. You can often tell that a person is in a good mood if he or she is humming or singing. Song is a true joy of life, no matter how you sing.

Song is often associated with spiritual experience. When I was in college, I attended Calvary Chapel, a large church in southern California. The music was magical. Listening to the choir was not just a pleasant experience, it was a wondrous experience that resonated through every cell in my body. The music uplifted both the soul and mood of the congregation. The pastor said the music was "blessed by God Himself." Several of my friends were choir members. They were often transformed when they started to sing. Shy people would become more extroverted, more alive. People in the congregation became more involved in the service during congregational singing. The church community glistened with the contagious joy of the music.

Preschool and kindergarten teachers have known for a long time that children learn best through songs. They remember the material better, and it is easier to keep them engaged in the activity. So why do we stop singing in as we progress through school? Perhaps we should continue the singing for much longer.

Interestingly, when I was in basic training in the military, we often sang when we marched. I still have those songs in my head. When we sang as a group, morale went up, and the tasks that we were doing (like twenty-mile road marches) didn't seem quite as bad.

Sing whenever and wherever you can. You may have to sing softly if your voice is like mine (my sixteen-year-old daughter is often embarrassed when I sing in church). It will have a healing effect on your temporal lobes, and probably your limbic system as well.

TL PRESCRIPTION 3:
USE HUMMING AND TONING TO TUNE UP YOUR BRAIN

In *The Mozart Effect*, Don Campbell, founder of the Institute of Music, Health, and Education, lists the benefits of using your voice to enhance mood and memory. He says that all forms of vocalization, including singing, chanting, yodeling, humming, reciting poetry, and simply talk can be therapeutic. "Nothing rivals toning," he concludes. The word *toning* goes back to the fourteenth century and means to make sounds with elongated vowels for extended periods of time. *Ah, ou* (as in *soup*), *ee, ay, oh,* and *om* are examples of toning sounds. Campbell writes that when people tone on a regular basis for five minutes a day, "I have witnessed thousands of people relax into their voices, become more centered in their bodies, release fear and other emotions, and free themselves from physical pain ... I have seen many people apply toning in practical ways, from relaxing before a dreaded test to eliminating symptoms of tinnitus or migraine headaches ... Toning has been effective in relieving insomnia and other sleep disorders ... Toning balances brain waves, deepens the breath, reduces the heart rate, and imparts a general sense of wellbeing." Campbell reports that in his experience certain sounds tend to have certain effects on the body and emotions:

Ahhh—immediately evokes a relaxation response

Ee or *ay*—is the most stimulating of vowel sounds; helps with concentration, releasing pain and anger

Oh or *om*—considered the richest of sounds; can warm skin temperature and relax muscle tension

Try toning for five minutes a day for two weeks to see if it will help you.

In a similar way, humming can also make a positive difference in mood and memory. Mozart hummed as he composed. Children hum when they are happy. Adults often hum tunes that go through their minds, lifting their spirits and tuning their mind. Consciously focus on humming during the day. As the sound activates your brain, you will feel more alive and your brain will feel more tuned in to the moment.

TL PRESCRIPTION 4:
LISTEN TO CLASSICAL MUSIC

Listen to a lot of great music. Music, from country to jazz, from rock to classical, is one of the true joys of life. Music has healing properties. Listening to it can activate and stimulate the temporal lobes and bring peace or excitement to your mind.

Music therapy has been a part of psychiatric treatment for decades. Certain music has a calming effect on patients. Fast-tempo, upbeat music can stimulate depressed patients in a positive way.

In highly publicized work, researchers at the University of California at Irvine (UCI) demonstrated that listening to Mozart's *Sonata for Two Pianos* (K448) enhanced visual-spatial learning skills. Frances H. Rauscher, Ph.D., and her colleagues conducted a study with thirty-six undergraduates from the department of psychology who scored eight to nine points higher on a spatial IQ test (part of the Stanford-Binet Intelligence scale) after listening to ten minutes of Mozart. Gordon Shaw, one of the researchers, suggested that Mozart's music may "warm up" the brain: "We suspect that complex music facilitates certain complex neuronal patterns involved in high brain activities like math and chess. By contrast, simple and repetitive music could have the opposite effect." In a follow-up study, the researchers tested spatial skill by projecting sixteen abstract figures similar to folded pieces of paper on an overhead screen for one minute each. The test looked at the ability of participants to tell how the items would look unfolded. Over a five-day period, one group listened to Mozart's *Sonata for Two Pianos*, another to silence, and a third to mixed sounds, including music by Philip Glass, an audio-taped story, and a dance piece. The researchers reported that all three groups improved their scores from day one to day two, but the group that listened to Mozart improved their pattern recognition scores 62 percent compared to 14 percent for the silence group and 11 percent for the mixed group. On subsequent days the Mozart group achieved yet higher scores, but the other groups did not show continued improvement. The researchers proposed that Mozart's music strengthened the creative right-brain processing center associated with spatial reasoning. "Listening to music," they concluded, "acts as an exercise for facilitating symmetry operations associated with higher brain function." Don Campbell gives a nice summary of this work in *The Mozart Effect*, along with many other examples of music enhancing learning and healing the body. Campbell writes that in his experience, Mozart's violin concertos, especially numbers 3 and 4, produce even stronger positive effects on learning.

In the context of the temporal lobes, this research makes perfect sense since the temporal lobes are involved in processing music and memory. Certain types of music may activate the temporal lobes and help them learn, process, and remember information more efficiently.

It is likely that certain types of music open new pathways into the mind.

Certain music may also be very destructive. I believe it is no co-incidence that the majority of teenagers who end up being sent to resi-dential treatment facilities or group homes listen to more heavy metal music than do other teens. Music that is filled with lyrics of hate and despair may encourage those same mind states in developing teens. What your children listen to may hurt them. Teach them to love classi-cal music when they are young.

Music is influential from a very early age. Dr. Thomas Verny in his book *The Secret Life of the Unborn Child* cites scientific experiments show-ing that fetuses preferred Mozart and Vivaldi to other composers in early as well as later stages of pregnancy. He reported that fetal heart rates steadied and kicking lessened, while other music, especially rock, "drove most fetuses to distraction," and they "kicked violently" when it was played to their mothers.

Classical music and other beautiful, soothing music can positively stimulate your brain.

TL PRESCRIPTION 5:
LEARN TO PLAY A MUSICAL INSTRUMENT

In a follow-up study by Rauscher and Shaw at UCI, thirty-four pre-schoolers were given piano keyboard training. After six months, all the children could play basic melodies from Mozart and Beethoven. They exhibited significant increases in visual-spatial skill—up to 36 percent improvement compared to other preschoolers who received computer lessons or other types of stimulation. Campbell cites the following studies: the College Entrance Examination Board in 1996 reported that students with experience in musical performance scored 51 points higher on the verbal part of the SAT and 39 points higher on the maths section than the national average. In a study of approximately 7,500 students at a university, music majors had the highest reading scores of any students on campus. Learning a musical instrument at any age can be helpful in the development and activation of temporal lobe neurons. As the temporal lobes are activated in an effective way, they are more likely to have improved function overall.

TL PRESCRIPTION 6:
MOVE IN RHYTHMS

The temporal lobes are involved with processing and producing rhythms. Chanting, dancing, and other forms of rhythmic movement can be healing. Many of us never learn about the concept of rhythm and how important it can be to healing and health.

Chanting is commonly used in Eastern religions and orthodox Western religions as a way to focus and open one's mind. Chanting has a special rhythm that induces a trancelike state, bringing peace and tranquillity and opening the mind to new experiences and learning.

Even for people with two left feet like myself, dancing and body movement can be very therapeutic. When I worked on a psychiatric hospital unit, the patients had dance therapy three to four times a week. I found that my patients were often more open and more insightful in psychotherapy after a dance therapy session. Dancing, like song and music, can change a person's mood and provide positive experiences to treasure throughout the day or week, or even longer.

Look for opportunities to move in rhythms.

TL PRESCRIPTION 7:
CONSIDER TEMPORAL LOBE MEDICATIONS

Abnormalities in the temporal lobes can cause serious problems, including seizures, visual changes, abnormal sensory experiences, and serious behavior changes. Medications can often be very helpful in temporal lobe dysfunction. Depakote (valproate semisodium), Neurontin (gabapentin), Lamictal (lamotrigine), and Tegretol (carbamazepine) are antiseizure medications that are very effective in stabilizing abnormal activity in the temporal lobes. They have been shown to be helpful for a wide variety of "psychiatric" problems, such as aggressiveness, intractable depression, manic-depressive disorder, migraine headaches, pain syndromes, and even learning disabilities. Dilantin, a classic antiseizure medication, has also been shown to help some patients with temporal lobe abnormalities. If you suspect you have temporal lobe problems, obtain an evaluation by a neurologist or neuropsychiatrist.

TL PRESCRIPTION 8:
GET ENOUGH SLEEP

Current research underscores the importance of sleep. A recent SPECT study demonstrated marked decreased perfusion in the temporal lobes in people who got less than six hours of sleep a night. Decreased sleep is also associated with mood instability, decreased cognitive ability, irritability, and periods of spaciness—all temporal lobe problems. When I was the chief psychiatrist at Fort Irwin in the Mojave Desert, I treated several people with severe sleep deprivation from military maneuvers. They often presented with symptoms of cognitive impairment, paranoia, and hallucinations. Sleep is essential to optimal brain function, especially temporal lobe function. Make sure you get at least six to eight hours every night.

TL PRESCRIPTION 9:
ELIMINATE CAFFEINE AND NICOTINE

In our experience and the experience of other brain researchers, caffeine and nicotine are powerful vasoconstrictors that decrease blood flow to the brain, especially to the temporal lobes. Eliminate these substances from your body, or at least cut down on the amount you consume. You will feel sharper and more in focus overall. Even though caffeine and nicotine may help in the short run, they will make things much worse in the long run. The overall decreased activity caused by the caffeine and nicotine makes people use more and more to get the same effect. They end up chasing a self-induced problem.

TL PRESCRIPTION 10:
WATCH YOUR NUTRITION

Nutritional support can be very helpful in temporal lobe problems. Many people with aggressive behavior become much worse after a high sugar load. If aggressiveness is present without features of depression or obsessive thoughts (more the explosive or short-fuse form of aggressiveness), then a higher-protein/lower-simple-carbohydrate diet is likely to be very helpful. If the aggressiveness is associated with ruminations, moodiness, and depression, then a balanced diet of equal amounts of carbohydrates and protein is likely to be best.

TL PRESCRIPTION 11:
TRY EEG BIOFEEDBACK

Given what we have learned from SPECT, my clinic often uses EEG biofeedback to enhance temporal lobe functioning. When we see over- or underactive areas on SPECT, we put electrodes over those areas, measure the activity, and train healthier brain-wave rhythms in that part of the brain. This can be very helpful for brain injury patients. One woman who was involved in a head-on collision had memory problems, irritability, and trouble reading after her accident. Her cognitive state prevented her from returning to work, which fed a growing depression. On SPECT she had decreased activity in the left temporal lobe. After twenty-five EEG biofeedback sessions over her left temporal lobe, she reported marked improvement in memory, was less irritable, and enjoyed reading once again. Her mood also improved, and she was able to return to work.

13

The Dark Side
Violence: A Combination of Problems

Violence is a complex human behavior. There has long been a passionate debate over whether violent behavior is the result of psychological, social, or biological factors. Current research indicates that violence in fact results from a combination of all three.

Because of the lack of specific biological studies to evaluate violent behavior, clinicians have had to rely on family history to look for genetic factors, along with a history of head trauma, seizures, or drug abuse to evaluate possible medical causes. One of the reasons underlying the lack of clear biological diagnostic tools in violence may be the diversity and variability of the reported findings in the scientific literature. Nonspecific and conflicting EEG findings have been reported. A wide variety of neurotransmitter abnormalities have been reported, including disturbances of noradrenaline, dopamine, serotonin, acetylcholine, and gamma-aminobutyric acid (GABA). Numerous neuroanatomical sites have also been implicated in violence, including the limbic system, temporal lobes, frontal lobe lesions, and prefrontal cortex.

Our SPECT studies provide a useful window into the brain of violent or aggressive patients and help bring together the diversity of biological findings. I have studied hundreds of children, teenagers, and adults who exhibited violent or aggressive behavior and compared them to people who have never been violent. The brain of the violent patient is clearly different from that of the nonviolent person. I have found clinically and statistically significant differences between aggressive groups and nonaggressive groups clustered around three major findings: decreased activity in the prefrontal cortex, increased cingulate activity, and increased or decreased activity in the left temporal lobe. Other significant findings included increased focal activity in the left basal ganglia and on the left side of the limbic system.

The brain SPECT profile of the violent or aggressive patient suggested by these findings is:

- *decreased activity in the prefrontal cortices (trouble thinking)*
- *increased cingulate activity (getting stuck on thoughts)*
- *focal increased or decreased activity in the left temporal lobe (short fuse)*
- *focal increased activity in the basal ganglia and/or limbic system (anxiety and moodiness)*

Case Histories

Paul

Paul, a twenty-eight-year-old gardener, came to my clinic for work-related problems. He had increasingly intense feelings of rage toward his boss. Paul said that his boss was prejudiced against him because he was Hispanic. He frequently thought about killing his boss, and he reported that only the thought of his wife and small daughter prevented him from doing so. He needed to maintain his job in order to support his family. Paul could not get the anger toward his boss out of his head.

He said that since childhood he had had many explosive outbursts. He imagined himself someday shooting down at people from the top of a tower. He described himself as having an extremely short fuse, especially while driving. At the age of seven, he had ridden his bike full speed into a brick wall and had been unconscious for several minutes.

Paul had no evidence of a psychotic disorder or significant depression, although he did complain of short periods of confusion, fear for no reason, and episodes of déjà vu. His EEG was within normal limits. A brain SPECT study was obtained in order to evaluate any underlying brain abnormalities that might have been contributing to his difficulties.

Paul's Aggression-Affected Brain

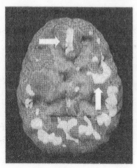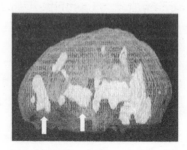

3-D underside active view   *3-D side active view*

Note markedly increased activity in left temporal lobe and cingulate (arrows).

Paul's brain SPECT study was significantly abnormal. It revealed normal activity in the prefrontal cortex at rest that worsened when he tried to concentrate (problems with impulsivity). There was also moderate marked increased uptake in the deep aspects of the left temporal lobe (short fuse) and the cingulate gyrus (stuck on thoughts).

Because of the clinical picture and information from the brain SPECT study, Paul was placed on the anticonvulsant Tegretol at therapeutic levels, along with Prozac several weeks later. After six weeks, he reported that he noted a sense of increased inner control and inner peace. His periods of confusion, déjà vu, and fearfulness diminished. His angry outbursts decreased, and he was able to go to work at a new job.

Steven

Steven, a thirty-nine-year-old radio station engineer, was admitted to hospital for suicidal thoughts. He had recently separated from his wife of eight years. During their relationship there had been mutual physical spousal abuse for which he had spent some time in jail. Steven also complained of having a very short fuse. He found himself frequently yelling at other drivers on the road and was easily upset at work. On admission he was depressed and tearful, and had problems sleeping and poor concentration. He reported short periods of confusion,

Steven's Aggression-Affected Brain

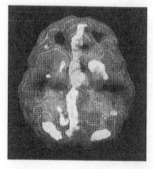
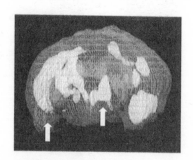

3-D underside active view   *3-D side active view*

Note markedly increased activity in left temporal lobe and cingulate (arrows).

feelings of intense rage with little provocation, and times when he would see shadows out of the corners of his eyes. His EEG was within normal limits. Steven's brain SPECT study revealed marked increased uptake in the deeper aspects of the left temporal lobe and marked increased activity in the cingulate gyrus.

With the clinical picture and information from the brain SPECT, it was decided to start Steven on an anticonvulsant in addition to an antidepressant. He was placed on Tegretol at therapeutic levels along with Prozac. Even though he continued to feel sad about the breakup of his marriage, he felt calmer and in better self-control, and his suicidal thoughts abated. He did report that he wished he had known about the dysfunction in his temporal lobe years earlier. He felt it might have changed the outcome of his marriage.

Mark

Mark, a thirty-four-year-old corporate employee, was referred by his counselor after he was discharged prematurely from a drug treatment program for psychotic thinking. Mark had gone into drug treatment voluntarily, trying to break a ten-year amphetamine addiction. Initially it seemed that Mark had an amphetamine psychosis, but after four months free from any drugs, his paranoia and aggressive behavior escalated. On three separate occasions he stormed out of my office,

Mark's Aggression-Affected Brain

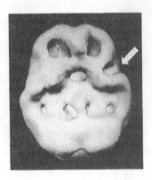

3-D underside surface view
Note markedly deaeased activity, especially in left temporal lobe (arrow).

cursing me as he left. He began to display dangerous behavior, express-ing homicidal and suicidal ideas along with grandiose thinking. He had gone through several similar episodes in the past. Mark refused medi-cation, suspecting that I was trying to control him or poison him. He did consent to having a brain SPECT study after much encouragement from his family.

The first time Mark went for his SPECT study, he ripped the IV out of his arm and ran from the clinic. He called me an hour later and swore at me, saying again that I was trying to poison him. I called his mother, who calmed him down and sat with him through the test. His brain SPECT study revealed significant decreased uptake in his left temporal lobe.

With the clinical picture and the SPECT information, Mark was started on the anticonvulsant Tegretol at therapeutic levels. Within ten days, he felt calmer and was obviously less paranoid. Within a month, he returned to work at full function and felt more in control of his temper than even before he had started using drugs. He was relieved to know about the temporal lobe dysfunction and felt it explained many of the problems he had had in the past. He continued his medication without incident.

Peter

Peter was a twelve-year-old boy with a history of oppositional behavior, emotional outbursts, increased activity level, short attention span, impulsiveness, school problems, frequent lying, and aggressive behavior. At age six, Peter had been placed on Ritalin for hyperactivity, but it had made him more aggressive and had been stopped. He was admitted to a psychiatric hospital at age eight for aggressiveness, where he was diagnosed with depression and started on an antidepressant, which had little effect. By the age of twelve, a psychiatrist in the Napa Valley had seen him for several years of psychotherapy, and his parents were seen in collateral sessions as well.

The psychiatrist frequently blamed the mother as the "biggest part of Peter's problem." He told her that if only she would get into psychotherapy and deal with her childhood issues, Peter's problems would lessen. Peter's behavior escalated to the point where he was frequently aggressive and uncontrollable at home. He was rehospitalized on the day he attacked a classmate with a knife.

I was on call the weekend Peter was hospitalized. To bond with the kids, sometimes I play football with them. Peter was on my team. On every single play, he tried to cheat. When we were on defense, he would move the ball back several feet and then turn around to look at me, as if he were trying to get me angry. I refused to play his conflict-seeking game, but I decided it was time to get a brain SPECT study to help me understand Peter's need for turmoil.

Peter's SPECT study was abnormal. There was significant left temporal lobe underactivity; in addition, when he tried to concentrate, his prefrontal cortex shut down. Peter was placed on Tegretol at a therapeutic level. Within three weeks, he was a dramatically different child. He was more compliant, better with the other children on the hospital ward, and less conflict-seeking with the hospital staff. On the weekend he was being discharged from the hospital, I was again on call. As I had the month before, I gathered the kids on the ward and we played football. Peter was on my team. On every single play, he talked to me about what we were going to do. There was no evidence of the prior conflict-seeking behavior. Peter was exhibiting socially effective behavior.

After Peter's discharge from the hospital, his mother no longer looked like "the problem." Even though Peter was emotionally more stable, he still had symptoms of attention deficit hyperactivity disorder, having trouble concentrating and following through on his schoolwork. Knowing about the drop-off in prefrontal cortex activity, I added Cylert (a brain stimulant) to the Tegretol, which helped him perform much better in school. Eight years after his hospitalization, Peter is stable and doing well at school and at home. When Peter was sixteen, I gave a lecture to the staff at his school. Peter saw me in the car park. He ran over to me and gave me a big hug (in front of his friends)!

Profile of Violence

These findings point to a brain SPECT profile of the aggressive patient that involves several specific areas of the brain, especially the left hemisphere. When these findings are taken together, they suggest that aggression is a complex process mediated by several different areas of the brain.

Decreased activity in the prefrontal cortex is a finding often cited in people who are having cognitive difficulty, such as in schizophrenia or major depression. The prefrontal cortex is involved in mediating concentration, impulse control, and critical thinking. Aggressive people often misinterpret situations and react in an impulsive manner.

As mentioned above, increased activity in the cingulate is frequently noted in people who become "stuck" on certain thoughts or behaviors. Aggressive people often become "stuck" on real or imagined injustices and think about them over and over. For example, in several of the case histories, the men often became enraged while driving. They reported that if someone accidentally cut them off on the road, they would think and think about it to the point where they would have to do something, such as honk, gesture, or even chase the other driver, in order to get the thoughts out of their minds. Studies have shown that medications that increase serotonin in the brain (such as Prozac or Anafranil) normalize activity in the cingulate.

Increased activity in the basal ganglia is often found in patients who have anxiety or panic disorders. People who are aggressive often report a baseline level of tension or anxiety, and many clinicians have seen a pattern with these patients where they become increasingly more anxious before they strike out.

Abnormalities in the limbic system have been associated with aggressiveness. Some researchers believe that affected people have limbic seizures. Studies consistently find that when the amygdala, a structure in the deep temporal lobes often considered part of the limbic system, is stimulated, a person becomes more agitated and aggressive. The limbic system is often cited as the part of the brain that sets the mood, and abnormal activity in this area may be associated with significant moodiness.

Aggression and abnormalities in the temporal lobes have been described in numerous studies. They are perhaps the most striking finding of our work. Medications such as Neurontin, Tegretol, and Depakote have been found helpful in decreasing abnormal activity in this portion of the brain.

In my experience with brain SPECT imaging, left-side brain abnormalities are associated with patients who are more irritable and aggressive. In addition, right-side brain abnormalities often correlate with patients who are more withdrawn, socially conscious, and fearful, and much less aggressive.

I was raised in a strong Catholic family. I was taught to believe that if you live a clean life and work hard, you will be successful. I believed that there was something the matter with the character of people who were drug addicts, murderers, child abusers, and even those who took their own lives. After being involved with about five thousand brain SPECT studies my mind has changed completely. I now believe that it is essential to evaluate the brain when behavior is out of bounds. The brain is an organ that dramatically influences behavior, thoughts, and feelings. These cases and many like them are yet further examples to me to press on studying the brains of people with abnormal behavior. What we need is more knowledge, more understanding, and less judgment.

Sometimes I want to cry when I think of all the children and teenagers who are in homes, residential treatment facilities, and young offenders' institutions, or who have run away from home because their families could not deal with them any longer. I know that many, many of them have brain problems that have never been properly evaluated. Perhaps they have seen a local counselor or doctor who looked at the abnormal behavior and told the parents that the child could behave if only he or she really wanted to. In today's "enlightened" society, that attitude is as prevalent as ever. No amount of trying would have changed Peter's behavior.

Here is an example of the impact that brain problems can have on a family.

Father-and-Son Study

Nine-year-old Phillip was frightened when the police came to his school to talk to him. His teacher had noticed bruises on his arms and legs and had called Child Protective Services. Phillip wasn't sure if he should tell them the truth—that his father, Dennis, had beaten him up—or if he should say that he had fallen down a flight of stairs or something like that. Phillip did not want to get his dad into trouble, and he felt responsible for the beating he had received. After all, he reasoned, his father had told him ten times to clean his room, but for some reason unknown to Phillip, he hadn't done it. Phillip and his father often fought, but it had never been apparent to people outside the home. Phillip decided to tell the truth, hoping that it would help his family get some help.

Indeed, Phillip's family did get help. The court ordered counseling for the family and a psychiatric evaluation for the father. The father was found to be impulsive and explosive in many different situations. He had begun to have problems with aggressiveness after sustaining a head injury in a car accident six years earlier. His wife reported that when Phillip had first been born, his father had been loving, patient, and attentive. After the accident, he had become irritable, distant, and angry.

In family counseling sessions, Phillip was very difficult—restless, overactive, impulsive, and defiant. He ignored his parents' request to stop his annoying behaviors. I soon discovered that the interaction between Phillip and his father was the problem and counseling alone would not be helpful. I believed there was some underlying biological or physical "brain problem" that contributed to the abusive interactions. In an effort to further understand the biology of this family's problems, I ordered brain SPECT studies on Phillip and his father.

The studies for both were abnormal. The father's clearly showed an area of increased activity in his left temporal lobe, probably a result of the car accident. Phillip's revealed decreased activity in the front part of his brain when he tried to concentrate. As we have seen, this is often found in children who have ADHD and are impulsive and overly active.

After taking a history, watching the family interact, and reviewing the SPECT studies, it was clear to me that Phillip's and his father's problems were, in part, biological. I placed both of them on medication. The father was put on an antiseizure medication to calm his left temporal lobe, and Phillip was placed on a stimulant medication to increase activity in the front part of his brain.

Once the underlying biological problems were treated, the family was able to benefit from psychotherapy and begin to heal the wounds of abuse. In counseling sessions, Phillip was calmer and more attentive, and his father was better able to learn how to deal with Phillip's difficult behavior in a constructive way.

Whenever abuse of a child occurs, it is a severe tragedy. The tragedy is compounded when the underlying brain problems that may be contributing to the abuse are ignored.

Suicide

Suicide is among the ten most common causes of death. It is often attempted when a person feels as though he or she has no other option. Suicide devastates a family, often leaving parents, spouses, and children feeling abandoned, guilt stricken, and depressed.

Brain SPECT studies have been useful in helping to understand suicidal behavior. I have scanned several hundred people who have attempted suicide. They frequently show the violent pattern described above. The majority of these patients had increased cingulate activity (tendency to get stuck on negative thoughts); increased or decreased activity in the temporal lobes, most commonly on the left side (short fuse and irritability); and decreased activity in the prefrontal cortex during a concentration task (impulsivity and poor judgment).

Most suicidal thoughts are brief in duration. Yet when someone who gets locked into negative thoughts also has a short fuse and problems with impulsivity—watch out! Here are several examples.

Danny

Danny was eight years old when his mother brought him to my clinic after he had twice tried suicide. He had attempted to jump out of a moving car, and he had put a rope around his neck and tied it to the wardrobe rail. Both times his mother had stopped him. She said that Danny had an obsession with death. He often complained that he hated his life and felt he'd be better off dead. At the age of three, Danny had fallen out of a motor home that was moving about thirty miles per hour and sustained a head injury with a brief loss of consciousness. Over the next year, he had changed from a happy, fun-loving child to a surly, negative, unhappy child who was subject to monumental temper tantrums. A neurologist had ordered an EEG on Danny when the parents complained he was having periods of spaciness. The EEG was normal. As part of my evaluation, I ordered a brain SPECT study to evaluate why a child so young would exhibit suicidal behavior (which is very unusual in children under ten).

Danny's SPECT study showed markedly increased activity in the deep aspects of his temporal lobes, markedly increased activity in the cingulate gyrus, and decreased activity in his prefrontal cortex during a concentration task. No wonder Danny was having so much trouble. Traditionally play therapy or psychotherapy is the first line of treatment for depressed or suicidal children. Given the seriousness of this case, I placed Danny on Depakote, an antiseizure medication, to stabilize his abnormal temporal lobe activity. Three weeks later, I added Lustral to help with his obsessive thinking. Within six weeks, Danny lost his anger, his suicidal thoughts had disappeared, and he was able to interact with his family in a more positive way. Danny was also seen twice weekly in psychotherapy for a few months. Three years later, Danny remains on lowered doses of his medication without any suicidal thoughts.

Mary

Sixteen-year-old Mary was admitted to hospital for recurrent suicide attempts. This was her fifth psychiatric hospitalization, and she was going to be transferred to a long-term residential treatment facility. Mary also had problems with obsessive thoughts about unusual sexual behaviors, and she compulsively took eight to ten showers a day and changed her clothes that many times during a day as well. Her mother could barely keep up with the laundry. On the day Mary was admitted to hospital, she had cut her wrists with broken glass. Mary had a paternal uncle who had multiple incarcerations for assaultive behavior. Her father's father was an alcoholic.

Mary's brain SPECT study revealed markedly increased cingulate activity, along with increased activity in the left side of her basal ganglia and the left side of her limbic system. The increased activity also spread into the deep aspects of her left temporal lobe. No wonder she was in so much pain! She had tried Prozac in the past, but it had made her more aggressive. Given her symptoms and SPECT findings, I put her on Depakote and Anafranil (an antiobsessive antidepressant). Over the course of the next month, Mary became more relaxed, and she was able to talk about her obsessive thoughts. Her suicidal thoughts diminished, and it was decided that she could return home rather than go to long-term treatment. She remained in therapy for several years and made no more suicide attempts. Her SPECT study was repeated eight months later to make sure we were on the right track. There was an 80 percent decrease in activity in the areas of her brain that had been overly active.

Randle

Randle had been hospitalized for two serious suicide attempts before he came to see me. He was the chief executive officer of a computer software company, and on the outside it appeared he was a man who had everything. He had a beautiful wife, three children, and a successful business. On the inside, however, he was tormented. He often went into rages at home over minor things. He drank too much, and he was obsessively jealous whenever any man looked his wife's way. Randle began having a repeat of his suicidal thoughts when he came to see me. Randle's father had killed himself when Randle was seventeen years old (suicide is often a modeled behavior). His father had been diagnosed as manic-depressive. Randle had an uncle who was an alcoholic, an aunt who was being treated for depression, and a nephew who was on Ritalin for ADHD.

On close questioning, Randle said he had "really dark days" even when he wasn't drinking. He also complained of seeing shadows and of frequent spacy periods. I ordered a brain SPECT study to help understand the patterns in Randle's brain. It showed left temporal lobe abnormalities, increased cingulate activity, and decreased activity in his prefrontal cortex when he tried to concentrate. Again, these findings are consistent with a short fuse, obsessive thoughts, and impulsivity. This symptom triad often leads to aggressive behavior, toward either oneself or others. Randle had a very positive response to a combination of Tegretol and Prozac.

Stalking

In my clinical practice I have studied four people who have been arrested for stalking. All four had the brain pattern I have described for violence with left temporal lobe problems, heavily increased cingulate activity, and decreased activity in the prefrontal cortex in response to a concentration task. These people would get stuck on negative thoughts, such as "I must have her," and they were unable to let go of those thoughts. In three of the four cases, medication helped these patients give up their obsessions. The fourth person went to jail. Cheryl was an example of successful treatment.

Cheryl

After seeing an interview on television, Cheryl, twenty-eight, became obsessed with a player on a professional baseball team. She started attending every home game. She wrote to him weekly. She couldn't stop thinking about him. She had a responsible job in a bank during the day, but at night and weekends she focused mostly on this one celebrity. When she didn't get any response to her letters, she began trying to contact him by telephone and in person. When this was unsuccessful the tone of her letters changed from admiration to irritation and then to subtle threats. After she sent a particularly hostile letter, the team reported her to the police. The police warned her to stop trying to contact the player.

Her brother Peter had been seeing me at the time for obsessive-compulsive disorder. He had had a nice response to the combination of Prozac and psychotherapy. When he heard what was going on with his sister, he insisted that she come to see me. Reluctantly she came to my office.

Cheryl was frightened by her own behavior. She had never before had any contact with the police. "I just couldn't get him out of my head," she said, referring to the player. Cheryl had for a long time had trouble getting certain thoughts out of her head. As a teenager, she had had problems with anorexia. As an adult she had gone through many relationships. Her boyfriends had complained that she worried too much and was too jealous. As part of my evaluation, I ordered a brain SPECT study. It revealed a significantly overactive cingulate, left temporal lobe changes, and decreased prefrontal cortex activity. Cheryl responded nicely to a combination of an antiobsessive antidepressant (Prozac), an anticonvulsant (Depakote), and psychotherapy. She said that the medication allowed her to be more flexible and not get locked into repetitive thoughts.

14

Brain Pollution:
The Impact of Drugs and Alcohol on the Brain

Robert

Robert, age thirty-nine, came to see me because he thought he had attention deficit hyperactivity disorder. He was forgetful, disorganized, and impulsive and had a very short attention span. However, he had not had these problems at school while he was growing up. They had come on gradually during his adult life. Most notably, he also had a twenty-year history of heroin abuse and had been in multiple treatment settings. It is hard to describe my personal feelings when I initially saw his SPECT study. This man was about my age, yet through abusing drugs his brain had assumed the functional pattern of an individual fifty years older with a dementialike condition.

When I showed Robert his SPECT study, he was horrified. Even though he had tried unsuccessfully to stop abusing heroin on many occasions, this time he went into treatment and was able to stop. Later he told me, "It was either the heroin or my brain. I wasn't giving any more of my brain to the drug."

Researchers consistently find that drug and alcohol abuse can cause serious brain damage. I often show Robert's studies and those of others like him to the teenagers I see in my office, as well as to groups of teenagers when I lecture around the country. I find these pictures much more powerful than pictures of fried eggs ("your brain on drugs").

Studying the effects of drugs and alcohol on the brain has been one of the most informative and fascinating parts of my work. While I was

Robert's Heroin-Affected Brain

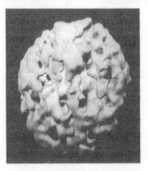

3-D top-down surface view
Notice the large holes of activity across the brain surface.

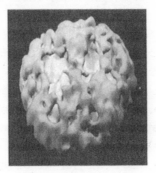

3-D front-on surface view
Notice markedly decreased activity across the brain surface.

growing up I had a sense that drugs and alcohol weren't beneficial to my overall health. This notion was solidified by the results of getting drunk on a six-pack of Michelob and half a bottle of champagne when I was sixteen years old—I was sick for three days. After that, I luckily stayed away from drugs and alcohol. After what I've seen in my work, there's no way you could get me to use marijuana, heroin, cocaine, methamphetamine,* LSD, PCP, or inhalants or to drink more than a glass or two of wine or beer. These substances damage the patterns

---

* Methamphetamines are in a class of drugs known as psychostimulants. These medications are used to treat attention deficit hyperactivity disorder. In therapeutic doses these medications are helpful and do not cause brain damage. Drug abuse and addiction doses are typically 10–50 times what doctors prescribe, and in those high doses these drugs are dangerous and highly addictive.

in your brain, and as you've gathered by now, without your brain, you are not you. In this chapter, I'll share with you some of the insights we have gained from SPECT about drug and alcohol abuse and tell you how I apply this information with my patients. In the next chapter I'll look at the connections between drug abuse, violence, and the brain.

There is quite a bit of scientific literature on the physiological effects of drugs and alcohol on the brain. The most common finding among drug and alcohol abusers is that their brain scans display an overall toxic look. In general, their brains look less active, more shriveled, less healthy overall. A "scalloping effect" is commonly seen in the brains of drug abusers. Normal brain patterns show smooth activity across the cortical surface; scalloping is a wavy, rough sea—like a pattern on the brain's surface. I see the same pattern in patients who have been exposed to toxic fumes or oxygen deprivation.

Cocaine and Methamphetamine

Cocaine and methamphetamine are rapidly taken up by the dopamine system in the basal ganglia, causing short-term brain activation. Over time, amphetamine and cocaine abusers show multiple perfusion defects across both hemispheres of the brain. On SPECT these areas look like mini-strokes across the surface of the brain. These effects appear both acutely and chronically. One study investigated the cerebral blood flow patterns and cognitive functioning in cocaine abusers. The patients had been drug-free for at least six months before evaluation. All showed regions of significant underactivity in the frontal and temporal-parietal areas. Deficits in attention, concentration, new learning, visual and verbal memory, word production, and visual-motor integration were observed. This study indicated that long-term cocaine use may produce sustained brain blood flow deficits and persistent intellectual compromise in some subgroups of cocaine-abusing patients. In another study, crack abusers showed a 23 percent decrease in cerebral blood flow compared to the control group, and crack users who were also cigarette smokers showed a 42 percent decrease overall compared to the control group. Cigarette smoking makes everything worse.

Jeff

Jeff, thirty-six, came to see me because he had severe problems abusing methamphetamines. Child Protective Services (CPS) had taken his three young children out of his home and placed them with his parents. He was also about to lose his job at a local warehouse because of chronic tardiness and erratic work performance. His parents had called CPS because they knew about the drug abuse and were afraid for the safety of the children. Jeff's wife, also a drug abuser, had left the family several years before and was nowhere to be found. His parents had tried to get Jeff help, but he had refused, denying that there were any problems. At first, when he was forced by the court to see me, he was in denial. It was everyone else's fault. He said that he used only a little bit and couldn't understand why everyone was so upset. To help break through his denial, I ordered a SPECT study. It showed multiple holes in activity across the surface of his brain. When I showed Jeff his brain on the computer screen, his mouth dropped open. He didn't say anything for about three minutes. "So much for denial," I said. "You have serious brain damage caused by this drug. Keep doing it and you won't have any choices about what you do. You won't have enough brainpower to make good decisions."

Through Jeff's history, it was clear that besides the drug abuse he had underlying attention deficit hyperactivity disorder. He had a childhood history of hyperactivity, restlessness, and impulse control problems, and a short attention span. He had barely finished high school, despite having a high IQ. He had been treated with Ritalin for a brief period as a child, but his parents had felt uncomfortable about "drugging" their son. When he had started using methamphetamines as an adult, he said, they had helped him concentrate, he had had better energy and initially he had been better at work. In fact, Jeff had the right class of medication, brain stimulants. Yet he didn't know how to use them to treat his problems. His estimated usage was approximately 500 milligrams a day—ten to twenty times higher than a therapeutic dose of a brain stimulant. And odds are, they were made in someone's garage and laced with other toxic chemicals. I knew that in order to really help him I had to treat his underlying brain disorder as well as get him into a drug treatment program. I told him, "Let me do your drugs for you. I'm a lot better at it than you are, and my drugs don't cause this damage." I put him on a low dose of Adderall, which is a combination

Jeff's Methamphetamine-Affected Brain

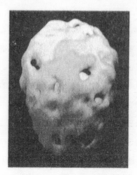

3-D top-down surface view

Notice the multiple holes in activity across the brain surface.

of amphetamine salts that are slowly released into the body and that, in prescribed doses, have little if any potential for abuse. I also saw him weekly and ensured that he attended a daily twelve-step program. After a year of maintaining sobriety and compliance with treatment, he was able to have his children come home.

Mark

Mark, twenty-four, was very different from Jeff. He had been abusing cocaine for two years when he decided he had had enough and came to my clinic. He told me, "When I first started using cocaine, I felt better around other people. I have always been shy and uncomfortable in group settings. From my first hit of cocaine, I felt more confident and was able to meet people without feeling anxious or uptight. But the more I used, the more I wanted to use. I want to stop." Mark was spending most of his salary on cocaine, and his parents were hassling him about never having any money, despite working full-time. As part of a research study I ordered a SPECT study on Mark. It showed increased activity in his basal ganglia on the right and left sides (corresponding to his anxiety) and multiple holes across the top surface of his brain (indicating multiple areas of decreased brain activity). He was very upset when he saw the scan. The first thing out of his mouth was "Will my brain get better if I stop?" I told him it was likely to get better,

Mark's Cocaine-Affected Brain

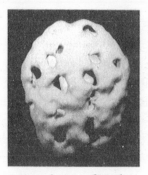

3-D top-down surface view

Notice the multiple holes in activity across the brain surface.

but there were no guarantees. One thing was certain: If he continued to use cocaine, things would get worse.

People frequently ask me what will happen if they stop abusing drugs. I answer, it depends. It depends on what drug you used, how long you used it, what other toxic substances might have been in what you used, and how sensitive your individual brain is. Some people are very sensitive to the effects of drugs and damage becomes evident after a short while. Other people have more resistance to drug damage and can use for longer periods of time without serious damage. It depends. But who is to know ahead of time? Seems to me like a stupid risk to take once you have this information!

I placed Mark in a drug treatment program and also saw him in individual psychotherapy. I taught him other ways to calm himself in social situations (using biofeedback and ANT therapy). Later Mark told me that seeing his brain had been the most powerful deterrent to doing cocaine. He said, "You could have told me all day long that cocaine was hurting me, but it felt so good. There was no getting around seeing my brain with holes in it." In my experience, having patients see their own drug-damaged brain is the most powerful way to break through the denial that typically accompanies drug abuse.

Alcohol

Alcohol abuse is also associated with cerebral blood flow abnormalities. Small doses of alcohol produce cerebral activation, while higher doses induce cerebral vasoconstriction and overall decreased brain activity. Chronic alcoholism is associated with reduced cerebral blood flow and cerebral metabolism, especially in the frontal and temporal regions of the brain. In one study, SPECT was used to study seventeen healthy volunteers and a sample of fifty patients dependent on alcohol, without other major physical or mental disorders. The SPECT studies were abnormal in thirty-four patients, but in only two volunteers. The main abnormality was decreased activity across the whole cortex. A genetic vulnerability to alcohol was suspected in the study because SPECT abnormalities were more frequent in patients with a family history of drinking problems.

Chronic alcohol abuse also decreases thiamine (a B vitamin essential for cognitive function) and puts patients at risk of Korsakoff's syndrome (KS). KS is an amnestic disorder in which the inability to record new memory traces often leads to confabulation (lying to make up for missed information) and a seemingly paradoxical situation in which the patient can carry out complex tasks learned before his illness but cannot learn the simplest new skills. In a study comparing alcoholics with and without KS, both had overall decreased activity, but the decreased activity in the KS group was much more severe. The study concluded that chronic alcohol abuse, in the absence of thiamine deficiency, reduces cerebral blood flow by causing direct toxic effects on the brain. If thiamine deficiency is also present, more severe blood flow reductions are superimposed.

"But, Dr. Amen," you might ask, "what about all of those studies that say that a little bit of alcohol is good for your heart?" A little bit of alcohol is probably good for your heart and maybe even for your brain. Some studies suggest that those who drink one to two drinks a day are psychologically healthier than those who don't drink at all. The operating phrase is "a little bit." Long term, "more than a little bit" of alcohol ingestion causes severe problems that on SPECT make the brain look shriveled. If you have any trouble at all stopping after one or two drinks, it is better not to drink at all.

Carl

Carl, a forty-six-year-old attorney, came to see me after his wife threatened to divorce him if he didn't stop drinking. He had been drinking for twenty-five years and heavily for the past ten years. Even though his drinking had just recently begun to affect his work, it had affected his family life for many years. His children stopped asking friends over because they never knew when Daddy would be drunk. They worried about him constantly. Carl fought regularly with his wife about his drinking. And his blood pressure had been elevated for several years. His doctor could not find a medicine to bring it down. Typical of many substance abusers, denial was part of Carl's problem, even when he was confronted by his whole family. I ordered a scan as part of his diagnosis. He reluctantly agreed. He saw the posters in my office about drug abuse and the brain. Before his scan he said, "Don't tell me if I have one of those brains with holes in it. I don't want to know." I thought to myself, "You better want to know. Otherwise you won't have enough brain left to care." Like many of my alcoholic patients, Carl had a shriveled brain that looked years older than it was. As Carl looked at the studies of his brain, he started to cry. His wife, sitting next to him, put her hand on his shoulder. I waited a few minutes for the impact to set in and then said, "Carl, you have a choice. You can look at your brain and think, 'Hell, I already have one screwed-up brain, I might as

Carl's Alcohol-Affected Brain

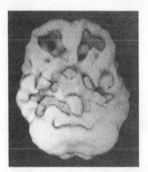

3-D underside surface view

Notice the shriveled appearance of the brain, especially in the prefrontal cortex and temporal lobes.

well go on drinking.' Or you can say to yourself, 'Thank God I have this information now. Thank God my wife forced me to get help. My brain has a chance to heal if I get away from this stuff now.' Alcohol is clearly toxic to your brain." Carl didn't need much more. He stopped drinking completely, attended a twelve-step program, and started to rebuild his relationship with his wife and children.

Rob's Brain, Affected by Alcohol, Cocaine, and Methamphetamine

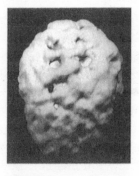

3-D top-down surface view

Notice the overall holes and shriveled appearance during abuse.

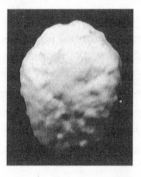

3-D top-down surface view

Notice marked improvement after a year of abstaining from drugs and alcohol.

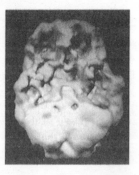

3-D underside surface view

Notice the overall holes and shriveled appearance during abuse.

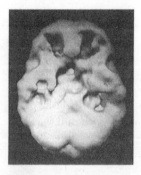

3-D underside surface view

Notice marked improvement after a year of abstaining from drugs and alcohol.

Rob

Rob had been a brilliant geneticist, but in recent years he had been tired all the time and unable to concentrate, and his work had suffered. He sought therapy. The psychologist who saw him quickly sent him to see me. Rob had been drinking alcohol heavily for the past five years, and he was also using cocaine and methamphetamines for energy. The psychologist told him she couldn't help him until he stopped drinking and using drugs. Clearly a bright man despite the substance abuse, Rob just didn't understand how these substances could be the problem. "What will I do without them? I feel terrible when I try to stop. I feel agitated, depressed, and very anxious." I wondered if Rob weren't using the alcohol and drugs to treat underlying brain abnormalities. I convinced him to stop drinking and using drugs for two weeks (I helped him detox from the alcohol with some medication) so that I could get some pictures of his brain. He clearly had a drug-affected brain with holes across the cortex and the shriveled appearance that comes from alcohol abuse. In addition, off his substances for two weeks, he had markedly increased activity deep in his basal ganglia and right temporal lobe. I thought that perhaps he was using the alcohol as a way to settle down his overactive basal ganglia and temporal lobe and then using the cocaine and methamphetamines as a way to counteract the alcohol. I showed Rob his scan. I was surprised at how nonchalant he was in viewing his brain. He said, "Do I really have to stop drinking? What am I going to do?" During our session I stressed the need for him to completely stop alcohol and drugs lest his brain deteriorate further. I also told him I would give him some medication to calm his overactive areas, and odds were that he would be feeling better shortly. Concerned that Rob didn't understand the seriousness of his situation, I called his therapist and reiterated how important it was for him to totally abstain from the drugs polluting his brain. She worked intensively with him. The more he stayed away from the drugs and alcohol (and the better he felt with his medication, which was more effective for his problems than alcohol mixed with cocaine and methamphetamines), the more he understood the importance of the scan and the need to stay away from the substances he had been abusing. A year later, he was dramatically improved. His work was better. His relationships were more stable, and his overall attitude toward life was very positive. In fact, he sent me many other people to treat. I decided to get a follow-up SPECT study on Rob to see what progress we made with his brain. It had dramatically improved, just as he had.

Karen

Karen, forty-eight, had waged a twenty-year battle with alcohol abuse. She had gone through three marriages, five alcohol treatment programs, and multiple medications. She complained of feeling tired, depressed, and angry. Without the alcohol she just didn't feel right. In addition, she had a terrible problem with impulsivity. Whenever she was placed on a new medication, her doctor could give her enough of it for only two or three days at a time. Otherwise she would take a whole month's worth of medication, no matter what it was for, within a few days. Surprisingly, no one had ever examined her brain to see if it held any keys to why Karen was so resistant to treatment. Her doctor, after hearing one of my lectures, sent her to see me for a scan. It showed overall decreased activity consistent with the alcohol abuse, but it also showed markedly decreased activity in the prefrontal cortex. The part of her brain that controlled impulses was damaged. On my intake form she reported that she had never had a head injury. I knew that many alcoholics, during blackouts, have head injuries they are not aware of. I asked her doctor to check further into her history for head injuries.

Karen's Brain, Affected by Alcohol and Head Injury

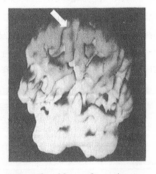 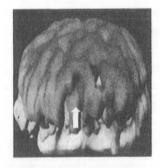

3-D underside surface view   *3-D front-on surface view*

Notice the overall shriveled appearance (scalloping) and markedly decreased activity in the prefrontal cortex (arrow).

When he asked her to check with her mother, her mother remembered a time when Karen had been kicked in the head by a horse at age seven and had been unconscious for about ten minutes. Given her history, I recommended that Karen be given a small dose of a slow-release stimulant medication to help her with impulse control. Slow-release stimulants, such as Ritalin-SR, enter the system slowly and are not associated with any sort of high, thus are not typically abused. I also made Karen poster-size pictures of her brain to put up on her wall, which effectively reminded her that she really didn't want to keep drinking.

Opiates

Opiate abuse has also been associated with severe blood flow abnormalities. Some of the worst brain damage I have seen was caused by heroin abuse. Robert's story at the beginning of this chapter illustrates how serious it can become. In my experience, heroin and other opiates (such as methadone, codeine, Pamergan [pethidine], Dilaudid [hydromorphone] and Oxycontin [oxycodone]) consistently cause overall decreased activity throughout the brain. These medications are very addictive and can literally take away your brain and your life. I often use the term "brain melt" to describe the SPECT appearance of opiate abusers. I have also seen similar serious brain damage in methadone users. Many heroin addicts are medically administered methadone as a way to help treat their addiction, decrease crime (if they get their drug legally, they don't need to commit crimes to get money to buy it), and eliminate the spread of infection from dirty needles. Even though I understand the logic behind methadone treatment centers, we must do a better job. Dosing drug addicts with methadone perpetuates the ongoing drug brain damage, and I fear these patients will be unable to ever get better.

Doug

Doug, age forty, was referred to me by a doctor who worked in a San Francisco drug treatment clinic. Doug had been addicted to heroin and had subsequently been in a methadone maintenance program for

Doug's Brain, Affected by Heroin and Methadone

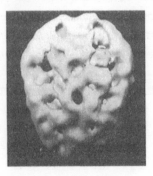

3-D top-down surface view

Notice the large holes of activity across the brain's surface.

seven years. The doctor continued to see Doug go downhill, despite treatment. He wondered what seven years of methadone had done to his brain. He had wanted to get him off the methadone, but Doug was panicked by the idea and other members of the treatment team were resistant. Doug's SPECT study showed significant overall decreased activity. As I showed Doug his brain, his attitude about methadone changed. "I need to get off this stuff," he said, "otherwise I won't have much brain left." He, and the treatment team, agreed to take him completely off opiates using a new rapid-detox protocol developed at Yale University. It worked for Doug, and he was grateful to be free of the drugs.

Marijuana

Marijuana use is common. Many teenagers and young adults believe that marijuana is safe, despite a number of studies demonstrating cognitive, emotional, and social impairment with chronic or heavy usage. Marijuana has also been described as a "gateway" drug by several researchers, with one study reporting that 98 percent of cocaine users started with marijuana. Despite these studies, there is controversy both in the mind of the general population and in the medical community about whether marijuana use is harmful. Legalizing marijuana has been a social/political topic for decades.

I am truly amazed by the nonchalant attitude our country has toward marijuana usage. Even my home state of California passed a law in 1996 legalizing marijuana as medicine. I think many people misunderstood Proposition 215, feeling that by voting for it they were allowing people dying from cancer to have marijuana to soothe their pain and increase their appetites. What they got was a law that basically says a doctor can write a prescription for marijuana for anything including anxiety, stress, moodiness, or irritability. The biggest problem with the law, as I see it, is that the perception of marijuana's dangerousness has gone way down. Teenagers tell me that it's medicine, not a problem. Drug abuse expert Mark Gold, M.D., put it succinctly: "As the perception of a drug's dangerousness goes down, its use goes up."

SPECT has been used to study both the short-term and long-term effects of marijuana on the brain. These studies report that inexperienced marijuana smokers had an acute decrease in cerebral blood flow and that chronic marijuana users had overall decreased perfusion when compared to a nonusing control group.

In performing many SPECT studies on marijuana abusers I noticed decreased temporal lobe activity that was not mentioned in the above studies, most likely because of the lesser sensitivity of the SPECT resolution in older scans. I wondered if our newer findings were the cause of the memory and motivation problems often associated with marijuana usage. I decided to study the effects of marijuana on the brain, comparing patients who had ADHD and chronic marijuana usage with people who had ADHD with no drug usage. I did this for three reasons: First, the functional brain-imaging studies of ADHD have not shown temporal lobe abnormalities. Utilizing a control group with the same diagnosis rather than a general psychiatric control group eliminates the possibility of contaminated findings. Even a normal control group adds an uncertainty because so many marijuana users have additional diagnoses. Second, I felt that comparing them to a population with the same, common diagnosis would give useful information. Finally, 52 percent of people with ADHD have been reported to have problems with substance abuse, a high number of them with marijuana abuse.

I compared the scans of thirty teenage and adult marijuana smokers (who had used it for a minimum of one year at least on a weekly basis) who had been diagnosed with ADHD, with ten control group subjects also diagnosed with ADHD, matched for age, sex, and handedness, who had never abused any drugs. In the marijuana/ADHD group, by clinical history, marijuana was the primary drug of choice and no other drugs of abuse had been used in the prior year; again by history, there was no significant alcohol use by these patients (significant alcohol use in this study meant more than three ounces of spirits or six beers a week). The interval between the most recent marijuana use and the SPECT scan was one to six months, by clinical history. Anyone who met the diagnostic criteria for alcohol or other substance abuse or dependence was eliminated from the study. Marijuana usage ranged from daily to weekly, and from one year to twenty-two years. All patients were medication-free at the time of the study, and participants reported being at least thirty days free from any marijuana usage. In addition, patients who were taking stimulant medication for ADHD had been medication-free for at least one week.

The only abnormality seen in the ADHD control group was decreased activity in the prefrontal cortex in eight of the ten subjects. A similar number of marijuana/ADHD subjects had decreased prefrontal cortex activity—twenty-five of thirty (83 percent)—but overall, this decreased activity in the prefrontal cortex was more severe. In addition, twenty-four marijuana/ADHD subjects showed decreased activity in the temporal lobes; five (21 percent) were rated as severe, seven (29 percent) were rated as moderate, and twelve (50 percent) were rated as mild. The severe and moderate ratings were in the heaviest users (use had been greater than four times a week in the preceding year), but not necessarily the longest users. One teenager who had been a daily user for two years showed some of the most profoundly poor temporal lobe perfusion among the group. Clinically, four patients had an amotivational syndrome (severe lack of interest, motivation, and energy). All four had decreased perfusion in their temporal lobes; three were rated as severe, one was rated as moderate.

This study was consistent with previous studies mentioned above demonstrating that frequent, long-term marijuana use has the potential to change the perfusion pattern of the brain. While prior studies showed global decreased brain activity, I found focal decreased activity in the temporal lobes. (This may be accounted for by the increased sophistication of the imaging camera used.) Abnormal activity in the temporal lobes has been associated with problems in memory, learning, and motivation—common complaints of teenagers (or at least their parents) and adults who chronically abuse marijuana. Amotivational syndrome, marked by apathy, poor attention span, lethargy,

Marijuana-Affected Brains

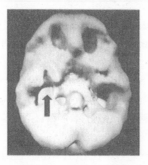

3-D underside surface view

Sixteen-year-old male with two-year history of daily usage; notice multiple areas of markedly decreased perfusion, especially in the temporal lobes (arrow).

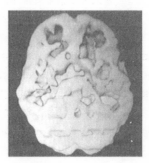

3-D underside surface view

Forty-four-year-old male with twelve-year history of daily usage; notice markedly decreased perfusion on undersurface of the brain.

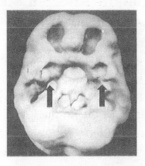

3-D underside surface view

Thirty-two-year-old female with a twelve-year history of mostly weekend usage; notice areas of decreased perfusion in medial temporal lobes.

social withdrawal, and loss of interest in achievement have been attributed to marijuana abuse for many years. One teenage male in the study, who had used daily for two years, had one of the most severe cases of temporal lobe underactivity. He had symptoms consistent with amotivational syndrome and had dropped out of school at seventeen.

Inhalants

Inhalants, such as petrol, correction fluid, paint thinner, lighter fluid, and glue are also seriously abused. I once had a four-year-old patient who was addicted to inhalants. His mother told me that he would go into the garage, take the petrol cap off the lawn mower, put his mouth over the opening, and take a deep breath, becoming intoxicated by the fumes. His mother reported that he inhaled many different substances. I first evaluated this child in the playroom of my office. He was very hyperactive. During the middle of our session he went over to a white marker board and took the top off a marker. He put the marker up to his nose and inhaled deeply. He then gave me a big smile like "Yeah, this feels good."

Inhalants are processed directly into the brain and can cause damage to the brain, lungs, and liver. They are dangerous! Most

Inhalant-Affected Brain

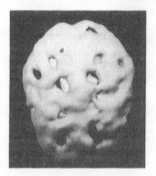

3-D top-down surface view

Notice the large holes of activity across the brain's surface.

inhalants and solvents are short-term vasodilators; chronic abuse, however, is often accompanied by serious decreased cerebral blood flow.

The accompanying SPECT scan shows the brain of a forty-nine-year-old patient who had used inhalants over a twelve-year period. It looks much like a cocaine- or methamphetamine-affected brain.

Caffeine and Nicotine

I know this next section may make many people uncomfortable, but I have to tell it as I see it. Published research indicates that caffeine, even in small doses, is a potent cerebral vasoconstrictor (decreases brain blood flow). My experience also suggests this to be true. The more caffeine you consume (caffeine is found in coffee, tea, most fizzy drinks, chocolate, and many cold remedies), the more underactivity occurs in your brain. Many people, especially my ADHD patients, use caffeine as a brain stimulant. They use it to get going and keep going through the day. The problem with caffeine is that even though in the short run it may help, in the long run it makes things worse. Then you begin chasing the underactivity caused by the caffeine with more caffeine, worsening an already tough brain condition. Periodic caffeine usage is probably not a big problem. Heavy daily usage (more than three cups of coffee a day) is a problem and needs to be stopped in order to maintain a healthy brain. Of interest, the brain stimulants such as Ritalin or Adderall in therapeutic doses to treat ADHD enhance brain activity.

There are so many reasons to stop smoking, you probably don't need another one. Yet in my experience, if you want to have full access to your brain, don't smoke. Shortly after you stop smoking, blood flow to the brain increases, although long-term smokers have overall marked decreased activity.

A successful businessman whom I knew socially came to visit me. He said that he had recently had trouble concentrating and his energy was low. I knew that he smoked three packs of cigarettes and drank at least three pots of coffee every day. For a long time I had suspected he had ADHD (he had underachieved in school, did impulsive things, and could never sit still) and that he was medicating himself with the stimulant effects of caffeine and nicotine. He was the CEO of a very successful corporation and not used to taking advice from others. I told him about ADHD and said that it would be a good idea to treat it and stop self-medicating with high-dose caffeine and nicotine. His first comment was that he didn't want to take medication. Didn't I have a natural treatment for it? A bit amazed, I said, "You are taking two 'natural' treatments for ADHD—caffeine and nicotine—but they might kill you. The medication I prescribe is more effective, and when it is used properly, it doesn't kill anyone."

I suggested that SPECT images of his brain might help him see the reality of the situation and encourage him to stop. Even I was surprised by how bad his brain looked. He had markedly decreased activity across the whole cortex, especially in the areas of the prefrontal cortex and temporal lobes. I told my friend that he needed to find some way other than using caffeine and nicotine to stimulate his brain or it was unlikely he would have much of a brain left to enjoy his success. He took my advice for a few weeks, but shortly went back to his old ways. I wondered whether his poor temporal lobe activity made him unable to hold the SPECT images in his memory or his very poor prefrontal cortex activity prevented sufficient impulse control. Even though I recommended he try a brain stimulant, such as Ritalin or Adderall, he maintained that he wanted to treat his ADHD "naturally."

Brain Affected by Heavy Caffeine and Nicotine Use

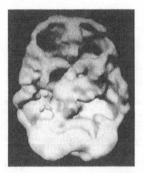

3-D underside surface view

Note markedly decreased activity overall, especially in prefrontal cortex and temporal lobes.

What Happens When You Stop Abusing Drugs?

Many people ask me what happens to the brain when alcohol or drug abuse is stopped. It depends. Generally, the longer a substance has been abused, the more toxic its effect. Certain drugs are clearly more toxic than others. It depends on what other toxic substances were also in the drug and on the sensitivity of the user's brain. There are rare individuals who can abuse drugs for a long time before stopping with few if any lasting ill effects. Others can incur brain damage after a very short period of time. In either case, the sooner you stop, the better chance your brain has to heal.

The Poster: Which Brain Do You Want?

In 1997 I developed a drug education poster titled "Which Brain Do You Want?" Based on my work with drug abusers and SPECT, it was intended to break through the perception that drugs are not danger-ous. The poster compares a normal brain to those of a heroin addict, a cocaine abuser, an alcoholic, and a chronic marijuana abuser. The damage caused by substance abuse is immediately apparent:

- *Normal brain is smooth, symmetrical, and full.*
- *The heroin brain shows massive areas of decreased activity throughout.*
- *The cocaine brain shows multiple small holes across the cerebral cortex.*
- *The alcoholic brain looks shriveled.*
- *The marijuana brain looks as though areas are eaten away, especially in the temporal lobe region, the seat of language and learning.*

After seeing these images, many of my patients tell me that they have no more interest in using drugs. They want the use of their whole brain. "Not one with holes in it," as a nineteen-year-old stated as he saw his brain scan after serving time in a young offenders' institution due to marijuana abuse.

I use these brain images day to day in my work with drug addicts, especially teenagers and young adults who are starting to experiment with drugs. Showing someone his or her own drug-damaged brain has a powerful impact. Many of my patients begin the process of recovery immediately.

In testing the effectiveness of the poster, one hundred people, ages twelve to forty, filled out a questionnaire. Over 50 percent of the people who participated in the study said that the poster had changed the way they thought about drugs. Sample comments from the study included:

"I had no idea marijuana could be harmful to the brain. Why did they just legalize it in California?"

"I don't want any holes in my brain. I'm staying away from drugs."

"Drugs affect your brain in a serious way."

"This really changed the way I think about alcohol use and marijuana."

"If they harm me, I want nothing to do with them."

"No one at school told me about this part. They just said drugs were cool to do. Seems pretty stupid to me."

The poster now hangs in over one hundred prisons, hundreds of schools across the country (the L.A. County School District bought one for each school), drug treatment centers, and hospitals. The criminal court system in Cleveland bought six hundred posters to give to people who came through the system. The chief judge said he needed to educate people on the real effects of drugs.

For more information on this poster see my website at www.amenclinic.com.

15

The Missing Links:
Drugs, Violence, and the Brain

There is a well-established connection between substance abuse and violence. Understanding the intricacies of this connection is essential to finding effective interventions and solutions. Much has been written about the psychosocial causes of drug abuse and violence, but there have been few studies of the biological relation of drugs and violence to the brain.

Through our brain-imaging work, we have recognized several clinical and SPECT patterns that may help further the understanding of the connection between substance abuse and violence and the brain. These observations have been made from our clinical database of over five thousand SPECT studies on a wide variety of neuropsychiatric patients, including more than 350 patients who had had problems with aggressive behavior during the six months before evaluation. (They had either destroyed property or physically attacked another person.) In addition, our clinic has been involved in approximately thirty forensic neuropsychiatric evaluations of violent offenders who have committed murder, rape, armed robbery, assault, torture, and stalking, many of whom had significant substance abuse problems as well. In this chapter, I examine the connection between substance abuse and violence through the lens of our work with SPECT.

In reviewing the literature on substance abuse it is important to note that substances traditionally linked with violence (e.g., cocaine, methamphetamine, and alcohol) cause abnormal perfusion patterns in the areas that have been associated with violent behavior. Nicotine and caffeine may also be involved and may magnify the negative effects of other substances.

Here are five patterns connecting the links between drugs, violence, and the brain.

1. Using drugs, especially alcohol, cocaine, methamphetamines, phencyclidine, and anabolic steroids, may directly elicit aggressive behavior.

This may be especially true when the user is prone to violence due to underlying brain vulnerabilities (such as a combination of problems in the prefrontal, cingulate, dominant temporal lobes, and dominant limbic and basal ganglia areas).

John

John, a right-handed seventy-nine-year-old contractor, had a long-standing history of alcohol abuse and violent behavior. He had frequently physically abused his wife over forty years of marriage and had been abusive to their children when they were living at home. Almost all of the abuse occurred when he was intoxicated. At age seventy-nine, John underwent open-heart surgery. After the surgery he had a psychotic episode that lasted ten days. His doctor ordered a SPECT study as part of his evaluation. The study showed markedly decreased activity in the left-outside frontal-temporal region, a

John's Brain

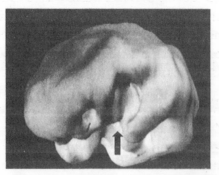

3-D left side surface view

Note area of markedly decreased activity in the left frontal and temporal region (arrow).

finding most likely due to a past head injury. When the doctor asked John if he had ever had any significant head injuries, John told him that at age twenty he'd been driving an old milk truck that was missing its side rear-view mirror. He had put his head out of the window to look behind him, and his head had struck a pole, knocking him unconscious for several hours. After the head injury he had more problems with his temper and memory. There was a family history of alcohol abuse in four of his five brothers. None of his brothers had problems with aggressive behavior.

Given the location of the brain abnormality (left frontal-temporal dysfunction), John was likely to exhibit violent behavior. Alcohol abuse, which did not elicit violent behavior in his brothers, did contribute to John's violence. If John had seen and understood his SPECT scan earlier, he could have sought help and prevented hurt to his family.

2. Drug or alcohol usage may impair executive function and increase the likelihood of aggression.

Bradley

Bradley was diagnosed with ADHD and left temporal lobe dysfunction (diagnosed by EEG) at the age of fourteen. Before then he had been expelled from eleven schools for fighting, frequently skipped school, and had already started drinking alcohol and using marijuana. He had a dramatically positive response to 15 milligrams of Ritalin three times a day. He improved three grade levels of reading within the next year, attended school regularly, and had no aggressive outbursts. His grandmother (with whom he lived) and his teachers were very pleased with his progress. However, Bradley hated taking medication. He said that taking it made him feel stupid and different, even though it obviously helped him. Two years after starting his medication, he decided to stop it on his own without telling anyone. His anger began to escalate again, as did his drinking and marijuana usage. One night while he was intoxicated, his uncle came over to his home and asked Bradley to help him "rob some bitches." Bradley went along with his uncle, who forced a woman into her car, then made her go to an ATM and withdraw money. The uncle and Bradley then raped the woman twice. Bradley was apprehended two weeks later and charged with kidnapping, robbery, and rape.

Bradley's Brain

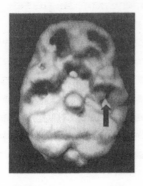 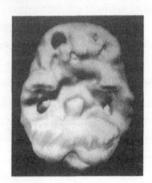

3-D underside surface view

| Bradley's concentration study (no medication); note decreased left prefrontal cortex and left temporal lobe activity (arrow). | Concentration study with Ritalin; notice overall improved activity. |

As the psychiatric forensic consultant, I agreed with the clinical diagnosis of ADHD and also suspected left temporal lobe dysfunction because of Bradley's chronic aggressive behavior and abnormal EEG. I ordered a series of brain SPECT studies: one while he was doing a concentration task without medication and one while he was doing a concentration task on Ritalin. The resting study showed mildly decreased activity in the left prefrontal cortex and the left temporal lobe. While he was performing a concentration task, there was marked suppression of the prefrontal cortex, a common finding in ADHD, and both temporal lobes. The third scan was done one hour after Bradley took 15 milligrams of Ritalin. This scan showed marked activation in the prefrontal cortex and both temporal lobes, although there was still some mild deactivation in the left temporal lobe.

It was apparent that Bradley already had a brain vulnerable to long-term behavioral and academic difficulties. His substance use may have further suppressed an already underactive prefrontal cortex and temporal lobe, diminishing executive abilities and unleashing aggressive tendencies. It is possible that if someone had explained the underlying metabolic problems to Bradley and provided him with brief psychotherapy to address the emotional issues surrounding the need to take medication, his crime spree might have been averted. In prison, he was placed on Cylert (a brain stimulant similar to Ritalin) and Depakote. He has had no aggressive outbursts in the past two years.

3. Drugs or alcohol may be used as self-medication for underlying brain problems involved in aggression.

Many substance abusers have dual psychiatric diagnoses, and we believe they may be using their substances as a way to medicate underlying psychiatric or neurological problems, such as depression, panic symptoms, post-traumatic stress anxiety, and even aggressive behavior.

Rusty

Twenty-eight-year-old Rusty was brought to see me by his parents. He had a severe methamphetamine problem that had wreaked havoc in his life. He was unable to keep steady work; he was involved in a physically abusive relationship with his girlfriend (he had been arrested four times for assault and battery); he was mean to his parents even though they tried to help him; and he had failed five drug treatment programs. In the last program the counselor had recommended a "tough love" approach: He had told the parents to let Rusty "hit bottom" so that he would want help. The parents read about my work and decided to do one more thing before going the "tough love" route. Rusty's lack of responsiveness to traditional treatments made me suspect an underlying brain problem. We scheduled a SPECT scan with the parents, but Rusty didn't know about it until the morning he was supposed to have it. He showed up at the clinic loaded on high-dose methamphetamine from the night before. Rusty told me about his drug abuse. He said, "I'm sorry for messing up the scan. I'll come back next week. I promise I won't use anything." I had often wanted to do SPECT studies on people intoxicated with illegal substances to see their effects on the brain, but due to ethical concerns I hadn't. But if a person shows up for the scan on drugs there isn't an ethical issue. I decided to scan Rusty that morning with the effects of the methamphetamine still in his system and then a week later off all drugs. It turned out to be a very fortuitous decision. When Rusty was under the influence of high-dose methamphetamine, his brain activity appeared suppressed. A week later, however, off all drugs, he had

Rusty's Brain

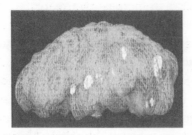

3-D active side view

While Rusty is on high-dose methamphetamine, the left temporal lobe appears relatively normal.

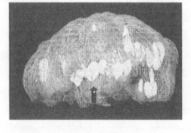

3-D active side view

When Rusty is drug-free, there is markedly increased activity in the left temporal lobe.

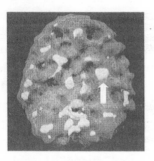

3-D underside active view
Notice hot area in deep left temporal lobe (arrow).

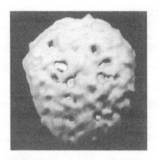

3-D top-down surface view
Notice multiple holes across cortex.

a terribly overactive left temporal lobe, probably causing his problems with violent behavior. In all likelihood, Rusty was unconsciously self-medicating an underlying temporal lobe problem with high-dose meth-amphetamine. I probed deeper into any history of a head injury, which initially both Rusty and his parents did not remember. When pressed, Rusty remembered a time when he had run full speed into a solid metal basketball pole and briefly been knocked unconscious. That could have caused his temporal lobe problem. Given this finding, I put Rusty on Tegretol (an antiseizure medication that stabilizes activity in the temporal lobes). Within two weeks Rusty felt better than he had in years. He was calmer, his temper was under control, and for the first time in his life, he was able to remain gainfully employed. An additional benefit of the scan was that I was able to show Rusty the serious damage he was doing to his brain by abusing the methamphetamines. Even though the drugs helped his temporal lobe problem, they were clearly toxic to his brain. Rusty, like others who abuse drugs, had developed holes in activity across the surface of his brain. Seeing these pictures was even more incentive to stay away from the drugs and get proper treatment for his problems. SPECT worked both as a powerful diagnostic tool to better assess one of the root causes of Rusty's problem and also as a therapeutic tool to address his denial. A picture is worth a thousand denials. Often, having this type of information is valuable in helping patients make a more positive move toward sobriety. I wondered how many people with severe nonresponsive drug problems are self-medicating an underlying problem, yet are labeled by their families and society in general as weak-willed or morally defective. "Tough love" for Rusty wouldn't have solved his problem.

4. Cingulate problems, in conjunction with prefrontal cortex and temporal lobe problems, can exacerbate addictions and potentially violent situations.

As mentioned, the cingulate part of the brain is associated with attention shifting and cognitive flexibility. When it is overactive, people can get locked into negative thoughts or behaviors.

Jose

Jose, a sixteen-year-old gang member, was arrested and charged with attempted murder after he and another gang member beat another teenager nearly to death. Their gang claimed the color red. One evening, when they were in an intoxicated state (from both alcohol and heavy marijuana usage), they approached a boy who was wearing a red sweater while walking his dog. They asked, "What colors do you bang?" (asking him about his gang affiliation). When the boy said he did not know what they were talking about, Jose replied, "Wrong answer," and he and his companion hit and kicked the boy repeatedly until he was unconscious. Other gang members described pulling Jose off the boy because once he had started, he wouldn't stop. They were afraid he would kill the boy.

The public defender ordered neuropsychological testing on Jose,

Jose's Brain

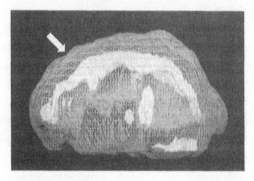

3-D active side view

Note markedly increased cingulate activity (arrow).

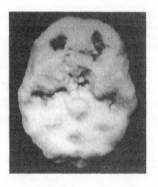

3-D underside surface view

At rest; note mildly decreased pfc activity.

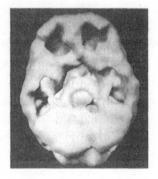

3-D underside surface view

During concentration; note markedly decreased pfc and temporal lobe activity.

which found frontal lobe dysfunction and evidence of ADHD, depression, and learning disabilities. The psychologist suggested a resting and concentration SPECT series for independent verification. The SPECT series was significantly abnormal. Both studies showed markedly increased activity in the cingulate gyrus, consistent with problems in shifting attention. At rest, Jose's SPECT study also showed mildly suppressed prefrontal cortex activity. While he was doing a concentration task, there was also marked suppression of the prefrontal cortex and both temporal lobes, consistent with ADHD, learning disabilities, and aggressive tendencies.

Jose had a long history of problems in attention shifting. He was described by others as brooding, argumentative, and oppositional. "Once he got a thought in his head," his father said, "he would talk about it over and over." In prison, he was placed on Lustral (a serotonergic antidepressant to calm his cingulate). He felt calmer, more focused, and less easily upset.

5. Drug or alcohol usage may be involved in poor decision-making processes or provocative behaviors that put a person in high-risk situations.

It may also decrease a person's ability to accurately perceive a threatening situation. The probability of aggression between two people is the greatest when both are intoxicated and least when both are sober.

Jonathan and Carol

Jonathan and Carol had been married for two years. Both were employed, and they had no children. Both drank heavily, and Jonathan also used marijuana and cocaine periodically. From the first month of marriage they had fought constantly, mostly over little things. Carol would start complaining about something over and over again, and Jonathan would react violently toward her. Drinking and drug use made their problems worse. On five occasions the police had been called to their home by neighbors because of fighting. On the last two occasions Jonathan had been arrested for striking his wife. Growing up, Jonathan had had difficulty in school, exhibiting both aggression and learning problems. Carol had grown up in an alcoholic home and had experienced periodic obsessiveness and depression. Through counseling it became clear that substance abuse increased Jonathan's aggressiveness and impulsivity and made Carol more irritable and more provoking.

As part of a research protocol on difficult couples, Jonathan and Carol underwent rest and concentration brain SPECT studies. Jonathan's scan showed decreased activity in his left temporal lobe at rest and marked deactivation of his prefrontal cortex when he performed a concentration task (consistent with ADHD, aggression, and learning problems). Both of Carol's scans showed markedly increased activity in the anterior cingulate gyms, consistent with problems in shifting attention and getting locked into negative thoughts or behaviors.

The information from the SPECT studies, along with their clinical history, proved to be helpful. In addition to couples counseling and substance abuse treatment, Jonathan was placed on Depakote (to stabilize his left temporal lobe) and sustained-release Dexedrine (for the impulsivity and ADHD symptoms), and Carol was placed on Lustral (for overfocus and depressive issues). Over the course of treatment, their relationship improved significantly and there were no more aggressive outbursts.

Strategies for effectively dealing with substance abuse and violence

This chapter highlighted some of the ways that brain dysfunction is intimately connected with violent behavior and substance abuse. Understanding this connection is critical to developing more effective treatment strategies and policies in dealing with this problem. Based on this work I offer several suggestions:

1. Consider the brain. Too often, brain dysfunction is thought of too late in the evaluation and treatment process. Evaluating brain function through clinical history, neurological examinations, and sophisticated brain-imaging studies when indicated is key to proper diagnosis and effective early intervention.

2. Violent individuals and substance abusers should be screened for a history of head injuries, since even minor ones can unleash aggressive tendencies (especially when they occur in the left frontal-temporal regions of the brain), and these conditions of the brain can and should be treated.

3. Violent individuals and substance abusers should be screened for underlying psychiatric and neurological conditions that may contribute to or exacerbate their problems (such as ADHD, bipolar disorder, learning disabilities, temporal lobe dysfunction, etc.). In Washington state, the criminal court system under Judge David Admire, in conjunction with the Learning Disability Association of Washington, set up a program for those convicted of crimes to be screened for ADHD and dyslexia. If they met a high level of suspicion for these disorders on screening, they were sent through a fourteen-week "Life Skills"

program to help them be more effective in dealing with these problems. Outcome data presented recently indicated that the recidivism rate had been decreased by 40 percent.

4. Do not be shy about obtaining medication for underlying medical and psychiatric problems when they are present with either substance abuse or violence. Effective medication is likely to make anger management programs and substance abuse treatment more effective. However, in our experience, many substance abuse treatment programs and anger management programs shy away from the use of medication, and patients are made to feel "inferior" for considering medication as an option. This attitude hampers appropriate treatment and leaves many individuals at higher risk of relapse.

5. Explore whether victims of crimes may be unwittingly contributing to their situation by their own substance use or underlying neuropsychiatric problems. I know this is a controversial suggestion, but it is my clinical experience that some victims have made bad decisions or exhibited provocative behavior based either on their own substance abuse or on their own underlying brain patterns. I am certainly not suggesting that victims are in any way responsible for what happened to them. It is my hope that by addressing any underlying problems, they won't become victims again.

6. In complicated cases, brain SPECT imaging may be an adjunctive diagnostic tool that can give more information than previously available. In my experience, SPECT can be helpful in the following ways:

- *by showing cerebral drug damage to abusers to enhance drug treatment compliance*
- *by uncovering past brain trauma that may be contributing to the clinical situation*
- *by providing help to clinicians in choosing appropriate medications (these include anticonvulsant medications for temporal lobe abnormalities, serotonergic medications for anterior cingulate hyperactivity, and stimulant medications for prefrontal cortex deactivation. SPECT is not a "doctor in a box," and the SPECT findings always need to be correlated with the clinical condition)*
- *by allowing family members and others (judges, probation officers, etc.) to see the medical contribution to problems so they will encourage appropriate treatment*

The brain of every individual has a violence "set point" determined by a large number of interconnected factors: brain system function, genetic factors, metabolic factors, psychodynamic and emotional issues, overall health, history of brain trauma, and the effects of prescribed medications and abused substances. These factors and their complex interplay, unique to each person, inhibit or encourage a person's responses to assaults on his or her equilibrium. Any drug—including doctor-prescribed—has an effect on this set point by either increasing or decreasing its reactivity to an insult. The degree of reactivity results from the unique response of any given brain to the metabolic changes induced by a chemical. The very short-term, moderately short-term, and long-term changes in brain function, combined with preexisting factors, result in a greater or lesser propensity for an individual to act on violent impulses.

When someone is healthy, he or she has a high degree of control and usually needs intense provocation to elicit a violent reaction. Over time actual changes in brain metabolism as a result of drug or alcohol abuse lead to a diminished ability to regulate aggressive impulses. Finally, a new and lower (more easily triggered) set point is reached, resulting in more violent, inappropriate behavioral responses.

16

I Love You and I Hate You, Touch Me, No, Don't, Whatever:

Brain Patterns That Interfere with Intimacy

Over the past eight years I have conducted a series of SPECT studies on couples who have had serious marital difficulties. I have been fascinated, saddened, and enlightened by this research. I now look at marriages and marital conflict in a whole new way, as involving compatible and incompatible brain patterns. I have come to realize that many marriages do not work because of brain misfires that have nothing to do with character, free will, or desire. Many marriages or relationships are sabotaged by factors beyond conscious or even unconscious control. Sometimes a little bit of medicine can make all the difference between love and hate, staying together and divorce, effective problem solving and prolonged litigation.

I realize many people, especially some marital therapists, will see the ideas in this chapter as radical, premature, and heretical. Frankly, I know of no marital therapy system or school of thought that seriously looks at the brain function of couples who struggle. But I wonder how you can develop paradigms and "schools of thought" about how couples function (or don't function) without taking into account the organ that drives behavior. Seasoned therapists who see couples day to day in their offices will recognize the truths in this chapter, and I hope they will gain new insights into their most difficult cases through the lens of the brain. The stories are real (although I've disguised identifying characteristics to protect patients' privacy). The problems are real. And the missing link in understanding the "couples from hell" is often the brain.

Mike and Gerry (A Couples' Guide)

Mike and Gerry had been in marital therapy for four years when they first came to see me. Their therapist had heard me lecture in their hometown. After my talk, she'd gone straight to her office, called Mike and Gerry, and told them to make an appointment to see me. "Mike," she said, "I think you need to take care of some biological brain problems before we can make any progress." This couple had been in trouble for most of their twelve-year marriage. They fought constantly. Mike had had two affairs, seemed prone to pick fights, and had to work excessively long hours because he performed inefficiently. Gerry had a tendency toward depression, was angry that their marriage was such a struggle, and would hold on to hurts from years in the past. The therapist had tried all the techniques she knew. She even went to a conference on "the resistant couple" as a way to find help for Mike and Gerry. She was frustrated because she couldn't make any progress with them.

When I first met with them, Mike was the IP (identified patient). The therapist felt that if she "fixed" Mike, they would make progress. Mike, in fact, had ADHD. He had underachieved in school. He was restless, fidgety, inattentive, disorganized, and impulsive. He had trouble listening to Gerry. His marital affairs had not been planned but impulsive. He tended to seek conflict from others and often inflamed situations by making thoughtless comments. In the first few meetings with the couple, however, I felt that Gerry also contributed to the marital turmoil. She tended to voice the same complaints over and over. She argued over insignificant things. She had a strong tendency toward repetitive worry, and when things weren't "just so," she'd be upset for hours.

I decided to scan both Mike and Gerry. Mike had markedly decreased activity in his prefrontal cortex (consistent with ADHD symptoms), and Gerry had a significantly overactive cingulate gyrus (consistent with overfocus issues). I placed Mike on Adderall (a brain stimulant to treat his ADHD) and Gerry on Lustral (a serotonergic antidepressant to decrease her tendency to overfocus). Within several days, Mike felt more focused. He was more organized at work, and he acted in a more positive, thoughtful way toward Gerry. Even Gerry noticed a difference. After several weeks (Lustral takes longer to be effective than Adderall), Gerry also felt a significant difference within herself. Her thoughts no longer tended to loop. She was better able to hold on to positive thoughts. She was more playful, less easily set off. Mike and Gerry could spend time together without fighting constantly. They began to use effectively the marital techniques they had learned in therapy.

Their therapist was ecstatic to see the couple's progress. She was initially surprised that both of them had brain misfires. Although she had at first attributed the failure solely to Mike, after seeing the brain pictures, she was struck by how "cingulate" Gerry had been, recalling how she overfocused and had trouble letting go of hurts.

The missing link for this couple was in their brain pattern and neurotransmitter irregularities. They continued in therapy for several more months to solidify their gains. It was important that they really understand the magnitude of the biological contribution to their problems and that they see each other through new eyes. This allowed them to be more forgiving of each other and to heal the painful memories associated with twelve years of marital struggle. If I had treated just Mike and not Gerry, she might very well have stayed stuck in the pain and frustration of the past, seeing herself as a victim of Mike and being unable to let go of the past.

In my work I have seen all of the five brain systems discussed in this book interplay within couples. I have found that by properly diagnosing which pattern or patterns are present I can develop proper medical and behavioral strategies to intervene effectively. *I want to emphasize that I do not scan every couple I see.* I am often able to pick out these patterns from the clinical presentation and will often intervene based on knowledge without a scan. My hope is that this book will help you be more effective in identifying these patterns in yourself or in those you love and get proper intervention, *not a scan.* When I have a particularly resistant couple, I'll order a scan because I want to know what their brain patterns look like, especially if there is violence in the relationship.

Since, as far as I know, this is the first time any psychiatrist has presented a model of marital discord based on brain misfires, you might want to share this book with your marital therapist and see if he or she is open to new ideas.

How do the five brain systems influence intimate relationships? How does one problem interact with another? What happens when multiple systems are involved in one or both couples? Is medication always necessary in this system of marital therapy? These are some of the questions addressed in this chapter.

Let's start by looking at the relational traits of each brain system when they work correctly and when they misfire.

Limbic Relational Traits

When the limbic system functions properly, people tend to be more positive and more able to connect with others. They tend to filter information in an accurate light and they are more likely to give others the benefit of the doubt. They are able to be playful, sexy, and sexual, and they tend to maintain and have easy access to positive emotional memories. They tend to draw people toward them with their positive attitude.

When the limbic system is overactive, people tend toward depression, negativity, and distance from others. They are more likely to focus on the most negative aspects of others, filter information through dark glasses, and see the glass as half empty, and less likely to give others the benefit of the doubt. They tend not to be playful. They do not feel sexy, and they tend to shy away from sexual activity due to a lack of interest. Most of their memories are negative, and it is hard for them to access positive emotional memories or feelings. They tend to push people away with their negativity.

Positive Limbic Relational Statements
"We have a lot of good memories."
"Let's have friends over."
"I accept your apology. I know you were just having a bad day."
"Let's have fun."
"I feel sexy. Let's make love."

Negative Limbic Relational Statements
"Don't look at me that way."
"All I can remember is the bad times."
"I'm too tired."
"Leave me alone. I'm not interested in sex."
"You go to bed. I can't sleep."
"I don't feel like being around other people."

"I don't want to hear you're sorry. You meant to hurt me."
"I'm not interested in doing anything."

Statements from the Partners of People with Limbic Problems
"She's negative."
"He's often depressed."
"She looks on the negative side of things."
"He doesn't want to be around other people."
"She tends to take things the wrong way."
"He's not interested in sex."
"She can't sleep."
"There's little playfulness in our relationship."

Sarah and Joe

Sarah's limbic system negatively affected her relationship. She and Joe had been married for five years. They both worked and did not have any children. At the end of the day, Sarah was frequently very tired. Most often she liked to be on her own and didn't want to do anything after work. She usually wasn't interested in sex, except for one or two days after she started her menstrual cycle. Sarah also tended to look at the negative side of any situation. Joe complained about the lack of companionship in their relationship. He was very upset by her lack of interest in sex and her nonchalant attitude toward it. He felt she was too negative, and their lack of connectedness made him feel lonely. Joe tried to talk to Sarah, but she said she didn't have any problems and he just expected too much from her. Joe made an appointment with me. He said, "I wanted to see if there was anything I could do before I saw a divorce attorney." I encouraged him to bring Sarah with him to see me. I first got Sarah's reading on the situation. She admitted to feeling chronically tired, overwhelmed, and negative. She just figured she had a low libido and was destined to live with it. She had experienced a major depression when she was a teenager. Her mother had been depressed, and her parents had divorced when she was five years old. I explained the limbic system to her and all about depression. I then placed her on the antidepressant Zyban (bupropion) and saw the couple in counseling. Over two months, Sarah felt much better. She had better energy and more focus, and she also felt more social. In addition, her libido increased and she was more sexually receptive to Joe.

Basal Ganglia Relational Traits

When the basal ganglia system functions properly, people tend to be calm and relaxed. They tend to predict the best and, in general, see a positive future. Their bodies tend to feel good, and they are physically free to express their sexuality. They are not plagued by multiple physical complaints. They tend to be relaxed enough to be playful, sexy, and sexual. They are able to deal with conflict in an effective way.

When the basal ganglia are overactive, people have a tendency toward anxiety, panic, fear, and tension. They tend to focus on negative future events and what can go wrong in a situation. They filter information through fear and seldom give others the benefit of the doubt. They tend to have headaches, backaches, and a variety of other physical complaints. They have lowered sexual interest because their bodies tend to be wrapped in tension. They often do not have the physical or emotional energy to feel sexy or sexual, and they tend to shy away from sexual activity. Most of their memories are filled with anxiety or fear. They tend to wear people out by the constant fear they project.

Positive Basal Ganglia Relational Statements
"I know things will work out."
"I can speak out when I have a problem. I don't let problems fester."
"I usually feel physically relaxed."
"I'm usually calm in new situations."

Negative Basal Ganglia Relational Statements
"I know this isn't going to work out."
"I'm too tense."
"I'm scared."
"I'm too afraid to bring up problems. I tend to avoid them."
"I can't breathe. I feel really anxious in this situation."
"I can't make love—I have a headache (chest pain, backaches, muscle aches, etc.)."
"You're going to do something to hurt me."

Statements from the Partners of People with Basal Ganglia Problems

"She's anxious."

"He's nervous."

"She's uptight."

"He cares too much about what others think."

"He predicts the worst possible outcomes to situations."

"She complains of feeling bad a lot (has headaches, stomachaches)."

"He won't deal with conflict."

"She won't deal with problems head-on."

Ryan and Betsy

Ryan was a nervous wreck. He tended to see the worst in situations and often predicted failure. He was anxious, nervous, and sickly (frequently complaining of headaches, backaches, and muscle tension). He had been married to Betsy for fifteen years. When they had first been married, Betsy had mothered him, taking care of his aches and pains and soothing his fears and negativity. She liked to feel needed. After years of this, however, she had got tired of Ryan's whining and his tendency to be afraid in even the most benign situations. Ryan's anxiety and medical problems were taking over their relationship. She felt isolated and alone. She became irritable, less understanding, and distant from him. Seeing the love go out of their relationship, she made an appointment for me to see them both. Ryan was angry with her about the appointment. He complained that they didn't have the money, counseling wouldn't help, his problems were physical and not psychological (actually he was right; this was a basal ganglia problem), and all psychiatrists were crazy anyway (I wouldn't say all of us are crazy, just a bit odd). When I first saw Ryan and Betsy, it was clear to me that Ryan's basal ganglia were overactive. The basal ganglia hyperactivity was interfering with their relationship. When I explained his behavior in medical/brain-physiology terms to Ryan, he relaxed. I helped the couple with communication and goal setting and then engaged Ryan in his own therapy. I taught him how to kill fortune-telling ANTs (his were very strong). I worked with him using biofeedback (teaching him how to warm his hands, relax his muscles, and breathe diaphragmatically). And I taught him self-hypnosis. Ryan was a very fast learner and quickly soaked up the basal ganglia prescriptions. He no longer used Betsy as his doctor; he began to work with his medical doctor to address his physical issues and started to predict positive things rather than fear in his conversations with his wife. Once we treated Ryan's basal ganglia problems, the marital therapy became more effective and the marriage improved.

Prefrontal Cortex Relational Traits

When the prefrontal cortex functions properly, people can engage in goal-directed behavior and effectively supervise their words and deeds. They are able to think before they say things and tend to say things that affect their goals in a positive way. They also tend to think before they do things, and their actions are consistent with their goals. They tend to learn from mistakes and don't make the same ones over and over. In addition, they are able to focus and attend to conversations, follow through on commitments and chores, and organize their actions. They are also able to be settled and sit still. They are able to express what they feel. And they tend not to like conflict, tension, and turmoil.

When the prefrontal cortex is underactive, people tend to be impulsive in what they say or do, often causing serious problems in relationships (such as saying hurtful things without forethought). They tend to live in the moment and have trouble delaying gratification ("I want it now"). They tend not to learn from their mistakes and to make repetitive mistakes. They also have trouble listening and tend to be easily distracted. They often have difficulty expressing thoughts and feelings, and their partners often complain of a lack of communication in the relationship. It is often hard for people with prefrontal cortex underactivation to sit still. They tend to be restless and fidgety. In addition, they tend to be especially sensitive to noise, smells, light, and touch. They have difficulty staying on task and finishing projects, commitments, and chores. They are often late. In addition, many people with prefrontal cortex problems have an unconscious tendency to seek conflict or to look for problems when none exist. I call this tendency the game of "let's have a problem." They also tend to seek stimulation or indulge in highly stimulating behaviors that upset or frighten their partner (driving too fast, bungee jumping, getting into the middle of a fight between strangers).

Positive Prefrontal Cortex Relational Statements

"You're important to me. Let's do something tonight."

"I love you. I'm glad we're together."

"I love to listen to you."

"I'll be on time for our date."

"Let's get these chores done so that we'll have more time together."

"I don't want to fight. Let's take a break and come back in ten minutes and work this out."

"I made that mistake before. I'm not making it again."

Negative Prefrontal Cortex Relational Statements

"I'm only a half hour late. Why are you so uptight about it?"

"I'll do it later."

"I find it hard to listen to you."

"Go ahead and talk to me. I can listen to you while I'm watching TV and reading this book."

"I can't express myself."

"My mind goes blank when I try to express my feelings."

"I didn't mean to have the affair (overspend, embarrass you at the party, make hurtful comments, etc.)."

"I just can't sit still."

"The noise bothers me."

"I get so distracted (while listening, during sex, when playing a game, etc.)"

"I need the answer now."

"I want it now."

"I'm so mad at myself I've made that mistake too many times."

Statements from the Partners of People with Prefrontal Cortex Problems

"He's impulsive."

"She blurts out and interrupts."

"He doesn't pay attention to me."

"She won't let me finish a comment. She says she has to say whatever thought comes into her head or she'll forget it."

"He has to have the fan on at night to sleep. It drives me crazy."

"She often seems to start a problem for no particular reason."

"He loves to challenge everything I say."

"She gets so distracted during sex."

"He teases the animals, and it makes me furious."
"She can't sit still."
"He puts things off and tends not to finish things."
"She's always late, rushing around at the last minute."

Ray and Linda

Ray and Linda came to see me on the advice of their marital counselor. Two of their three children had been diagnosed with ADHD, and the counselor felt that Ray had it as well. Even though Ray owned a very successful restaurant, he was restless, impulsive, and very easily distracted. He spent excessive time at work due to inefficiency, and he had frequent employee problems (often because he hired impulsively without adequate screening). Marital counseling was Ray's idea, because he saw his wife turning away from him. He told the counselor that his wife was chronically stressed, tired, and angry. "She's not the woman I married," he said to their counselor. In my first session with this couple, Linda clearly explained that it was true; she had changed. It was an all-too-familiar story to me. She had married Ray because he was fun, spontaneous, thrill-seeking (she was actually a bit reserved), and hardworking. She now felt her life had been taken from her. Her ADHD children were a handful, and she felt she had no support from Ray. She said, "When he's home, he's not with me. He's always working on projects that don't get finished. He stirs up the kids after I get them settled down. And I can't get him to pay attention to me. He's so restless. When I try to talk with him, I have to follow him around the house." In addition, Ray had made several bad financial business decisions and the family was struggling with debt, despite Ray's successful business. He had had an affair several years before they entered counseling, and Linda didn't believe she could trust him. She felt isolated, alone, and angry.

There was no question in my mind that Ray had ADHD. As a child and teenager he had been restless, impulsive, hyperactive, and disorganized. He had underachieved in school and barely finished high school, despite obviously being very bright. The chronic stress of living in an ADHD home was beginning to change Linda's personality. She had gone from being a relaxed, happy person to being depressed, angry, and withdrawn. Something had to change. I put Ray on

Adderall, a stimulant medication, which helped him be more thoughtful, more attentive, and more efficient at work. I encouraged the couple to continue to see their counselor to work on healing the hurts from the past. I got involved with the children's treatment to make sure they were on the right dosages of medication and that Ray and Linda used effective parenting strategies (many of Ray and Linda's fights were over disciplining the children). I encouraged Linda to use St John's wort (the herbal antidepressant discussed in the cingulate prescription chapter) to reset her limbic system back to normal. Over the next four months, this couple dramatically improved; even the kids noticed a big difference.

Cingulate Relational Traits

When the cingulate functions properly, people are able to shift their attention easily. They tend to be flexible and adaptable. They are likely to see options in tough situations. They are usually able to forgive the mistakes of others and tend not to hold on to hurts from the past. They encourage others to help but do not rigidly control situations. They tend to have a positive outlook and see a hopeful future. They are able to roll with the ups and downs of relationships.

When the cingulate is overactive, people have a tendency to get locked into thoughts, thinking them over and over. They tend to hold grudges, hold on to hurts from the past, and be unforgiving of perceived wrongs. They tend to be inflexible, rigid, and unbending. They often want things done a certain way (their way), and they may get very upset when things do not go their way. They have difficulty dealing with change. They tend to be argumentative and oppositional.

Positive Cingulate Relational Statements
"It's okay."
"I can roll with this situation."
"How would you like to do this?"
"Let's collaborate."
"Let's cooperate."
"What would you like to do?"
"That was in the past."

Negative Cingulate Relational Statements

"You hurt me years ago."

"I won't forgive you."

"It'll never be the same."

"I'm always worried."

"I get stuck on these bad thoughts."

"Do it my way."

"I can't change."

"It's your fault."

"I don't agree with you."

"No. No. No."

"I won't do it."

"I don't want to do it."

"I have a lot of complaints about you."

"I've never hated anyone more than you."

"This will never change."

Statements from Partners of People with Cingulate Problems

"Nothing gets forgiven or let go."

"She brings up issues from years and years ago."

"Everything has to be the way he wants it."

"He can't say he's sorry."

"She holds on to grudges forever."

"He never throws anything away."

"She's rigid."

"If things aren't perfect, he thinks they are no good at all."

"I don't help her because I have to do it exactly her way or she goes ballistic."

"He argues with everything I say."

"She tends to be oppositional."

"He doesn't like to try new things."

Rose and Larry

Rose and Larry had been married for twenty-two years. They had been unhappy for twenty-one of them. I was the sixth marriage counselor they had seen. They were a very persistent couple. Larry had heard me speak in San Francisco at a local conference on children of alcoholics.

He said when I talked about problems associated with the cingulate gyrus, I was talking about things that affected his wife. He bought one of my videotapes and took it home for Rose to see. Rose was stunned when she recognized herself when I talked about some of my work with couples who had incompatible brains. She had grown up in an alcoholic home. As a teenager she had also had problems with alcohol and marijuana. As an adult she had periodic bouts of depression. More damaging to the marriage was her inflexibility: She had to have things a certain way or she'd explode (even though she didn't know it and even though she didn't want to be that way). She was "the world's worst worrier" according to her husband. Her house looked perfect. "The president could visit any time of the day or night," her husband said. "I don't know why she cleans so much. It's not like we're dirty people." She held grudges. Things would get brought up multiple times over the years. If she liked someone, she was a wonderful friend. If someone rubbed her the wrong way, she would write that person off and never let go of her anger. She hadn't talked to her own mother for eighteen years because of a trivial fight one Christmas. Rose never said she was sorry. She tended to oppose whatever Larry wanted to do, and their arguments were frequently over nothing. Larry said, "We argue just to argue." Sex was often an ordeal. The setting had to be just right in order for anything to happen. "God help me if I ask for it directly," Larry said.

When I asked Larry what kept him in the relationship, he said he didn't know. He had grown up Catholic and felt it was his obligation to stay. He found gratification at work and just spent more and more time away. Plus, he felt Rose really tried. She always set up the counseling appointments, and she was committed to staying with him. I was very surprised that no one had sent Rose to see a psychiatrist. None of her previous therapists had considered the brain to be an important factor in this couple's struggles. They wanted to help this couple with their behavior and never wondered if the hardware that runs behavior was working properly. Amazing.

Before I tackled this couple, I wanted to see how Rose's brain functioned. This couple had long-term marital dissatisfaction and multiple failures at marital counseling. I was betting there were brain patterns interfering with intimacy. As I suspected, Rose had one of the most active cingulates I had ever seen. No wonder she had so many problems shifting her attention! Her brain's gearshift was stuck, unable to shift into new and different modes of thinking. I put her on Lustral (a serotonergic antidepressant) to help her mood and flexibility. I taught the couple about how the brain works and how it can interfere with intimacy. I taught them the functions and problems of this part of the brain, along with cingulate prescriptions. In addition, I worked with them on developing a new perspective about their past behavior and healing the memories of pain. After four months of medication and therapy, they were much better. They were able to have fun together. Larry was able to ask for sex without fear of rejection. He no longer had to play "cingulate games." He spent more time at home, because the atmosphere was so much more relaxed. Rose called her mother and reconnected with her. Ultimately Rose stayed on Lustral for three years and then slowly tapered off. When some of her problems resurfaced, she resumed taking it.

Temporal Lobe Relational Traits

When the temporal lobes function properly, people tend to be emotionally stable. They are able to process and understand what others say in a clear way. They can retrieve words for conversations. They tend to read the emotional state of others accurately. They have good control over their temper. They have access to accurate memories. Because of their memory, they have a sense of personal history and identity.

When the temporal lobes do not function properly, people tend to have memory struggles. They don't have clear access to their own personal history and identity. They are often emotionally labile (up and down). They tend to be temperamental and have problems with anger. They often have violent thoughts and express their frustration with aggressive talk. They often take things the wrong way and appear to be a little paranoid. They may have periods of spaciness or confusion and misinterpret what is said to them.

Positive Temporal Lobe Relational Statements
"I remember what you asked me to do."
"I have a clear memory of the history of our relationship."
"I feel stable and even."
"I can find the words to express my feelings."
"I can usually tell when another person is happy, sad, mad, or bored."

"I have good control over my temper."
"My memory is good."

Negative Temporal Lobe Relational Statements
"I struggle with memory."
"I blow things way out of proportion."
"I get angry easily. I have a bad temper."
"My moods tend to be volatile."
"I tend to get scary, violent thoughts in my head."
"It's hard for me to read."
"I often misinterpret what others say."
"I tend to be too sensitive to others or feel others are talking about me."
"I tend to misread the facial expressions of others."
"I frequently have trouble finding the right words in a conversation."

Statements from Partners of People with Temporal Lobe Problems
"He can be physically or verbally very aggressive."
"She's volatile."
"His memory is very poor."
"She misreads situations."
"He's very moody."
"She takes things the wrong way."
"He spaces out easily."
"She doesn't seem to learn by reading something or hearing directions. You have to show her what to do."

Don and Shelley

Don and Shelley had been married for only four years when they sought therapy. Don had a terrible problem with his temper. He had physically abused Shelley on three occasions and had been charged with assaulting her. During one of those times he had been drunk, but during the other two he had not been drinking at all. Shelley's family and friends thought she was crazy for staying with him. Shelley said she loved Don and wanted the marriage to work. She was afraid when she thought about staying and sad when she thought about leaving, but she knew the violence had to stop. Don was always so sorry after the attacks. He always cried for a long time and seemed truly sorry.

When the therapist learned that Don had had a significant head injury from a motorcycle accident at the age of seventeen, he suggested that Don see me as part of his evaluation. Don and Shelley seemed to truly love each other. Don did not have a good explanation for his problems, and he denied that he ever wanted to hurt Shelley. "I just get out of control," he said. I found out that Don saw shadows. He had many periods of spaciness. He had difficulties finding the right words. He was very forgetful. He was moody, volatile, and temperamental, and he had odd sensations of déjà vu. Don often took things the wrong way, and he thought many other people were out to hurt him. In Don's motorcycle accident, he had swerved to avoid a deer and fallen against the left side of his helmet. His helmet (with head inside) had slid for approximately eighty feet. I was convinced he had temporal lobe problems (probably on the left), which was confirmed by his SPECT scan. I placed Don on Tegretol (an antiseizure medication) to stabilize the activity in his left temporal lobe. Within three weeks, he reported he was calmer, less angry, and less easily agitated. "It takes much more to get me upset," he said. Shelley noticed an almost immediate difference. "He is more relaxed. He's calmer, and he's much more mellow. Things don't upset him like before." Their therapist continued to see Don and Shelley for several more months and taught them about forgiveness and understanding based on this new information.

It is important to remember that there's no rule that says people get only one problem. Some of the toughest couples have multiple system problems in both partners. It is always important to consider the brain when thinking about couples who struggle.

Better Relationships Through Biochemistry?

One of the underlying messages of this chapter is that many couples struggle not because they want to, but because they have underlying brain patterns that interfere with intimacy. Sometimes medication can help alleviate these problems. The appropriate medications for each of the brain systems have been discussed in the chapters on individual brain system prescriptions. I have seen many relationships literally saved by the use of medication. Here are several additional tips about the use of medication in couples:

1. Be aware of when the medications will wear off and be especially cautious about conflict then. Some medications, such as stimulants, work for defined periods of time. If the medication's effectiveness wears off around 8:00 p.m., do not bring up emotionally loaded topics at 10:30 p.m. Be sensitive to the effectiveness cycle of the medication.

2. Be sensitive to the sexual side effects of medication. Some of the medications we use to treat brain abnormalities can alter sexual function and libido. Medications that enhance serotonin production in the brain, such as Prozac, Seroxat, Lustral, Anafranil, Efexor, and Faverin, often decrease libido or delay the ability to achieve orgasm. If this occurs, there are strategies your doctor can use to counteract these problems, such as adding gingko biloba or the antidepressant Zyban. Talk these problems over with your doctor. Also, let your partner know that there may be medication side effects and not to take them personally.

3. Be persistent when medication is required. Too often people will try medication, then abandon it too early if it isn't immediately effective. Sometimes it takes several trials of medication for prolonged periods of time. Be patient.

Relational Therapy Brain Prescriptions

It is clear that using medications is only part of the solution to people's problems. Based on my brain-imaging work, I have developed a number of effective nonmedication brain system prescriptions to help couples. I break them into the different systems we've discussed. Of course, there is overlap between systems, but I think this is a useful way to think about helping couples. The "Self" prescriptions here are for those affected by these problems, and the "Partner" prescriptions are for the partners of those affected.

Limbic Relational Prescriptions for Self

1. Spend time together: Bonding is essential to all human relationships. You need to spend physical time with your partner. The less you are around each other, the less bonded or limbically connected you become.

2. Smell good: Choose scents your partner likes and wear them. The limbic system directly processes the sense of smell, and it can have a positive or negative effect on your relationship.

3. Build positive memories: Focus on the times you have enjoyed each other. The limbic system stores highly charged emotional memories. When you focus on the negative in a relationship, you feel more distant from each other. When you focus on the positive in your relationship, you feel more connected.

4. Touch each other: Touch is healing, and couples need to have their hands on each other. Sexual and nonsexual touching is essential to intimacy. It is likely that touch cools the limbic system and is involved with the stabilization of mood.

5. Kill the ANTs: Automatic negative thoughts (ANTs) infest and destroy relationships (see chapter 4). Do not believe every thought you have. Focus on positive, uplifting, nurturing thoughts about your partner. It makes a difference to your brain function and subsequently affects your relationship.

Limbic Relational Prescriptions for Partner

1. Don't let your partner isolate himself or herself. Even though isolation is a natural tendency in depression, it makes the situation worse. Encourage activity and togetherness.

2. Touch your partner. Back rubs or a touch on a shoulder or hand can be very reassuring to someone who feels alone. Connectedness is very important.

3. If your partner has a loss of sexual interest, do not take it personally. Often depression is accompanied by sexual problems. Work on getting him or her help.

4. Help your partner around the house, with the children, and so on. Often limbic problems are associated with low energy and poor concentration. Your partner may feel overwhelmed and need your help. Many partners, not properly understanding the reality of the situation, become critical and make the situation much worse. Your partner needs understanding, love, and support, not criticism.

5. Make sure you help get your partner to the doctor if the limbic problems interfere with functioning. Limbic problems are often very treatable.

6. Take care of yourself. It is stressful to be married to someone who is depressed. Take time to replenish yourself.

Basal Ganglia Relational Prescriptions for Self

1. Kill the fortune-telling ANTs: Predicting failure, pain, or an unhappy outcome often causes erosion in relationships. Clear thinking is essential in relationships. Do not believe every thought you have.

2. Predict the best: Looking to the future in a positive manner is a key to happiness. Your mind helps to make happen what it sees. People with basal ganglia issues have a natural tendency to predict the worst and thus help to make bad things happen by their predictions. Fight that tendency. When you see good things happening in your relationship, act in ways to make them even more likely to happen. Hope for the best.

3. Get control of your breathing: Anxiety, tension, and out-of-control behavior are often preceded by shallow, rapid breathing. Before responding to your partner in an anxious or tense situation, take a deep breath, hold it for three seconds, and then very slowly exhale (taking up to five to eight seconds to exhale). After three or four deep breaths of this type, your brain will be filled with oxygen, you will feel more relaxed, and you will be much more likely to make better decisions.

4. Deal with conflict: Effectively dealing with conflict is one of the keys to relationship health. Whenever couples bury their differences or put off dealing with conflict, anxiety, tension, and subversive behavior result. It is important to develop both negotiation and conflict resolution skills in relationships (see the basal ganglia prescription chapter). It is also important to deal with conflict in a kind, respectful manner.

Basal Ganglia Relational Prescriptions for Partner

1. Help your partner look at the positive side of things. Help him or her predict good things rather than bad things. Join forces to kill the fortune-telling ANTs.

2. Do not get irritated with your partner's anxiety or negative predictions. Soothe him or her with gentle words or a touch.

3. Pace your breathing to help your partner's breathing. Often

people unconsciously mirror their partner. When you breathe slowly and deeply, your partner is likely to pick up a more relaxed breathing pattern, automatically calming his or her anxiety.

4. Encourage your partner to face conflict in an effective way.

Prefrontal Cortex Relational Prescriptions for Self

1. Focus on what you want: Clear focus is essential to relationships. I have many of my couples develop a "two-minute focus statement." In this statement they write down, on one piece of paper, the major goals they have for their relationship in the areas of communication, time together, money, work, parenting, and sexuality. Then they post this statement where they will see and read it every day. This helps to keep their behavior on track.

2. Focus on what you like about your partner more than what you don't like: This encourages your partner's positive behavior. Think about how we train pets. Do you smack them every time they do something wrong (this will not train them to do anything but avoid you), or do you praise them every time they do something right (this encourages new behavior)? Focus on what you like, and you are more likely to get it. Many couples with prefrontal cortex problems are conflict-seeking as a way to stimulate themselves. Naturally they tend to notice the problems in their relationships, which makes them more upset and unconsciously gives them stimulation. The problem with focusing on negative behavior is that you drive the other person away. The negativity kills the relationship.

3. Positive stimulation is helpful: Look for new, exciting ways to stimulate the relationship. The prefrontal cortex seeks stimulation. It is important to have new, exciting, stimulating experiences to keep the relationship fresh and alive. Look for ways to do new things together, such as sharing a hobby, going to new places, or trying new sexual experiences.

4. Learn to say "I'm sorry": Admitting mistakes and saying you're sorry are essential to relational health. When the prefrontal cortex doesn't work hard enough, people don't have access to good internal supervision, and they may say or do things impulsively. When that happens, it is important to apologize and let your partner know you're sorry. Unfortunately, many people aren't good at saying they are sorry, and they try to justify why they did or said hurtful things. Learn to

apologize and take responsibility for your mistakes.

5. Think about what you say or do before you say or do it: Thoughtfulness and forethought are essential to effective relationships. Before you say or do something in a relationship, ask yourself if what you say or do fits with the goals you have for the relationship. Will your behavior help or hurt the relationship? Supervising your thoughts and actions is essential to relational health.

Prefrontal Cortex Relational Prescriptions for Partner

1. Do not be your partner's Ritalin: Because the prefrontal cortex seeks stimulation, many partners unconsciously seek stimulation in a negative way. Without knowing it (unconsciously), they try to upset you. They try to get you to yell. They try to make you angry. It is very important if you feel this is happening to have a calm demeanor. Do whatever you can to not yell or become emotionally intense. When you feel as if you are going to blow, take a deep breath or a break until you can get yourself under control.

2. Notice the positive. You change behavior by focusing on what you like a lot more than what you don't like. Often people with prefrontal cortex problems have low self-esteem and need encouragement and positive input from those they love.

3. Help your partner with organization. Disorganization is often a hallmark of prefrontal cortex problems. Rather than complain about the disorganization, it is generally much more effective to help your partner become more organized—if he or she will allow you to.

4. Make the appointment and drive your partner to the doctor. Often forgetfulness, procrastination, and denial accompany prefrontal cortex problems. Help may be put off for many years, even when it is obviously needed. Professional help can make a big difference in these problems, and I often see partners bring their loved ones in for evaluation and treatment. Don't wait for your partner to have the desire, will, or commitment to change; you may wait too long.

5. If medication is necessary, help your partner remember to take it. Do not do this in a condescending way, such as "Did you take your medicine? Your behavior is way off." Instead, help your partner with a gentle (nonsarcastic) reminder, or help your partner come up with a reminder system, such as weekly pill organizers or calendars.

Cingulate Relational Prescriptions for Self

1. Notice when you are stuck: The first step in breaking negative cycles is for you to notice when you are in them. Being aware of repetitive negative patterns of behavior allows you to do something different. Notice these patterns when you have the same argument over and over and just do something different than you usually would. If you would usually just go on and on trying to make your point, stop and say, "I'm finished. What do you have to say?" Then be quiet long enough to really hear what your partner is saying.

2. Take a break when things get hot: When you notice things are getting into a negative "cingulate" loop, take a break. When you notice tension in your voice, your body, or your conversation, find a way to distract yourself or take a break from the situation.

3. Stop nagging: Nagging erodes a relationship and needs to stop. Nagging—complaining about something over and over—is very common in cingulate people. It often has a seriously negative impact on a relationship. When you find yourself going over the same material again and again, stop it. Beating someone over the head who is not listening to you is ineffective and irritating. Try to find new ways to deal with your frustrations.

4. Use good problem-solving techniques: When you are stuck in an impasse, write out the problem, options, and solutions to the problem. Writing down the issues that bother the relationship can often be very helpful. Use the following problem-solving model: Write out the issue (such as spending too much money), write out the options and solutions to the problem (spending less, budgeting, cutting up credit cards), and then choose among the options. Writing problems down often helps to get them out of your head and out of repetitive relational arguments.

5. Exercise together: Exercise enhances serotonin production in the brain and often helps a person (maybe even a couple) to become more flexible and less cingulate.

6. Have a carbohydrate snack. Carbohydrates (whole-grain bread, crackers, yogurt, etc.) often improve mood and help cingulate people be more flexible. Low blood sugar often correlates with anger and irritability.

Cingulate Relational Prescriptions for Partner

1. Notice when your partner is stuck: The first step to breaking negative cycles is for couples to notice when they are in them. Being aware of repetitive negative patterns in your partner allows you to be helpful in the situation rather than inflame it. For example, if you notice your partner is not listening to you but holding firmly on to his or her own position, take a breath and really try to listen to your partner. Do something different to break the negative cycle.

2. Take a break when things get hot: When you notice your partner is getting into a negative "cingulate" loop, change the pace. If you see your partner going over and over the same territory, or when his or her anger is escalating, find a way to distract your partner or take a break from the situation. As I've said, one of the most helpful things I tell people to do is learn how to go to the bathroom when things get hot.

3. Deal effectively with nagging. Nagging may be caused by an overactive cingulate, or it may arise because you're not listening to your partner. When someone has repetitive complaints about you, let him or her know you hear what they are saying. Ask your partner what steps you can take to make the situation better. Also, make it clear that you have heard about the issue and would appreciate not hearing about it again. In a kind way, ask what you can do to make that happen.

4. Exercise together: Exercise enhances serotonin production in the brain and often helps people (couples included) become more flexible and less cingulate.

Temporal Lobe Relational Prescriptions for Self

1. Use memory helpers to keep the relationship fresh: Reminders can make all the difference between your partner knowing you care and feeling he or she is not important. Given the busy pace of our lives, we often forget to notice the people who are most special to us. Use notes, signs, computer reminder systems, ticklers, and so on to keep your attention focused on making the person you love feel loved. Flowers (limbic smells), cards, CDs, and loving notes help your partner remember you love and care for him or her. Temporal lobe partners need constant reminders to keep you lovingly in their memory banks.

2. Listen to beautiful music together: Music is healing and often has a positive impact on relationships. As we have seen, music can enhance moods and sharpen learning and memory. Use beautiful music to enhance your connection to your partner.

3. Move in rhythms together: Moving together helps maintain connection. Dancing, walking hand in hand, and loving are movements that promote bonding in a relationship. They promote connectedness and provide rhythms that help to solidify memories of togetherness.

4. Remember the best times. Develop a positive sense of the history of the relationship. Reread loving cards and letters on a regular basis to maintain an overall happy sense of the relationship.

5. Deal effectively with anger. When you know that you have a temporal lobe problem and anger is a serious issue for you, practice effective anger management strategies. Deep breathing, correcting negative thoughts, and clear communication are some anger management strategies that work. In addition, be sure to stay away from alcohol and drugs. They can unleash a vulnerable temporal lobe, uncorking anger and causing serious problems.

6. Know you have a tendency to be extremely sensitive to the behavior of others. Mild paranoia often accompanies a temporal lobe problem. When you feel others are being negative toward you, check it out. Do not automatically believe your negative thoughts or feelings. Check them out.

7. Protein snacks may be helpful. Often, stabilizing blood sugar with a protein snack (cheese, nuts, meat, hard-boiled eggs) helps to settle down the situation caused by temporal lobe irregularities.

Temporal Lobe Relational Prescriptions for Partner

1. Do not take this problem personally. Often people with temporal lobe problems struggle in relationships because of their negativity, anger, and mild paranoia. Help your partner see situations clearly, but do not take the negativity personally.

2. Take anger seriously. Sometimes temporal lobe rage can get out of control. Do not escalate the situation when you see your partner is escalating, especially if substance abuse is involved. Talk in a soft voice. Take a break. Actively listen. Offering food may also help. Do not use addictive substances around the temporal lobe partner. The more

you use, the more likely your partner will use. Then things can really get out of control.

3. Keep protein snacks around.

4. Make sure you help get your partner to the doctor if the temporal lobe problems interfere with functioning. Such problems are often very treatable.

Use these prescriptions to enhance the love in your life. Love makes life worth living.

17

HELP!
When and How to Seek Professional Care

This chapter will attempt to answer four questions that I am frequently asked:

When is it time to see a professional about these problems?
What should I do when a loved one is in denial about needing help?
How can I find a competent professional?
When do you order a SPECT study?

When To Seek Help

This is relatively easy to determine. I recommend that people seek professional help when their attitudes, behaviors, feelings, or thoughts interfere with their ability to be successful in the world, whether in their relationships, in their work, or within themselves, and when self-help techniques have not helped them fully understand or alleviate the problem. Let's look at all three situations.

As seen in the last chapter, underlying neurobiological problems can truly sabotage relationships. *If you or someone you know suffers these problems and they interfere with the quality of relationships, get help.* Often it is necessary to address psychobiological problems first, before working on the psychology of the partners. I often use a computer analogy: you need to first fix computer hardware before it can effectively run sophisticated software. Let's take another look at how each brain system can interfere with relationships.

- *Depression can cause a person to feel distant, uninterested in sex, irritable, unfocused, tired, and negative. Unless the partners understand this disorder, they often have severe relational problems. People who suffer from depression have a divorce rate six times higher than those who are not depressed.*
- *Anxiety causes sufferers to feel tense, uptight, physically ill, and dependent, and to avoid conflict. Partners often misinterpret the anxiety or physical symptoms as complaining or whining and do not take seriously the level of suffering.*
- *Obsessive or overfocus tendencies, as we have seen, cause rigid thinking styles, oppositional or argumentative behavior, holding on to grudges, and chronic stress in relationships. Seeking help is essential to establishing a new ability to relate effectively.*
- *Prefrontal cortex problems, such as ADHD, often sabotage relationships because of the impulsive, restless, and distractible behavior involved. Without help there is a high degree of relational and family turmoil.*
- *Temporal lobe problems may be associated with frequent attacks of rage, angry outbursts, mood swings, hearing things wrong, and low frustration tolerance. I have seen these problems ruin otherwise good relationships.*

These underlying brain problems often need treatment in order for relationships to heal.

The workplace is also affected by underlying and often unrecognized brain system problems. *If you or someone you know suffers these problems and they interfere with work, it is often essential to get professional help.* Addressing these problems can literally change the whole atmosphere at work.

- *Depression can cause people at work to be negative, unfocused, tired, and unmotivated, and to take things too personally or the wrong way. Such employees may negatively affect others' morale and unknowingly skew everyone's perceptions at work so they see positive things in a bad light. Depressed people have more sick days than people without depression.*
- *People with anxiety are often tense, physically sick, and conflict-*

avoidant. Their level of anxiety often causes them to be dependent and require too much supervision. Their anxiety tends to be contagious, and those around them may also begin predicting negative outcomes to situations. They can negatively affect a work group and tend to be fearful rather than hopeful.

- *Obsessive or overfocus tendencies cause rigid thinking styles, and employers or employees tend to be more irritable, oppositional, or argumentative. They often hold grudges and can be unforgiving, causing long-term workplace problems.*

- *Prefrontal cortex problems, such as ADHD, cause many problems at work, including chronic lateness, inefficiency, missing deadlines, impulsive decision making, and conflict-seeking behavior.*

- *Temporal lobe problems often affect work. I am willing to bet that most workplace violence is associated with temporal lobe disorders. More commonly, temporal lobe problems are manifested at work by mood swings or unpredictable behavior, low frustration tolerance, misperceptions, auditory processing problems, and memory problems. The anger, misperceptions, and mild paranoia can wreak havoc in a work group.*

Ben

Let me give an example of how brain system problems can affect the workplace. Ben was on the verge of being fired. He was frequently late to work, disorganized, forgetful, late on deadlines, and off task. His boss let his behavior slide because she felt that Ben had a good heart and wanted to do well. His boss's boss, however, wanted Ben fired. He thought Ben was bad for unit discipline and morale. Ben's boss was my patient. I was treating her for ADHD. She saw many of her own characteristics in Ben. One day she asked Ben to come into her office. She told him her own story, about her problems in school and with timeliness, organization, distractibility, and procrastination. She told him she had ADHD and that her treatment had made a big difference for her. She said that her boss wanted her to fire him, but she had convinced him to give Ben another chance. She suggested that Ben seek professional help if he could relate to her story. Ben started to cry. His history was a carbon copy of hers. He had done poorly in school and had trouble with concentration, organization, completing assignments, and underachievement. He did not expect his boss to care enough about him to try to help. Other employers would just fire him, as the boss's boss wanted to do. Ben came to see me. He had a classic case of ADHD. With medication and structured therapy, his behavior improved dramatically. His boss and those higher up in the company saw a wonderful turnaround in Ben. The company saved money by not having to hire and retrain someone to take Ben's place, and Ben was deeply grateful that he was given another chance, along with the information he needed to heal. The odds are that he will always be a loyal employee of this company.

All of these brain systems can have a significantly negative effect on internal life, self-esteem, emotional health, and physical health.

- *Depression (limbic system) clouds a sense of accomplishment (even with incredible accomplishment) and causes intense sadness and internal pain. Depression is not the absence of feeling, but rather the presence of painful feelings. Depression is one of the most common precursors to drug abuse and suicide. Depression often compromises immune system function, leaving people more prone to illness.*
- *The tension and panic associated with anxiety (often a result of basal ganglia problems) can feel like torture. I have known many patients with panic attacks who become suicidal in hope of escaping their fear. Anxiety is often associated with physical tension and an increase in illness. Many anxious people self-medicate by drinking alcohol, taking drugs, overeating, engaging in inappropriate sex, and other potentially addictive behaviors.*
- *Overfocus (cingulate) issues cause repetitive thoughts and worries that are often self-medicated with drugs or alcohol. Internal torture by constant worry is common. When someone says one negative thing, they may hear it in their minds five hundred times. They cannot get away from negative thoughts.*
- *People with prefrontal cortex issues, such as ADHD, often feel a tremendous sense of underachievement, repetitive failure, and low self-esteem. People with prefrontal cortex issues may use internal problems for self-stimulation and be chronically upset. The stress associated with these problems is often accompanied by increased illness.*

■ *Temporal lobe problems can wreak internal havoc. The internal violent mood swings and thoughts often torment the soul. Unpredictable behavior, low frustration tolerance, misperceptions, and memory problems are often associated with an internal sense of damage. Anger often alienates others, and loneliness is common.*

Gaining Access to your Own Good Brain

The internal problems associated with these brain system difficulties can ruin lives, relationships, and careers. It is essential to seek help when necessary. It is also critical for people not to be too proud to get help. Pride often devastates relationships, careers, and even life itself. Too many people feel they are somehow "less than others" if they seek help. I often tell my patients that, in my experience, *it is the success-ful people who seek help when they need it.* Successful business people hire the best possible outside consultants when they are faced with a problem that they cannot solve or when they need extra help. Unsuccessful people tend to deny they have problems, bury their heads, and blame others for their problems. If your attitude, behavior, thoughts, or feelings sabotage your chances for success in relationships, work, or within yourself, get help. Don't feel ashamed; feel as though you're being good to yourself.

In thinking about getting help, it is important to put these brain system problems in perspective. I tell my patients to get rid of the concept of "normal versus not normal." "What is normal anyway?" I ask. I tell my patients who worry that they are not normal that "normal" is the setting on a dryer. Or that Normal is a city in Illinois. Actually, I spoke in Normal, Illinois, at a major university several years ago. I got to meet Normal people, shop at the Normal grocery store, see the Normal police department and fire department. I even met Normal women. They were a very nice group, but really not much different from folks in California. The Normal people seemed to have all of the problems I mention in this book. I also tell my patients about a study published in 1994, sponsored by the National Institutes of Health, in which researchers reported that 49 percent of the U.S. population suffer from a psychiatric illness at some point in their lives. Anxiety, substance abuse, and depression were the three most common illnesses. At first, I thought this statistic was too high. Then I made a list of twenty people

I knew (not from my practice). Eleven were taking medication or were in therapy. Half of us at some point in our lives will have problems. It's just as normal to have problems as not to have problems. Again, it is the more successful people who will get help first. The same NIH study reported that 29 percent of the population will have two separate and distinct psychiatric diagnoses and 17 percent of us will have three. In my experience, very few people are completely without these problems. In fact, in doing research, one of the most difficult challenges is finding a "normal control group."

Most of us have traits of one or more brain system misfires. Sometimes the problems associated with each section are subclinical (they don't get in your way much), and sometimes they are severe enough that they significantly interfere with your life. When they do, it is time to get help. I see many of the problems I treat as medical with significant psychological and social consequences. This classification is, I believe, accurate, and a lot less stigmatizing for patients.

One of the most persuasive statements I give patients about seeking help is that I am often able to help them have *more access* to their own good brain. When their brain does not work efficiently, they can't be efficient. When their brain works right, they can work right. I will often show them a number of brain SPECT studies to show them the difference on and off medication or targeted psychotherapy, as a way to help them understand the concept. As you can imagine after looking at the images in this book, when you see an underactive brain versus one that is healthy, you want the one that is healthy.

What to Do when a Loved One is in Denial about Needing Help

Unfortunately, the stigma associated with "psychiatric illness" prevents many people from getting help. People do not want to be seen as crazy, stupid, or defective, and they often don't seek help until they (or their loved one) can no longer tolerate the pain (at work, in their relationships, or within themselves).

Jerry and Jenny

When Jerry and Jenny started to have marital problems early in their marriage, Jenny wanted to get help. Jerry refused. He said that he didn't want to air his problems in front of a stranger. It wasn't until Jenny threatened to leave him that he finally agreed to go for counseling. Initially, Jerry listed many reasons why he wouldn't go for help: He didn't see that the problems were that bad; it was too much money; he thought all counselors were "messed up"; and he didn't want to be perceived as crazy by anyone who might find out about the counseling.

Unfortunately, Jerry's attitude is common among men. Many men, when faced with obvious problems in their marriages, their children, or even themselves, refuse to see the issue. Their lack of awareness and strong tendency toward denial prevent them from seeking help until more damage has been done than necessary. In Jerry's case, he had to be threatened with divorce before he would go. Another factor in Jerry's case was that he had ADHD. As a child he had been forced to see a counselor for behavioral problems at school. He hated feeling different from the other kids and resented his mum for making him talk to the doctor.

Some people may say it is unfair for me to "pick on" men. And indeed, some men see problems long before some women. Overall, however, in my experience mothers see problems in children before fathers and are more willing to seek help, and many more wives call for marital counseling than husbands. What is it in our society that causes men to overlook obvious problems, to deny problems until it is too late to deal with them effectively or until more damage is done than necessary? Some of the answers may be found in how boys are raised, the societal expectations we place on men, and the overwhelming pace of many men's daily lives.

Boys most often engage in active play (sports, war games, video games, etc.) that involves little dialogue or communication. The games often involve dominance and submissiveness, winning and losing, and little interpersonal communication. Force, strength, or skill are used to handle problems. Girls, on the other hand, often engage in more interpersonal or communicative types of play, such as dolls and storytelling. When my wife was a little girl, she used to line up her dolls to teach them. Fathers often take their sons out to throw the ball around, rather than to go for a walk and talk.

Many men retain the childhood notions of competition and that one must be better than others to be any good at all. To admit to a problem is to be less than other men. As a result, many men wait to seek help until their problem is obvious to the whole world. Other men feel totally responsible for all that happens in their families; to admit to a problem is to admit that they have in some way failed.

Clearly, the pace of life prevents some men from being able to take the time to look clearly at the important people in their lives and their relationships with them. When I spend time with fathers and husbands and help them slow down enough to see what is really important to them, more often than not they begin to see the problems and work toward more helpful solutions. The issue is not one of being uncaring or uninterested; it is not seeing what is there.

Many teenagers also resist getting help even when faced with obvious problems. They worry about labels and don't want yet another adult judging their behavior.

Here are several suggestions to help people who are unaware or willing to get the help they need:

1. Try the straightforward approach first (but with a new brain twist). Clearly tell the person what behaviors concern you. Tell him or her that the problems may be due to underlying brain patterns that can be tuned up. Explain that help may be available—help not to cure a defect but rather help to optimize how the brain functions. Tell the loved one that you know he or she is trying to do his or her best, but unproductive behavior, thoughts, or feelings may be getting in the way of success (at work, in relationships, or within themselves). Emphasize access, not defect.

2. Give the loved one information. Books, videos, and articles on the subjects you are concerned about can be of tremendous help. Many people come to see me because they read a book of mine, saw a video I produced, or read an article I wrote. Good information can be very persuasive, especially if it is presented in a positive, life-enhancing way.

3. When a person remains resistant to help, even after you have been straightforward and given him or her good information—plant seeds. Plant ideas about getting help and then water them regularly. Drop an idea, article, or other information about the topic from time to time. However, if you talk too much about getting help, people become resentful and won't get help, just to spite you. Be careful not to go overboard.

4. Protect your relationship with the other person. People are more receptive to people they trust than to people who nag and belittle them. I do not let anyone tell me something bad about myself unless I trust him or her. Work on gaining the person's trust over the long run. It will make him or her more receptive to your suggestions. Do not make getting help the only thing that you talk about. Make sure you are interested in the person's whole life, not just potential medical appointments.

5. Give new hope. Many people with these problems have tried to get help and it either didn't work or made them worse. Educate them on new brain technology that helps professionals be more focused and more effective in treatment efforts.

6. There comes a time when you have to say enough is enough. If, over time, the other person refuses to get help, and his or her behavior has a negative impact on your life, you may have to separate yourself. Staying in a toxic relationship is harmful to your health, and it often enables the other person to remain sick. Actually, I have seen that the threat or act of leaving can motivate people to change, whether it is about drinking, drug use, or treating underlying ADHD or manic-depressive disorder. Threatening to leave is not the first approach I would take, but after a time it may be the best approach.

7. Realize that you cannot force people into treatment unless they are dangerous to themselves, dangerous to others, or unable to care for themselves. You can do only what you can do. Fortunately, today there is a lot more we can do than even ten years ago.

Finding a Competent Professional

At this point, I must get thirty to forty calls, faxes, or e-mails a week from people all over the world who are looking for competent professionals in their area who think in ways similar to myself and utilize the principles outlined in this book. Because these principles are still on the edge of what is new in brain science, such professionals may be hard to find. Still, finding the right professional for evaluation and treatment is critical to the healing process. The wrong professional can make things worse. There are a number of steps you can take to find the best person to assist you:

1. Get the best person you can find. Saving money up front may cost you a lot in the long run. The right help not only is cost-effective but saves unnecessary pain and suffering. Don't rely on a therapist solely because he or she is on your managed care plan. That person may or may not be a good fit for you. Search for the best. If he or she is on your insurance plan or authorised by your private healthcare provider—great. Just don't let that be the primary criterion.

2. Use a specialist. Brain science is expanding at a rapid pace. Specialists keep up with the latest developments in their fields, while generalists (GPs) have to try to keep up with everything. If I had a heart arrhythmia, I would see a cardiologist rather than a general medical practitioner. I want to be treated by someone who has seen hundreds or even thousands of cases like mine.

3. Get information about referrals from people who are highly knowledgeable about your problem. Hopefully your GP will be able to recommend the right specialist to help you. He or she should know who in your area is the appropriate doctor to refer you to. However, well-meaning GPs sometimes give very bad information. I have known many doctors and teachers who make light of brain system problems, such as ADHD, learning disabilities, or depression, and discourage people from getting help. One family doctor told one of my recent patients: "Oh, ADHD is a fad. You don't need help. Just try harder." In searching for help, contact people who are likely to give you good information, such as specialists in the field, people at major research centers, people in support groups about your specific problem. Check out Internet medical support groups. Support groups often have members who have visited the professionals in the area, and they can give you important information about the doctor, such as his or her bedside manner, competence, responsiveness, and organization.

4. Once you get the names of competent professionals, check their credentials. Preferably he or she will have consultant qualifications—such as membership of the Royal College of Physicians, Paediatricians or Psychiatrists—and be involved in a clinic specializing in brain problems. His or her medical school doesn't matter: in the United Kingdom there is a system of external examiners that ensures that the standards throughout the whole country are the same. What you need is a forward-thinking and caring doctor.

5. At your first appointment with the doctor you will know whether or not you want to work with him or her. It is worth spending time

getting to know the people you will rely on for help. If you sense the fit isn't good, keep looking.

6. Many professionals write articles or books or speak at meetings or local groups. If possible, read their writings or hear them speak to get a feel for the kind of people they are and their ability to help you.

7. Look for a person who is open-minded, up to date, and willing to try new things.

8. Look for a person who treats you with respect, who listens to your questions, and who responds to your needs. Look for a relationship that is collaborative and trusting.

I know it is hard to find a professional who meets all of these criteria and who also has the right training in brain physiology, but it is possible. Be persistent. The right caregiver is essential to healing.

How Can I Tell if I Need a SPECT Study?

I order SPECT studies only for very specific reasons. Because of our very large database, I actually order fewer studies now than I did several years ago. Our extensive SPECT work has given me the clinical experience to diagnose more readily brain patterns that are responsive to certain treatments. I have included many of these patterns in this book. Here are several common questions and answers about SPECT.

Will the SPECT study give me an accurate diagnosis? No. A SPECT study by itself will not give a diagnosis. SPECT studies help the clinician understand more about the specific function of your brain. Each person's brain is unique, which may lead to unique responses to medicine or therapy. Diagnoses about specific conditions are made through a combination of clinical history, personal interview, information from families, diagnostic checklists, SPECT studies, and other neuropsychological tests. No study alone is a "doctor in a box" that can give accurate diagnoses on individual patients.

Why are SPECT studies ordered? Some of the common reasons include:

1. *Evaluating seizure activity*
2. *Evaluating cerebral vascular disease*
3. *Evaluating dementia and distinguishing between dementia and pseudodementia*

4. *Evaluating the effects of mild, moderate, and severe head trauma*
5. *Suspicion of underlying organic brain condition, such as seizure activity contributing to behavioral disturbance, prenatal trauma, or exposure to toxins*
6. *Evaluating atypical or unresponsive aggressive behavior*
7. *Determining the extent of brain impairment caused by drug or alcohol abuse*

In this book I have listed other examples of SPECT's use, such as in difficult marital situations. I must emphasize that this is a very sophisticated use of SPECT and not likely to be found in clinics outside our own.

Do I need to be off medication before the study? This question must be answered individually between you and your doctor. In general, it is better to be off medication until they are out of your system before a scan, but this is not always practical or advisable. If the study is done while on medication, let the technician know so that when the doctor reads the study, he or she will include that information in interpreting the scan. In general, we recommend that patients try to be off stimulants at least four days before the first scan and remain off them until after the second scan if one is ordered. Medications such as Prozac (which lasts in the body four to six weeks) are generally not stopped because of practicality. Check with your doctor for specific recommendations.

What should I do the day of the scan? On the day of the scan decrease or eliminate your caffeine intake, and try to not take cold medication or aspirin (if you do, please write it down on the intake form). Eat as you normally would.

Are there any side effects or risks to the study? The study does not involve a dye, and people do not have allergic reactions to the study. The possibility exists, although in a very small percentage of patients, of a mild rash, facial redness and edema (swelling), fever, and a transient increase in blood pressure. The amount of radiation exposure from one brain SPECT study is approximately the same as from one abdominal X-ray.

How is the SPECT procedure done? The patient is placed in a quiet room, and an intravenous (IV) line is started. The patient remains quiet for approximately ten minutes with eyes open to allow his or her mental state to equilibrate to the environment. The imaging agent is then injected through the IV. After another short period of time, the patient lies on a table and the SPECT camera rotates around his or her head (the patient does not go into a tube). The time on the table is approximately fifteen minutes. If a concentration study is ordered, the patient returns on another day to repeat the process; a concentration test is performed during the injection of the isotope.

Are there alternatives to having a SPECT study? In our opinion, SPECT is the most clinically useful study of brain function. There are other studies, such as electroencephalograms (EEGs), positron emission tomography (PET) studies, and functional MRIs (fMRIs). PET studies and fMRIs are considerably more costly, and they are performed mostly in research settings. EEGs, in our opinion, do not provide enough information about the deep structures of the brain to be as helpful as SPECT studies.

Does insurance or private healthcare cover the cost of SPECT studies? Reimbursement by insurance companies varies according to your plan. It is a good idea to check with the company ahead of time to see if it is a covered benefit.

Is the use of brain SPECT imaging accepted in the medical community? Brain SPECT studies are widely recognized as an effective tool for evaluating brain function in seizures, strokes, dementia, and head trauma. There are literally hundreds of research articles on these topics. In our clinic, based on our experience over eight years, we have developed this technology further to evaluate aggression and nonresponsive psychiatric conditions. Unfortunately, many doctors do not fully understand the application of SPECT imaging and may tell you that the technology is experimental, but over one hundred doctors in the United States have referred patients to us for scans.

18

Who Is Andrew Really?

Questions About the Essence of Our Humanity

In the introduction, I told the story of Andrew, my nephew who became violent because of a brain cyst occupying the space in his left temporal lobe. When the cyst was removed, he returned to his kind, caring, inquisitive self. In subsequent chapters I have also discussed:

- *Michelle, a woman who attacked her husband with a knife several days before her period and who, when treated with Depakote, became her normal, nonviolent self.*
- *Samuel, a negative, oppositional ten-year-old who was failing in school and isolated from friends and who, on 10 milligrams of Prozac daily, became successful at school, at home, and with friends.*
- *Rusty, a man who was arrested four times for assault and failed five drug treatment programs for methamphetamine abuse and who, since his underlying temporal lobe disorder was diagnosed and properly treated, has been able to remain personally more effective as well as gainfully employed.*
- *Sally, a woman admitted to the hospital as suicidal, depressed, and anxious and who, when properly diagnosed with adult ADHD and effectively treated, felt less depressed and more focused, and was able to be the mother and wife she had always wanted to be.*
- *Willie, a college student who experienced "minor" head injuries in two car accidents and whose whole personality subsequently changed. He became aggressive and depressed, and nearly killed his roommate. With the proper treatment he was able to return to his funny, happy, effective self.*

- Rob, "the anger broker of the Valley" who had severe family problems and suicidal ideas and actions. On the antiobsessive antidepressant Anafranil, he became pleasant, effective, and someone his family wanted to be around.
- Linda, a woman who had been raped on two occasions and who suffered from anxiety, depression, worrying, and drug abuse. With St John's wort and EMDR psychotherapy, her brain normalized and she was able to be much more effective in her life.
- John, a retired contractor, who had been physically and emotionally abusive to his wife during most of their marriage, and emotionally abusive to his children. At the age of seventy-nine, after a psychotic episode following open-heart surgery, it was discovered that he had had a serious head injury at the age of twenty that had damaged his left frontal-temporal region. The head injury may have changed his behavior and affected three generations of his family.

These stories and many others in the book and in my practice have caused me to question the very essence of who we are. Who are we really? Are we really who we are when our brain works right? Or are we really who we are when our brain misfires?

I believe, after seeing five thousand SPECT studies (along with the patients and stories that go with them), that we are really who we are when our brain works right. When our brain works right, we are more thoughtful, more goal-oriented, and more interested in other people. We are kinder, our moods are more stable, and we are more tolerant. Anxiety doesn't rule us, although we have enough anxiety to get out of bed in the morning and go to work. Even though we may have negative thoughts from time to time, they do not rule our internal life. Even though we may have graphic, violent thoughts, they are not common and we do not act them out. When our brain works right, our spouse may make a mistake, but we do not hold on to that mistake for twenty or thirty years. We feel sexual, but we are not ruled by our sexual desires. Our children may still drive us crazy, but we act toward them in a positive, helpful way the vast majority of the time. When our brain works right, we are more able to be who we really want to be.

Other questions that this work has stimulated me to ask are:

- *What choices do we really have about our behavior? Probably not as many as we think.*
- *Does our relationship with God depend on brain function? Probably it is easier to see a kind, loving, involved God when our brain works right. And it is probably easier to imagine a harsh, punitive God when we have an overactive cingulate and limbic system coloring the world in a negative way. (This will probably get a few people mad at me—I am not trying to be conflict-seeking.)*
- *Do we make bad choices as a result of bad training, in defiance of God's will, as a result of poverty, because of a moral or character defect? Perhaps, but again, we are more likely to make bad choices when our prefrontal cortex is underactive as a result of brain trauma or having ADHD. Of course this doesn't mean we cannot make bad choices as a result of bad training, defiance of God, poverty, and the like, but doing so will be more likely when our internal supervisor is less active than necessary.*
- *Do we make better choices when our brains work right? Of course we do, is the obvious answer from this book.*
- *Is our personality a collection of neurons, neurotransmitters, and hormones? Yes and no. Our personality is intimately connected to brain function, but as we have seen, brain function is also intimately connected to our thoughts and environment. They work in a circle and cannot be separated.*
- *What does Mike Tyson's brain look like? Did he bite Evander Holyfield's ear in the heavyweight championship fight in 1997 because he wanted to embarrass himself and seem like an animal? Or did his brain misfire after a head butt and did his cingulate and temporal lobes consequently go haywire with little prefrontal cortex supervision? I bet on the latter.*
- *What does Saddam Hussein's brain scan look like? What about Adolf Hitler's brain scan?*
- *Should we scan our political leaders? My guess is that we would gain great insight into the political process. Odds are President Ronald Reagan's brain would have demonstrated blood flow patterns indicating Alzheimer's disease in the early part of his presidency. His forgetfulness became obvious during his second term. If we had known about his impending Alzheimer's disease, what then?*

■ *Should I scan my son's and daughters' romantic interests? I think so. My kids are not thrilled about the idea.*

The questions could go on and on. The main point is that the brain matters in all we do. The brain is one of the first things we should think about when we try to understand abnormal behavior. Self-help programs need to consider the brain. To prevent relapse from substance abuse, to cut down on violence in our society, and to curtail the alarming rates of divorce and family discord, we need to think about the brain.

Of course, the brain doesn't function in a vacuum—we always need to think about the psychological and social underpinnings of behavior as well—but all behavior starts in the actual physical functioning of the brain. Your brain matters.

19

Brain Dos and Brain Don'ts:

A Summary of Ways to Optimize Brain Function and Break Bad Brain Habits

Based on my research and that of many other neuroscientists, here is a list of brain dos and don'ts to optimize your own brain function and begin to break bad brain habits that hold you back from getting what you want in life.

Brain Dos:

1. *Wear a helmet in high-risk situations.*
2. *Drink lots of water (six to eight glasses daily) to stay well hydrated.*
3. *Eat healthfully, adjusting the proportion of protein and carbohydrate to your brain needs.*
4. *Take gingko biloba as necessary under your doctor's supervision.*
5. *Think positive, healthy thoughts.*
6. *Love, feed, and exercise your internal anteater to rid yourself of ANTs (automatic negative thoughts, see page 57).*
7. *Every day, take time to focus on the things you are grateful for in your life.*
8. *Watch the Disney movie Pollyanna.*
9. *Spend time with positive, uplifting people.*
10. *Spend time with people you want to be like (you are more likely to become like them).*
11. *Work on your "people skills" to become more connected and to enhance limbic bonds.*
12. *Talk to others in loving, helpful ways.*

13. *Take fish oil daily.*
14. *Build a library of wonderful experiences.*
15. *Make a difference in the life of someone else.*
16. *Exercise.*
17. *Regularly connect with your loved ones.*
18. *Learn diaphragmatic breathing.*
19. *Learn and use self-hypnosis and meditation on a daily basis.*
20. *Remember the "18/40/60 Rule"; see page 108.*
21. *Effectively confront and deal with situations involving conflict.*
22. *Develop clear goals for your life (relationships, work, money and self) and reaffirm them every day.*
23. *Focus on what you like a lot more than what you don't like.*
24. *Collect penguins, or at least send them to me.*
25. *Have meaning, purpose, excitement, and stimulation in your life.*
26. *Establish eye contact with and smile frequently at others.*
27. *Consider brain wave biofeedback or audiovisual stimulation to optimize brain function.*
28. *Notice when you're stuck, distract yourself and come back to the problem later.*
29. *Think through answers before automatically saying no.*
30. *Write out options and solutions when you feel stuck*
31. *Seek the counsel of others when you feel stuck (often just talking about feeling stuck will open new options).*
32. *Memorize and recite the Serenity Prayer (see page 180) daily and whenever bothered by repetitive thoughts* (God, grant me the serenity to accept the things I cannot change, the courage to change the things I can, and the wisdom to know the difference).
33. *Take a break and come back later when you're unsuccessfully trying to convince someone who is stuck.*
34. *Use paradoxical requests in dealing with cingulate people.*
35. *Make naturally oppositional children obey you the first time (through a firm, kind, authoritative stance).*
36. *Learn something new every day.*
37. *Enhance your memory skills.*
38. *Sing and hum whenever you can,*
39. *Make beautiful music a part of your life.*
40. *Make beautiful smells a part of your life.*
41. *Touch others often (appropriately).*
42. *Make love with your partner.*

43. *Move in rhythms.*
44. *Use a skilled psychotherapist when needed.*
45. *Use an EMDR (eye movement desensitization and reprocessing) therapist to deal with trauma.*
46. *Take head injuries seriously, even minor ones.*
47. *Take medication when needed, under your doctor's supervision.*
48. *Take herbal remedies when needed, under your doctor's supervision.*
49. *Consider underlying brain problems in substance abusers.*
50. *Do full brain evaluations for people who do terrible things.*

Brain Don'ts

1. *Isolate a developing baby.*
2. *Use alcohol, tobacco, drugs, or much caffeine when pregnant.*
3. *Ignore erratic behavior.*
4. *Lie around the house and never exercise.*
5. *Ignore concussions.*
6. *Smoke.*
7. *Drink much caffeine.*
8. *Drink much alcohol.*
9. *Do drugs (NO heroin, inhalants, mushrooms, PCP, marijuana, cocaine, methamphetamines [unless in prescribed doses for ADHD]).*
10. *Eat without forethought about what foods are best for your brain.*
11. *Drive without wearing a seat belt.*
12. *Ride a motorcycle, bicycle, skateboard, in-line skates, snowboard, and so forth without a helmet.*
13. *Hit a football with your head.*
14. *Bang your head when you're frustrated (protect the heads of children who are head bangers).*
15. *Bungee jump.*
16. *Hang out with people who do drugs, fight, or are involved in other dangerous activities.*
17. *Allow your breathing to get out of control.*
18. *Think in black-or-white terms.*
19. *Think in words like always, never, every time, everyone.*
20. *Focus on the negative things in your life.*
21. *Predict the worst.*
22. *Think only with your feelings.*

23. Try to read other people's minds.
24. Blame other people for your problems.
25. Label yourself or others with negative terms.
26. Beat up yourself or others with guilt (very ineffective).
27. Personalize situations that have little to do with you.
28. Feed your ANTs.
29. Use sex as a weapon with your partner.
30. Talk to others in a hateful way.
31. Push people away.
32. Be around toxic smells.
33. Be around toxic people.
34. Focus too much on what other people think of you (odds are they aren't thinking about you at all).
35. Allow your life to just happen without you directing and planning it.
36. Take the "stimulant bait" from other people.
37. Be another person's stimulant.
38. Allow thoughts to go over and over in your head.
39. Automatically say no to others; think first if what they want fits with your goals.
40. Automatically say yes to others; think first if what they want fits with your goals.
41. Argue with someone who is stuck.
42. Isolate yourself when you feel worried, depressed, or panicky.
43. Allow naturally oppositional children to be oppositional.
44. Listen to toxic music.
45. Blame substance abusers as morally defective.
46. Refuse to take medication when needed.
47. Self-medicate; when you have problems, get help from professionals.
48. Deny you have problems.
49. Refuse to listen to the people you love who are trying to tell you to get help.
50. Withhold love, touch, and companionship from those you love as a way to express anger.

Appendix

Medication Notes

1. Stimulants

In my opinion these are the first-line medications for treating ADHD without hyperactivity. They are also used to treat narcolepsy, help in some postconcussive syndromes, and are used in resistant depression. Our current understanding of these medications is that they increase dopamine output from the basal ganglia and increase activity in the prefrontal cortex and temporal lobes.

GENERIC NAME	BRAND NAME	MILLIGRAMS A DAY/ AVAILABLE STRENGTHS	TIMES A DAY	NOTES
amphetamine salt combination	Adderall (sustained-release)	5–80/ 5, 10, 20, 30	1–2	my first stimulant of choice for teens and adults
methylphenidate	Ritalin	5–120/ 5, 10, 20	2–4	watch rebound when wears off
methylphenidate sustained-release	Ritalin-SR (sustained-release)	10–120/ 20	1–2	may be erratic in effect
dexamfetamine sulphate	Dexedrine	5–80/ 5	2–4	watch rebound when wears off
dexamfetamine sulphate slow-release caps	Dexedrine Spansules (sustained-release)	5–80/ 5, 10, 15	1–2	

Continued

GENERIC NAME	BRAND NAME	MILLIGRAMS A DAY/ AVAILABLE STRENGTHS	TIMES A DAY	NOTES
pemoline	Cylert	18.75–112.5, up to 150 for adults/ 18.75, 37.5, 75	1–2	routine liver screening essential

- Contrary to popular belief, these are considered very safe medications when taken as prescribed under a doctor's supervision.
- The PDR (Physicians Desk Reference) lists 60 milligrams as the top dosage for Ritalin and 40 milligrams as the top dosage for Adderall and Dexedrine. Many clinicians, like myself, feel the range of effectiveness may be much higher for some individuals.
- With Cylert it is very important to monitor liver function tests, as 2 to 3 percent of people taking this medication may develop chemical hepatitis.
- Do not take stimulants with citrus juices (orange, grapefruit, lemon). They lessen the effect.
- Decrease caffeine intake when taking a stimulant. Caffeine and these stimulants together tend to overstimulate the nervous system.
- The common side effects of stimulants tend to be decreased appetite, sleep problems (if taken too late in the day), and transient headaches or stomachaches.

2. Tricyclic Antidepressants (TCAs) and Bupropion (Zyban)

These medications are effective antidepressants. They tend to decrease overactive limbic activity. These medications increase various neuro-transmitters, including noradrenaline (imipramine, desipramine, doxepin), dopamine (bupropion), serotonin (clomipramine), or a combination of these (amitriptyline, nortriptyline). They tend to be more stimulating than the others listed. Many of these are now considered second-line medications for depression because they tend to have more side effects than the SSRIs (next section). Yet some of them also have significant advantages. When depression is mixed with anxiety, imipramine and desipramine may be a better choice. When depression is mixed with ADHD, desipramine, imipramine, bupropion, and ven-lafaxine (see next section) seem to be the most effective. Bed-wetting and depression or anxiety may best respond to imipramine. A skilled psychopharmacologist can help you sort through these medications.

GENERIC NAME	BRAND NAME	MILLIGRAMS A DAY/ AVAILABLE STRENGTHS	TIMES A DAY	NOTES
desipramine (TCA)	Norpramin	10–300/ 10, 25, 50, 75, 100, 150	1–2	stimulating; often helps ADHD in adults, not currently used in children
imipramine (TCA)	Tofranil	10–300/ 10, 25, 50, 75, 100, 125, 150	1–2	also used for anxiety, panic disorder, bed-wetting
bupropion	Zyban	50–450/ 75, 100	1–3	never > 150 mg a dose; do not use if prone to seizures
bupropion sustained-release	Zyban SR	150–450/ 50, 100, 150	1–3	never > 150 mg a dose; do not use if prone to seizures
amitriptyline (TCA)	Triptafen	10–300/ 10, 25, 50, 75, 100, 150	1–2	often used to help with sleep problems, headaches, fibromyalgia, and pain syndromes
nortriptyline (TCA)	Allegron	10–150/ 10, 25, 50, 75	1–2	often used to help with sleep problems, headaches, fibromyalgia, and pain syndromes
doxepin (TCA)	Sinepin	10–300/ 10, 25, 50, 75, 100, 150	1–2	often used to help with sleep problems
clomipramine (TCA)	Anafranil	10–200 for a child, 10–300 for an adult/ 25, 50, 75	1–2	also used for OCD

- These medications need to be monitored more closely than stimulants, especially their effect on heart function.
- Many adults respond to very low doses of these medications for ADHD symptoms. This is important because the low doses often produce far fewer side effects than the higher "antidepressant" doses.
- Unlike stimulants, these may take several weeks to a month to become effective.
- When Zyban was first released in the United States, a number of people developed seizures while taking it. It was pulled from the market in the early 1980s. The manufacturer figured out that the dosage pattern was wrong, and the FDA allowed it to rerelease it with

a different dosage regimen. Do not take more than 150 milligrams at a time.

- *These medications are usually not first-line treatments for ADHD. I use these medications to treat depression, anxiety disorders, bedwetting, and the limbic subtype of ADHD, often in conjunction with one of the stimulants.*

3. Antiobsessive or 'Antistuck' Medications

These medications increase the availability of serotonin in the brain, and they are often helpful to calm down cingulate hyperactivity. They are typically marketed as antidepressants. They also tend to calm down limbic hyperactivity. Except for Efexor, these medications are not first-line treatments for ADHD and, in fact, they may make ADHD worse. These serotonin-enhancing medications are also used to treat eating disorders, obsessive-compulsive disorder, oppositional defiant disorder, PMS (overfocused type), excessive worrying, temper problems associated with things not going a person's way, and other cingulate problems listed in this book.

GENERIC NAME	BRAND NAME	MILLIGRAMS A DAY/ AVAILABLE STRENGTHS	TIMES A DAY	NOTES
fluoxetine (SSRI)	Prozac	10–80/ 10, 20	1	long acting; do not use if temporal lobe symptoms present
clomipramine (TCA & SSRI)	Anafranil	10–200 in children, 10–300 in adults/ 25, 50, 75	1–2	tends to have more side effects, so not used as a first-line drug
sertraline (SSRI)	Lustral 25,50,100	25–200/ 25, 50, 100	1	often my first choice of these meds
paroxetine (SSRI)	Seroxat	10–60/ 10, 20, 30, 40	1	
fluvoxamine (SSRI)	Faverin	25–200/ 50, 100	1	
venlafaxine	Efexor	37.5–300/ 18.75, 25, 37.5, 50, 75, 100	2–3	best of these meds for ADHD symptoms
mirtazapine	Zispin	15–60/ 15, 30	1	smaller doses cause drowsiness

- Contrary to the negative media attention, Prozac is generally a very safe medication. In our experience, however, people who have temporal lobe problems may experience an intensification of angry and aggressive feelings on Prozac or other serotonin-enhancing medications. Therefore, we are careful to screen for these before placing someone on these medications. If you have side effects on any medication, it is important to contact your doctor and discuss them.
- Unlike stimulants, these may take several weeks to several months in order to be effective and even three to four months to become optimally effective.
- The most common side effect of these medications is sexual dysfunction. Sometimes adding gingko biloba or bupropion counteracts these problems.

4. Anticonvulsants or Antiseizure Medications

These medications are used to treat temporal lobe dysfunction, seizures, aggression, emotional instability, headaches, resistant depression, and bipolar disorder. They are often very effective in resistant psychiatric conditions where all else has failed.

GENERIC NAME	BRAND NAME	MILLIGRAMS A DAY/ AVAILABLE STRENGTHS	TIMES A DAY	NOTES
carbamazepine	Tegretol	100–200/ 100, 200	2	essential to monitor white blood cell count and blood levels
valproic acid	Depakene	125–3,000/ 250	1–2	monitor liver function and blood levels
valproate semisodium	Depakote	125–3,000/ 125, 250, 500	1–2	monitor liver function and blood levels
gabapentin	Neurontin	100–4,000/ 100, 300, 400	1–2	tends to have the smallest number of side effects
lamotrigine	Lamictal	25–500/ 25, 100, 150, 200	1–2	start slow, watch for rash
phenytoin	Epanutin	30–300/ 30, 100	1–2	monitor blood levels

- *Tegretol and Depakote/Depakene are used as primary treatments for manic-depressive disorder. Neurontin and Lamictal are now also being used for this as well.*
- *These are often helpful for people with ADHD and violent outbursts or those who have experienced head trauma.*

5. Blood Pressure Medications

The following blood pressure medications have been used to help with tic disorders, hyperactivity, aggressiveness, and impulsivity. They are not usually helpful with the attentional symptoms, and they are often mixed with a stimulant medication when ADHD is present.

GENERIC NAME	BRAND NAME	MILLIGRAMS A DAY/ AVAILABLE STRENGTHS	TIMES A DAY	NOTES
clonidine	Catapres	0.05–0.6/ 0.1, 0.2, 0.3 tabs and patches	1–2	watch rebound hypertension and sedation
propranolol	Inderal	10–600/ 10, 20, 40, 60, 80	2–3	helpful with hand tremors as well

- *Clonidine is also used as a primary treatment for tic disorders such as Tourette's syndrome.*
- *When I use clonidine in addition to a stimulant medication, I order a screening EKG. There have been several reports that this combination may cause problems, even though I have found it to be effective and safe.*
- *These medications are also used to treat insomnia, which is very common in ADHD.*

6. Combination Medications

People can have more than one problem or more than one brain system involved in their symptoms. Sometimes one medication seems to be able to treat a number of problems, as mentioned above, and sometimes a combination of medications is needed to obtain full therapeutic benefit.

Here are four common combinations I use in my practice.

- *A stimulant plus an antiobsessive antidepressant (such as Adderall plus Efexor) for patients with ADHD plus depression, obsessiveness,* or severe oppositional behavior. In my clinical experience I have seen many people who are children or grandchildren of alcoholics benefit from this combination. Frequently, this population presents with cingulate (overfocus symptoms) and prefrontal cortex problems (attentional symptoms).

- An anticonvulsant plus an antiobsessive antidepressant (such as Depakote plus Lustral) for patients with temper problems and excessive worrying or depression.
- A blood pressure medication, plus a stimulant and an antiobsessive antidepressant (such as Catapres, Adderall, plus Efexor) for patients with Tourette's syndrome, ADHD, and OCD.
- A tricyclic antidepressant plus a blood pressure medication (such as Tofranil plus Inderal) for patients with depression, anxiety, and hand tremors in social situations.

Bibliography

Abdel-Dayem HM, Abu-Judeh H, Kumar M, Atay S, NADHDaf S, El-Zef-tawy H, Luo JO: SPECT *brain* perfusion abnormalities in mild or moderate traumatic *brain* injury. *Clin. Nucl. Med.* 23 (5), May 1998, 309–17.

Alavi A, Hirsch LJ: Studies of central nervous system disorders with single photon emission computed tomography and positron emission tomography: evolution over the past 2 decades. *Semin. Nucl. Med.* 21 (1), Jan. 1991, 58–81.

Amen DG: New directions in the theory, diagnosis, and treatment of mental disorders: The use of SPECT imaging in everyday clinical practice. In *The Neuropsychology of Mental Disorders,* ed. Koziol and Stout (Springfield, IL: Charles C Thomas, 1994), 286–311.

Amen DG, Stubblefield MS, Carmichael B: Brain SPECT findings and aggressiveness. *Annals of Clinical Psychiatry* 8 (3), 1996, 129–37.

Amen DG, Carmichael B: High resolution brain SPECT imaging in ADHD. *Annals of Clinical Psychiatry* 9 (2), 1997, 81–86.

Amen DG: Three years on clomipramine: Before and after brain SPECT study. *Annals of Clinical Psychiatry* 9 (2), 1997, 113–16.

Amen DG, Waugh M: High resolution brain SPECT imaging in marijuana smokers with AD/HD. *Journal of Psychoactive Drugs* 30 (2), April–June 1998, 1–13.

Amen DG, Yantis S, Trudeau J: Visualizing the firestorms in the brain: An inside look at the clinical and physiological connections between drugs and violence using brain SPECT imaging. *Journal of Psychoactive Drugs* 29 (4), 1997, 307–19.

Amen DG: Brain SPECT imaging in psychiatry. *Primary Psychiatry* 5 (8), August 1998, 83–90.

Andreason NC (ed.): *Brain Imaging: Applications in Psychiatry* (Washington, D.C.: American Psychiatric Press, 1989).

Bavetta S, Nimmon CC, White J, McCabe J, Huneidi AH, Bomanji J, Birkenfeld B, Charlesworth M, Britton KE, Greenwood RJ: A prospective study comparing SPET with MRI and CT as prognostic indicators following severe closed head injury. *Nucl. Med. Commun.* 15 (12), Dec. 1994, 961–68.

Bonte FJ, Weiner MF, Bigio EH, White CL: Brain blood flow in the dementias: SPECT with histopathologic correlation in 54 patients. *Radiology* 202 (3), Mar. 1997, 793–97

Ceballos C, Baringo T, Carrero P, Ventura T, Pelegr n C: Chronic schizophrenia: validity of the study of *regional cerebral blood* flow through *cerebral SPECT. Rev. Neurol.* 25 (145), Sep. 1997, 1346–49.

Costa DC: The role of nuclear medicine in neurology and psychiatry. *Curr. Opin. Neurol. Neurosurg.* 5 (6), Dec. 1992, 863–69.

Friberg L: Brain mapping in thinking and language function. *Acta Neurochir. Suppl. (Wien)* 56, 1993, 34–39.

George MS, et al.: *Neuroactivation and Neuroimaging with SPECT* (Berlin, Heidelberg, New York: Springer-Verlag, 1991).

George MS, Trimble MR, Costa DC, Robertson MM, Ring HA, Ell PJ: Elevated frontal cerebral blood flow in Gilles de la Tourette syndrome: a 99Tcm-HMPAO SPECT study. *Psychiatry Res.* 45 (3), Nov. 1992, 143–51.

George MS, Ketter TA, Post RM: SPECT and PET imaging in mood disorders. *J. Clin. Psychiatry* 54 Suppl., Nov. 1993, 6–13.

George MS, Ketter TA, Parekh PI, Horwitz B, Herscovitch P, Post RM: Brain activity during transient sadness and happiness in healthy women. *Am. J. Psychiatry* 152 (3), Mar. 1995, 341–51.

Gunther W, Müller N, Knesewitsch P, Haag C, Trapp W, Banquet JP, Stieg C, Alper KR: Functional EEG mapping and SPECT in detoxified male alcoholics. *Eur. Arch. Psychiatry Clin. Neurosci.* 247 (3), 1997, 128–36.

Hoehn-Saric R, Pearlson GD, Harris GJ, Machlin SR, Camargo EE: Effects of fluoxetine on regional cerebral blood flow in obsessive-compulsive patients. *Am. J. Psychiatry* 148 (9), Sep. 1991, 1243–45.

Holman BL, Devous MD Sr: Functional brain SPECT: the emergence of a powerful clinical method. *J. Nucl. Med.* 33 (10), Oct. 1992, 1888–904.

Holman BL, Garada B, Johnson KA, Mendelson J, Hallgring E, Teoh SK, Worth J, Navia B: A comparison of brain perfusion SPECT in cocaine abuse and AIDS dementia complex. J. Nucl. Med. 33 (7), July 1992, 1312–15.

Iyo M, Namba H, Yanagisawa M, Hirai S, Yui N, Fukui S: Abnormal cerebral perfusion in chronic methamphetamine abusers: a study using 99MTc-HMPAO and SPECT. Prog. Neuropsychopharmacol Biol. Psychiatry 21 (5), July 1997, 789–96.

Jacobs A, Put E, Ingels M, Bossuyt A: Prospective evaluation of technetium-99m-HMPAO SPECT in mild and moderate traumatic brain injury [see comments]. J. Nucl. Med. 35 (6), June 1994, 942–47.

Kao CH, Wang SJ, Yeh SH: Presentation of regional cerebral blood flow in amphetamine abusers by 99Tcm-HMPAO brain SPECT. Nucl. Med. Commun. 15 (2), Feb. 1994, 94–98.

Kuruoíglu AC, Arikan Z, Vural G, Karatas M; Arac M; Isik E: Single photon emission computerised tomography in chronic alcoholism. Antisocial personality disorder may be associated with decreased frontal perfusion. Br. J. Psychiatry 169 (3), Sep. 1996, 348–54.

Legido A, Price ML, Wolfson B, Faerber EN, Foley C, Miles D, Grover WD: Technetium 99mTc-HMPAO SPECT in children and adolescents with neurologic disorders. J. Child Neurol. 8 (3), July 1993, 227–34.

Levin JM, Holman BL, Mendelson JH, Teoh SK, Garada B, Johnson KA, Springer S: Gender differences in cerebral perfusion in cocaine abuse: technetium-99m-HMPAO SPECT study of drug-abusing women. J. Nucl. Med. 35 (12), Dec. 1994, 1902–9.

Machlin SR, Harris GJ, Pearlson GD, Hoehn-Saric R, Jeffery P, Camargo EE: Elevated medial-frontal cerebral blood flow in obsessive-compulsive patients: a SPECT study. Am. J. Psychiatry 148 (9), Sep. 1991, 1240–42.

Masdeu JC, Abdel-Dayem H, Van Heertum RL: Head trauma: use of SPECT. J. Neuroimaging 5 Suppl. 1, July 1995, S53–57.

Mathew RJ, Wilson WH: Substance abuse and cerebral blood flow. Am. J. Psychiatry 148 (3), Mar. 1991, 292–305.

Mena I, Giombetti RJ, Miller BL, Garrett K, Villanueva-Meyer J, Mody C, Goldberg MA: Cerebral blood flow changes with acute cocaine intoxication: clinical correlations with SPECT, CT, and MRI. NIDA Res. Monogr. 138, 1994, 161–73.

Messa C, Fazio F, Costa DC, Ell PJ: Clinical brain radionuclide imaging studies. Semin. Nucl. Med. 25 (2), Apr. 1995, 111–43.

Miller BL, Mena I, Giombetti R, Villanueva-Meyer J, Djenderedjian AH:

Neuropsychiatric effects of cocaine: SPECT measurements.
J. Addict, Dis. 11(4), 1992, 47–58.

Newberg AB, Alavi A, Payer F: Single photon emission computed
tomography in Alzheimer's disease and related disorders. Neuroimaging Clin. N. Am. 5 (1), Feb. 1995, 103–23.

O'Connell RA, Sireci SN Jr, et al.: The role of SPECT brain imaging in
assessing psychopathology in the medically ill. Gen. Hosp.
Psychiatry 13 (5), Sep. 1991, 305–12.

O'Connell RA, Van Heertum RL, et al.: Single photon emission computed tomography (SPECT) with [123I]IMP in the differential diagnosis of psychiatric disorders. J. Neuropsychiatry Clin. Neurosci. 1 (2),
Spring 1989, 145–53.

O'Connell RA, Van Heertum RL, Luck D, Yudd AP, Cueva JE, Billick SB,
Cordon DJ, Gersh RJ, Masdeu JC: Single-photon emission computed
tomography of the brain in acute mania and schizophrenia.
J. Neuroimaging 5 (2), Apr. 1995, 101–4.

O'Tuama LA, Treves ST: Brain single-photon emission computed
tomography for behavior disorders in children. Semin. Nucl. Med. 23
(3), July 1993, 255–64.

Raine A, Buchsbaum MS, Stanley J, et al.: Selective reductions in prefrontal glucose metabolism in murderers. Biol. Psychiatry 36 (6), Sep.
1994, 365–73.

Rose JS, Branchey M, Buydens-Branchey L, Stapleton JM, Chasten K,
Werrell A, Maayan ML: Cerebral perfusion in early and late opiate
withdrawal: a technetium-99m-HMPAO SPECT study. Psychiatry Res.
96 (1), May 1996, 39–47.

Rubin RT, Villanueva-Meyer J, Ananth J, Trajmar PG, Mena I: Regional
xenon 133 cerebral blood flow and cerebral technetium 99m
HMPAO uptake in unmedicated patients with obsessive-
compulsive disorder and matched normal control subjects.
Determination by high-resolution single-photon emission
computed tomography. Arch. Gen. Psychiatry 49 (9), Sep. 1992,
695–702.

Rubin P, Holm S, Madsen PL, Friberg L, Videbech P, Andersen HS,
Bendsen BB, Stromso N, Larsen JK, Lassen NA, et al.: Regional
cerebral blood flow distribution in newly diagnosed
schizophrenia and schizophreniform disorder. Psychiatry Res. 53 (1),
July 1994, 57–75.

Rumsey JM, Andreason P, Zametkin AJ: Right frontotemporal

activation by tonal memory in dyslexia, an O15 PET Study. *Biol. Psychiatry* 36 (3), Aug. 1994, 171–80.

Schlosser R, Schlegel S: D2–receptor imaging with [123I]IBZM and single photon emission tomography in psychiatry: a survey of current status. *J. Neural Transm. Gen. Sect.* 99 (1–3), 1995, 173–85.

Semple WE, Goyer PF, McCormick R, Compton-Toth B, Morris E, Donovan B, Muswick G, Nelson D, Garnett ML, Sharkoff J, Leisure G, Miraldi F, Schulz SC: Attention and regional cerebral blood flow in posttraumatic stress disorder patients with substance abuse histories. *Psychiatry Res.* 67 (1), May 1996, 17–28.

Trzepacz PT, Hertweck M, Starratt C, Zimmerman L, Adatepe MH: The relationship of SPECT scans to behavioral dysfunction in neuro-psychiatric patients. *Psychosomatics* 33 (1), Winter 1992, 62–71.

Tunving K, Thulin SO, Risberg J, Warkentin S: Regional cerebral blood flow in long-term heavy cannabis use. *Psychiatry Res.* 17 (1), Jan. 1986, 15–21.

Van Heertum RL, Miller SH, Mosesson RE: Spect brain imaging in neurologic disease. *Radiol. Clin. North. Am.* 31 (4), July 1993, 881–907.

Van Heertum RL and Tikofsky RS (eds.): *Advances in Cerebral SPECT Imaging* (New York: Trivirun Publishing, 1995).

Wolfe N, Reed BR, Eberling JL, Jagust WJ: Temporal lobe perfusion on single photon emission computed tomography predicts the rate of cognitive decline in Alzheimer's disease. *Arch. Neurol.* 52 (3), Mar. 1995, 257–62.

Wu J, Amen D: The clinical use of functional brain imaging. In *The Comprehensive Textbook of Psychiatry*, ed. Kaplan and Sadock, 1999.

Zametkin AJ, Nordahl TE, et al.: Cerebral glucose metabolism in adults with hyperactivity of childhood onset. *N. Eng J. Med.* 323 (20), Nov. 1990, 1361–66.

Index

Please note that page references to SPECT photographs will be in *italic* print

absentmindedness, 21
abuse
    of children, 227
    and SPECT, 23–24
    see also substance abuse
accidents, and basal ganglia system, 84–85, 86
adaptability, 157
ADD *see* attention deficit hyperactivity disorder (ADHD)
Adderall
    for ADHD, 86, 96, 126, 266
    for caffeine use, 250
    for substance abuse, 235–36
addictions, 165, 167
    see also alcohol abuse; substance abuse
ADHD *see* attention deficit hyperactivity disorder (ADHD)
adrenaline, 124
aggressiveness
    atypical behaviour, 17
    in children, 30, 110, 111
    impulsiveness in, 224
    left-side abnormalities, 225
    and nutrition, 216–17
    substance abuse in, 254–57
    temporal lobes in, 9, 198–99, 201, 225
        relational traits, 278
    see also violence
agoraphobia, 91
alcohol abuse, 29, 238–43

case histories, 239–43
and cingulate system, 172
eliminating alcohol, 113
as self-medication for underlying brain problems, 257–59
support for, 70
and violence, 229, 254–55
and work, 111
see also substance abuse
Alice's Adventures in Wonderland (Carroll), 207
alpha brain waves, 148
alprazolam (Xanax), 112
always/never thinking, 62, 65
Alzheimer's disease
    and depression, 22
    living with patient, 21
    SPECT of, *205*, *206*
    and temporal lobe dysfunction, 204–5
amantadine (Symmetrel), 134
Amen Clinic for Behavioral Medicine, Brain Imaging Division, 15
amino acids, examples, 83, 113, 190–91
amphetamines, 128
anabolic steroids, and violence, 254
Anafranil (clomipramine)
    for cingulate system, 164, 165, 166, 186–87
    for intimate relationships, 281
    for suicidal tendencies, 229
anatomical studies, 14
anger

in ADHD, 124
automatic negative thoughts, 58
basal ganglia system in, 93
breathing, effect on, 103
and divorce, 47
head injuries, 135
in partner, taking seriously, 288–89
personality changes, 34
in PMS, 54
in PTSD, 93
road rage, 161–62
animals
bonding disruption, 45
deep limbic system of, 41
antidepressants, 79
antiobsessive, 35, 165
for basal ganglia system, 112–13
benefits versus side-effects, 49–50
coming off too soon, 28, 173
for manic-depression, 52
MAOs, 91
new, on market, 80
and people skills, 73
and physical exercise, 81
sensationalism, 49
see also specific drugs
antisocial personality disorder, x
anxiety, 3–4
and alcohol, eliminating, 113
of author, 9, 25–26
automatic negative thoughts, 57, 101
basal ganglia system in, 87, 91
case histories, 6
in children, 131
and conflict avoidance, 94
in delusional thinking, 130
diaphragmatic breathing for, 102–04
prefrontal cortex in, 119
and professional care, 291, 293
in PTSD, 93
in workplace, 292
appetite
changes in, following head injuries,
34
deep limbic system in, 41, 45, 47
and divorce, 47
and physical exercise, 81
see also nutrition
aromatherapy, 77, 113
Ascher, L. M., 182
assertiveness, 111–12
lack of in conflict avoidance, 94, 95
Ativan (lorazepam), 112
attention deficit disorder (ADD) see
attention deficit hyperactivity

disorder (ADHD)
attention deficit hyperactivity disorder
(ADHD), 6–8, 119–29
in adults, 6, 32, 33, 123
attention spans, 120–21
basal ganglia system in, 85, 86
and biofeedback, 148–49
and caffeine use, 249, 250
case histories, 32, 33, 126–29
in children, 6, 30, 32, 123
concentration problems, 120
and depression, 123
disorganization in, 124–25
distractability and distraction, 121–22
genetic factors, 32, 127–29
impulsiveness, 30, 122
incidence of, 125
as medical problem, 15
medication for, 6, 86, 151
moodiness and negative thinking, 125
music for, 154
and nutrition, 153–54
and OCD, 95–96
prefrontal cortex in, 6, 7, 118
and professional care, 296
projects, failure to finish, 125
SPECT of, 6–7, 120, 126, 128, 129, 151
and substance abuse, 235
symptoms of, 6, 30, 145
terminology, 119n
worrying, 123
see also prefrontal cortex (pfc)
attention spans, 117, 120–21
audiovisual stimulation, 149
autistic children, bonding with, 75–76
automatic negative thoughts (ANTs),
57–68
always/never thinking, 62, 65, 67
bad thoughts, as pollution, 60
blaming, 65, 66, 67
body, effect on, 58–59
effects of, 57
examples, 57
extermination/extinguishing of,
61–66, 100–101, 177, 282
examples, 67–68
feeding them to your anteaters,
66–68
focusing on the negative, 62–63, 65
fortune-telling, 63, 67
see also fortune-telling
guilt, 64, 66
inaccuracies of, 60
labeling, 64–65, 66, 67
mind reading, 63–64, 66, 67

personalizing, 65, 66
summary of species of, 65–66
talking back to, 61, 66
thinking with your feelings, 64, 66
writing down, 61, 67, 101
see also negativeness
automatic no, 160–61, 178
see also negativeness

"baby blues", 45
basal ganglia system
and accidents, 84–85, 86
checklist for, 98–99
conflict, dealing with, 109–12
and deep limbic system, 113
diaphragmatic breathing for, 102–04
18/40/60 rule, 108–09
fortune-telling, eliminating, 100–101
functions of, 9, 84–89
guided imagery, 102
medication for, 112–13
meditation/self-hypnosis for, 104–08
motor problems, 86, 87, 97
overactive/underactive, 85, 87, 241,
271
in author, 9, 25–27, 105
panic and panic disorder, 89, 90–92
partners of people with basal ganglia
problems, 271
prescriptions for, 26, 92, 100–113
for partner, 283–84
for self, 283
problems with, 89–99
relational traits, 270–72
and romantic love, 88–89
soothing, 104
SPECT of, 85
and violence, 224
behavior
abnormalities interfering with, 7
brain as seat of, 35
brain patterns that correlate with,
3–4
modeled, suicide as, 229
provocative, 261–62
violent *see under* violence
behavior therapy, 164, 172
behavioral shaping, 144
Benson, Herbert, 104
benzodiazepines, 112
bereavement, 46, 47, 78
binge eating, 167
biofeedback, 92, 103
brain-wave, 147–49
description of, 147–48

relationship problems, 271
for temporal lobes, 217
bipolar disorder *see* manic-depression
blaming, 21, 65, 66
body, effect of automatic negative
thoughts on, 58–59
body dysmorphic disorder, 165
body language, 31, 33
bonding
with children, 41, 75
failure to bond, 45
deep limbic system in, 8, 41
disruption, 45–48
positive, surrounding yourself with
people providing, 69–70
and smell, 42
two-way nature of, 75
brain
anatomical studies, 14
as body's computer, 36
dissemination of information on, 4
and genetic factors, 25, 27
as hardware of soul, 3
identifying own brain type, 9
impact of abnormalities on families,
225, 226–27
infections of, 204
interconnectedness of systems, 9
and marriage, 30–37
optimization of physical functioning
of, 7–8, 307–10
own good, gaining access to, 294–95
and oxygen, 103
physiology of, 3, 8–10
abnormal, 36
in PMS, 27–28
"reptilian", 38
rescanning following treatment, 53
as seat of feelings/behavior, 35
substance abuse, effect of, 232–52
brain-waves/brain-wave biofeedback,
147–49
breakfasts, recommended, 153
Breaking Through (Amen), 5
breast cancer, support for sufferers, 70
breathing exercises, 106, 283
see also diaphragmatic breathing
breathing rates, 104
bulimia, 166
bullying, 110, 111
bupropion, 22, 153, 269, 281
buspirone (BuSpar), 112

caffeine, 216, 249–50
Campbell, Don, 211–12

cancer, fear of, 90
carbamazepine see Tegretol
  (carbamazepine)
carbohydrates, 82, 83, 216, 217, 286
  simple, eliminating, 153
  see also nutrition
Carlson, Tucker, ix, x
Carroll, Lewis, 207
Carter, John, 149
Cartesian thinking, x
cerebral cortex, 39
chamomile, oils of, 113
chanting, 215
children
  ADHD in, 6, 30, 32, 123
  aggressiveness in, 30, 110, 111
  anxiety in, 131
  autistic, 75–76
  bonding with, 41, 75
    failure to bond, 45
    protecting with limbic bonding,
      71–72
  bullying, 110, 111
  and divorce, 31
  home, leaving, 48
  homicidal thoughts in, 9, 13
  music, benefits for, 214
  OCD in, 172
  oppositional, dealing with, 183–86
    see also oppositional defiant
      disorder (ODD)
  school problems, 30
  suicidal tendencies in, 9, 13
  violent behavior, 9, 13, 201
  women as main caretakers of, 43
  see also parents
cigarette smoking, 216, 234, 249–50
cingulate system, 155–75
  and addictions, 259–61
  and ADHD, 32
  "attack and retreat" model, 181–82
  automatic no, 160–61
  checklist for, 175
  cognitive inflexibility, 159–60
  and deep limbic system, 54
  in dementia, 21
  distractability and distraction,
    177–78, 181, 183
  exercise for, 190–91
  family therapy, 173–75
  functions of, 9, 155–57
  future-oriented thinking, 156–57
  as "gear shifter", 9
  and head injuries, 35
  hurts, holding on to, 159

  medications for, 186–88
  nutrition for, 189–90
  obsessive-compulsive disorder,
    29–30, 162–64
  overactive/underactive, 32, 159
  overfocus issues, 32, 190, 291, 293
  paradoxical requests, making, 182–83
  parental behavior recommended,
    184–86
  partners of people with cingulate
    problems, 276
  and prefrontal cortex, 259–61
  prescriptions for, 176–91
    for partner, 287
    for self, 286
  problems with, 157–75
  relational traits, 275–76
  road rage, 161–62
  sections of, 156
  seeking counsel of others when
    stuck, 179–80
  Serenity Prayer, memorizing/reciting,
    180
  SPECT of, 189
  and stress, 171–73
  thinking through before saying no, 178
  vulnerability of, 197
  worrying, 158
  writing out options and solutions,
    178–79
cinnamon, 77
classical music, 212–14
cleaning, obsessive, 162
clinical depression see depression
clomipramine see Anafranil
  (clomipramine)
clonazepam see Rivotril (clonazepam)
cocaine, 87–88, 89, 234–37, 241, 254
  case histories, 240, 241
codeine, 243
cognitive flexibility, 155–56
  inflexibility, 54, 159–60, 190
cognitive impairment, and sleep
  deprivation, 216
cognitive therapy, 73
Colt, George Howe, 76
communication skills, 74
complex carbohydrates, 83
compulsions, 162, 174
  examples of, 163–64
  paying too much attention to, in
    OCD, 95
  and SPECT, 29–30
computerized axial tomography (CAT)
  scans, 14, 17

concentration, in ADHD, 120
conduct disorder, x, xi
confabulation, 238
conflict avoidance
  of author, 26–27
  basal ganglia system in, 94–95
  fearing conflict, examples, 110–11
  in intimate relationships, 111
  learning to deal with conflict, 109–12,
    283
conflict seeking, in ADHD, 122–24
confusion, 103, 219, 220
cooperativeness, 156
coordination, basal ganglia system in,
  86
counting compulsion, 164
cyclic mood disorders, 28, 51, 53
  see also manic-depression;
    premenstrual syndrome (PMS)
Cylert (pemoline), 224
cysts, xi, xii, 9–13

dancing, 215
deaths
  bonding disruption, 46–47
  obsession with, 227
  positive memories, building, 78
  by suicide see suicidal tendencies
debt problems, in OCD spectrum
  disorders, 165, 168–69
decision-making, 3, 261–62
deep limbic system, 8–9
  of animals, 41
  and appetite, 45
  automatic negative thoughts see
    automatic negative thoughts
    (ANTs)
  and basal ganglia system, 113
  and bonding, 8, 41
    see also bonding
  checklist for, 55
  and cingulate system, 54
  and diet, 82–83
  emotional stability, tone, and color,
    39–41
  estrogen receptors in, 28
  exercise, benefits of, 80–82
  functions of, 38–44
  gender differences in, 43
  inflammation in, 49
  left side, hotter activity in, 54
  and limbic system, 38n
  location of, 38
  medications for, 79–80
  and memories, 40

memories, building library of, 77–79
and nervous system, 43–44
nutrition, 82–83
overactive/underactive, 27, 39, 40, 41,
  42, 49, 53, 268
people skills for, 73–74
and physical bonding, 74
physical contact for, 74–76, 282
positive bonding, people providing,
  69–70
and prefrontal cortex, 44, 117
prescriptions for, 50, 56–83
  for partner, 282–83
  for self, 281–82
problems in, 44–54
relational traits, 268–70
and sexuality, 42
and sleep, 45
smell, sense of, 41
SPECT of, 22
views of, 39
déjà vu, 203, 219, 220
delta brain waves, 148
delusional thinking, 51, 130
dementia
  Alzheimer's disease see Alzheimer's
    disease
  and functional brain images of
    sufferers, 5
  SPECT of, 17, 22
Depakote (valproate semisodium), 28,
  113, 204
  for headaches, 203
  for manic-depressive disorder, 53
  for motor problems, 97
  for PMS, 54
  for post-traumatic stress disorder, 93
  for prefrontal cortex, 130
  for suicidal tendencies, 229
  for temporal lobes, 198, 207, 208, 215
  for violence, 225
depression, 3–4, 29, 48
  in ADHD, 123
  and Alzheimer's disease, 22
  atypical, 45
  and automatic negative thoughts, 58
  bonding disruption, 48–51
  case histories, 6
  deep limbic system in, 22, 39
  and divorce, 47
  dopamine levels, 83
  eating and sleeping difficulties, 45
  empty nest syndrome, 48
  and functional brain images of
    sufferers, 5

gender differences in, 43
as medical problem, 15
and motivation, 41
negative thinking, 57
noradrenaline levels, 83
and people skills, 73
in PMS, 27
postnatal, 45
and professional care, 291, 293
selective memory in, 78
and serotonin, lack of, 49, 83
and sexuality, 42
SPECT of, 20
treatable nature of, 49
at work, 110, 111, 291
desipramine (Norpramin), 152
Dexedrine (dextroamphetamine), 86, 96, 149
diaphragmatic breathing, 26, 102–04, 271
diazepam (Valium), 91, 112
addiction to, 92
Dilaudid (hydromorphone), 243
disorganization see organization
distractability and distraction, 3–4
in ADHD, 120, 121–22
cingulate system in, 177–78, 181, 183
oppositional children, dealing with, 183
prefrontal cortex in, 119
divalproex see Depakote (valproate semisodium)
divorces
and alcohol problems, 239
as bonding disruption, 47–48
and effects on children, 31
and PTSD, 92
see also intimate relationships; marriages
dopamine
and ADHD, 96
low levels of, 82
medications increasing, 86, 87, 88, 151
see also Ritalin (methylphenidate)
and motivation, 97
and nutrition, 153–54
and Parkinson's disease, 87
and serotonin, 96
see also serotonin
Dostoyevsky, Fyodor, 205–06
drive see motivation
drug abuse see substance abuse
DSM-IV (diagnostic bible), xii
dyslexia, 200

eating disorders, 165, 166–67, 169
ecstasy see pleasure/ecstasy
EEG see electroencephalograms (EEGs)
Efexor (venlafaxine), 153, 164, 186
for intimate relationships, 281
18/40/60 rule, 108–09
electroencephalograms (EEGs), 3
limitations of, 14
and prefrontal cortex, 148
and temporal lobes, 217
and violent behavior, 219, 221, 228
EMDR (eye movement desensitization), 188
emotional shading, in deep limbic system, 39–41
emotional stability, and temporal lobes, 195
empty nest syndrome, 48
encephalitis, 204
endorphins, 80
energy, 83, 109, 191
entrainment, 149
essential oils, 77, 113
estrogen receptors, in deep limbic system, 28
exercise, physical
for cingulate system, 190–91
for deep limbic system, 80–82
in intimate relationships, 286, 287

family therapy, 173–75
fats, 82
Faverin (fluvoxamine), 97, 164, 186
fear
basal ganglia system in, 87, 91
of public speaking, 109
right-side abnormalities, 225
and violent feelings, 219
feelings, thinking with, 64, 66
fight-or-flight response, 44
finger agnosia, 86
flexibility, cognitive, 155–56
fluoxetine see Prozac (fluoxetine)
fluvoxamine, 97, 164, 186
focus
developing and maintaining, 138–41
focusing problems, in deep limbic system, 83
in pfc, 138–44
on positive, 142–44
and professional care, for overfocus tendencies, 291
relational prescriptions, 284
forgetfulness, 21, 22

fortune-telling, 63, 66, 92
  overcoming, 100–101, 271, 283
  pessimism, 44
fragrances, effect on mood, 77
Frederick II, German Emperor, 75
free will and brain, ix–x
frontal lobes see cingulate system
Fueloep-Miller, Rene, 205
functional MRI (fMRI) scans, 15

GABA (amino acid), 113
gabapentin see Neurontin (gabapentin)
Gage, Phineas P., 132–33
gambling, pathological, 165, 167, 168
gamma rays, SPECT, 16
gender differences, 43, 296, 297
genetic factors
  ADHD in, 30, 127–29
  and brain, 25, 27
  dyslexia, 200
  Tourette's syndrome in, 95
George, Mark, 59
getting stuck see compulsions;
  obsessive-compulsive disorder (OCD)
Glad Game, 62–63
goal setting, 138
Gold, Mark, 245
good qualities, noticing, 74
grape seeds, 154
grief, 46, 47, 78
Gualtieri, Thomas, 116
guided imagery, 102
guilt
  automatic negative thoughts, 64, 66
  in impulsive behavior, 122

Haldol (haloperidol), 96, 113
hallucinations, and sleep deprivation, 216
handwriting
  basal ganglia system in, 86
  see also hypergraphia
head injuries, 4–5
  biofeedback for, 217
  cingulate system in, 23–24
  cognitive ability, effect on, 201
  and functional brain images of sufferers, 5
  personality changes, 34
  prefrontal cortex in, xi, 131–36
  SPECT of, 17, 134
  and substance abuse, 243
headaches
  basal ganglia system in, 97
  cingulate system in, 158

in PTSD, 93
temporal lobes in, 203
help, when to seek, 290–94
  denial about needing help, 295–98
herbal treatment, 79, 113, 281
  St John's Wort, 80, 188
heroin, 243
highway hypnosis, 104
Hollister, Anne, 76
homicidal thoughts, in children, 9, 13
humanity, 8
  loss of, in Vietnam, 93
  questions about essence of, 303–06
  touch, importance of, 76
humming, 212
hyperactivity
  in ADHD, 30
  Ritalin for, 223
  see also attention deficit hyperactivity disorder (ADHD)
hypergraphia, temporal lobe dysfunction, 203–04
hypochondria, 90, 165
hypothalamus, 38n, 41, 43–44

The Idiot (Dostoyevsky), 205–06
illusions, 203
imipramine see Tofranil
immune system, 124, 142
impulsiveness
  in ADHD, 30, 122
  in aggression, 224
  and breathing, 103
  and nutrition, 83
  prefrontal cortex in, 117, 119
infections, brain, 204
inhalants, 248–49
inositol, 83, 190
Insel, Thomas, xi
interpersonal psychotherapy, 73
interpretive cortex, temporal lobes as, 195
intimate relationships
  automatic no, 161, 178
  basal ganglia relational traits, 270–72
  and biochemistry, 280–81
  brain systems influencing, 267–68
  cingulate relational traits, 275–76
  conflict avoidance in, 111
  exercising together, 286, 287
  limbic relational traits, 268–70
  losing spouse or lover, 46
  love, 76, 88–89
  mind reading, 63–64
  nagging, avoiding, 33, 286, 287

positive memories, building, 79
prefrontal cortex relational traits, 272–78
prescriptions for, 281–89
temporal lobe relational traits, 278–80
see also marriages
irritability
and automatic negative thoughts, 58
basal ganglia system in, 93
and breathing, 103
cingulate system in, 158
and divorce, 47
in intimate relationships, 110, 111
in PMS, 27, 54
and serotonin, lack of, 83

jamais vu, 196

Kaczynski, Ted (Unabomber), 203
Kinkel, Kip, xi
kleptomania, 165
Korsakoff s syndrome (KS), 238

labeling
antidepressants, use of, 50
automatic negative thoughts, 64–65, 66, 101
of parents with autistic children, 75–76
Lamictal (lamotrigine)
in PMS, 54
for temporal lobes, 215
language understanding and processing, 194, 200
lavender flowers, 77, 113
learning, 117, 200
lethargy, 83
libido
cingulate problems, 161
diminished, 110, 111
and smell, 42
see also sexuality
lie detector tests, 59
limbic bonding
protecting children with, 71–72
support groups, 70
limbic system
and aggressiveness, 224–25
and bonding, 71–72
and deep limbic system, 38n
partners of people with limbic problems, 269
and prefrontal cortex, 117
lithium, xi, 113

for manic-depression, 52
for post-traumatic stress disorder, 93
locking compulsion, 174
loneliness see social isolation
lorazepam (Ativan), 112
low fat diets, 82
l-tryptophan (amino acid), 83, 190–91
Lubar, Joel, 147, 148
Lustral (sertraline)
for addiction, 167
for cingulate system, 186, 266
for intimate relationships, 281
and motivation, 97
for OCD, 30, 163, 164
for PMS, 54

magnetic resonance imaging (MRI)
scans, 9, 17
functional, 15
standard, 14
manic-depression, 51–53
case histories, x, xi
medication for, 28, 79
SPECT of, 52
marijuana, 244–48
effect on brain, 247
as "gateway" drug, 244
legalization as medicine, 245
SPECT of affected abusers, 245, 246
marriages
body language, 31, 33
and brain, 30–37
communication problems, 94
control in, 110
and empty nest syndrome, 48
marital counseling, 31, 32, 33, 181–82
memories, effect on, 194–95
SPECT of couples in difficulties, 265
violence in, 23–24
see also divorces
Martin, Steve, 81
massage, 76
medication, 5–6
for ADHD, 6, 86, 96
for Alzeimer's disease, 22, 205
antianxiety, 52, 112
anticonvulsant, 97
antipsychotic, x, 96, 113
antiseizure, x, 28, 35
see also Depakote (valproate semisodium)
for basal ganglia system, 112–13
for cingulate system, 186–88
coming off too soon, 28, 173
for depression see antidepressants

limbic, 79–80
for manic-depression, 53
for OCD, 30, 163, 164, 166
physical functioning of brain
  optimized through, 7
for prefrontal cortex, 151–53, 285
psychostimulants, 96, 233n
refusal to take, 174
serotonergic, 186, 188, 281
side effects, 188
for temporal lobes, 215
see also specific medications
meditation, 104–08
melatonin, 81
Mellaril (thioridazine), 113
memory and memories
  in Alzeimer's disease, 21
  attention spans, 117
  deep limbic system in, 40
  music therapy, 211–12
  positive, building, 77–79, 282
  prefrontal cortex in, 119
  and smell, sense of, 77
  temporal lobes in, 193–94
menstrual periods *see* premenstrual
  syndrome (PMS)
methadone, 243
methamphetamines, 233n, 234–37
  case histories, 240, 241, 257–59
  and violence, 254
methylphenidate *see* Ritalin
  (methylphenidate)
migraines, 97
mind reading, 63–64, 66
mirtazapine (Zispin), 164, 186
mistakes, learning from, 116, 284–85
moodiness and moods
  in ADHD, 125
  and automatic negative thoughts,
    58
  deep limbic system in, 9
  fragrances, effect on, 77
  music therapy, 211–12
  and serotonin, lack of, 83
  smell, effect on, 77
  SPECT, in mood disorders, 17
mother-infant bond *see under* bonding
motivation
  basal ganglia system in, 97–98
  deep limbic system in, 41
  excessive, 97–98
motor control, basal ganglia system in,
  86, 87, 97
movement
  in Parkinson's disease, 87

in rhythms, 215, 288
Mozart, Wolfgang Amadeus, 154, 212
The Mozart Effect (Campbell), 211–12,
  213
muscle tension and pain
  basal ganglia system in, 97
  medication for, 112
  thoughts, effect on body, 59, 60
music therapy, 154
  classical music, 212–14
  in intimate relationships, 288
  singing, benefits of, 211
musical instrument, learning to play,
  214

Napoleon I, Emperor of France, 42
Nardil (phenelzine), 91, 112–13
negativeness
  in ADHD, 125
  and breathing, 103
  changing of patterns, 78
  deep limbic system in, 9, 39
  and emotional shading, 40
  focusing on the negative, 62–63, 65
  and head injuries, 35
  labeling, 64
  life as obstacle course, 69
  and nutrition, 83
  in PMS, 54
  in thoughts, 4, 26, 35, 60, 102, 227
  see also automatic negative thoughts
    (ANTs); automatic no
nervous system, and deep limbic
  system, 43–44
nervousness
  of author, 9
  medication for, 112
Neurontin (gabapentin), 215, 225
neurotransmitters
  lack of in depression, 49
  proteins as building blocks of, 82
  Tourette's syndrome and OCD, 96
nicotine, 216, 234, 249–50
Niebuhr, Reinhold, 180
noradrenaline, 49, 83, 152
Norpramin (desipramine), 152
nuclear medicine, 16–17
nutrition
  and basal ganglia system, 113
  and cingulate system, 189–90
  and deep limbic system, 82–83
  physical functioning of brain
    optimized through, 7
  and prefrontal cortex, 153–54
  and temporal lobes, 216–17

see also appetite; *specific nutritional components*

obsessions
  examples of, 163
  paying too much attention to, in OCD, 95
obsessive-compulsive disorder (OCD), 3–4
  and ADHD, 95–96
  in children, 172
  and cingulate system, 29–30, 162–64
  compulsions, 163
  incidence of, 163
  intensity of, 164
  obsessions, 163
  and professional care, 291
  psychostimulants, effect on, 96
  sexual thoughts, 164
  SPECT of, 29–30, 162, 164
  spectrum, 165–73
  in workplace, 292
occupational setting
  depression in, 110, 111, 291
  violent feelings in, 219
OCD *see* obsessive-compulsive disorder (OCD)
olfactory system, 41, 76–77
  see also smell and smells
oligomeric procyanidius, 154
omega-3 fatty acids, 82
One-Page Miracle (OPM), 139–41
onychophagia (nail biting), 165
opiates, 243–44
oppositional behavior *see* negativeness
oppositional defiant disorder (ODD), 165, 169–71
  SPECT of, 170
optimism, 283
Orap (pimozide), 96
organization
  in ADHD, 124–25
  becoming organized, 146–47
  helping partner, 285
  poor skills, 30, 146
oxazepam, 112
Oxycontin (oxycodone), 243
oxygen, in brain cells, 103

pain, chronic, 165, 166
Paldi, Jack, 5, 15
Pamergan (pethidine), 243
panic and panic disorder
  agoraphobia in, 91
  of author, 26

basal ganglia system in, 89, 90–92
  conflict avoidance, 95
  diaphragmatic breathing for, 102–04
  as medical problem, 15
  medication for, 112, 113
  suicidal tendencies, 293
paradoxical requests, making, 182–83
paranoia
  following death of pet, 47
  and head injuries, 34, 35
  in manic-depressive disorder, 52
  and sleep deprivation, 216
  and temporal lobe abnormalities, 200
parasympathetic nervous system, 43
parents
  and ADHD, 30, 124, 150
  of autistic children, 75–76
  of cingulate children, 184–86
  empty nest syndrome, 48
  father-and-son study, 226–27
  see also children
parietal lobes, SPECT of, 21, 22
Parkinson's disease (PD), 87
paroxetine *see* Seroxat (paroxetine)
pemoline *see* Cylert (pemoline)
people skills, 73–74
personality, 5
  brain's role in, 3
  head injuries, effect on, 34
  worrying, 158
personalizing, 65, 66
pessimism *see* negativeness
pets, deaths of, 46–47
phencyclidine, and violence, 254
phenelzine (Nardil), 91, 112–13
dl-phenylalanine, 83
phobias
  agoraphobia, 91
  conflict, 110
  social, 109
physical contact, 74–76, 282
Pies, Ronald, 165
pleasure/ecstasy
  basal ganglia system in, 84, 87–88
  see also sexuality
pollution, negative thoughts as, 60
Pollyanna (Porter), 62–63
polygraphs, 59
Porter, Eleanor, 62–63
positive bonding, people providing, 69–70
positive thinking
  body, effect on, 59
  building library of happy memories, 77–79

deep limbic system, cooling, 59
enhancing, 56–83
seminars in, 70
and senses, 79
see also automatic negative thoughts
(ANTs); negativeness; thoughts
and thinking
positron emission tomography (PET)
scans, use of, 5–6, 15, 75, 176
postnatal depression, 45
post-traumatic stress disorder (PTSD),
92–94
Pratt, Rosalie Rebollo, 154
predictions, pessimistic *see*
fortune-telling
prefrontal cortex (pfc), 114–37
in ADHD *see* attention deficit
hyperactivity disorder (ADHD)
audiovisual stimulation, 149
brain-wave biofeedback for, 147–49
calmness, achieving, 150
checklist for, 136–37
and cingulate system, 259–61
and deep limbic system, 44, 117
dorsolateral, 117
focus
developing and maintaining, 138–41
on positive, 142–44
functions of, 114–18
head injuries, xi, 131–36
inferior orbital cortex, 119
meaning, purpose, stimulation and
excitement for, 145–46
medications for, 151–53
music therapy, 154
nutrition, 153–54
organizational skills, 146–47
overactive/underactive, x, 5–6, 9, 131,
242
partners of people with prefrontal
cortex problems, 273–74
penguin collecting, by author, 142,
143
prescriptions for, 138–54
for partner, 285
for self, 284–85
problems with, 118–19
and professional care, 291, 293
psychotic disorders, 129–31
relational traits, 272–78
sections of, 114, 115
SPECT of, 117–18, 143
stimulation for, 284
and violence, 224
vulnerability of, 197

workplace problems, 292
pregnancies, teenage, 71
premenstrual syndrome (PMS)
deep limbic system in, 54
and emotional shading, 40
medication for, 79
SPECT of, 27–28
prescriptions
for basal ganglia system, 26, 92,
100–113
for partner, 283–84
for self, 283
for cingulate system, 176–91
for partner, 287
for self, 286
for deep limbic system, 50, 56–83
for partner, 282–83
for self, 281–82
for intimate relationships, 281–89
need for, 9
for prefrontal cortex, 138–54
for partner, 285
for self, 284–85
for sleep, 105
for temporal lobes, 210–17
for partner, 288–89
for self, 287–88
problem solving, in intimate
relationships, 286
professional care
credentials, checking, 299
denial about needing help, 295–98
finding competent professional,
298–300
GP referrals, 299
own good brain, gaining access to,
294–95
seeking of help, 290–94
specialist, using, 299
SPECT study, need for, 300–302
see also psychotherapy
progressive relaxation, 106
prosopagnosia, 195
proteins, 82–83, 153, 216, 217
see also amino acids, examples
Prozac (fluoxetine), 32–33, 50, 143
for ADHD, 96, 127
for cingulate system, 32–33, 186
for eating disorders, 166
for gambling, 168
for intimate relationships, 281
in media, 49
and motivation, 97
for OCD, 164, 174
for PMS, 54

and St John's Wort, 188
with Tegretol, 230
for violent behavior, 220
see also smell and smells
Prozac Bulimia Nervosa Collaborative
Study Group, 166–67
pseudodementia, 22, 23
psychiatric illness
hospitalization for, 228
medical problems, 15
stigma of, 295
temporal lobe medications, 215
psychiatric illness, stigma of
psychological exercises, physical
functioning of brain optimized
through, 7
psychosis, in postnatal depression, 45
psychostimulants, 96, 233n
psychotic disorders, 129–31
PTSD (post-traumatic stress disorder),
92–94
public speaking, fear of, 109

radiopharmaceuticals, 16
relapse, following coming off
medication too quickly, 28
relational traits
basal ganglia system, 270–72
cingulate system, 275–76
limbic system in, 268–70
prefrontal cortex, 272–78
temporal lobes, 278–80
relationships
and grief, 46
interpersonal psychotherapy for, 73
intimate see intimate relationships
limbic bonding, enhancing, 73–74
One-Page Miracle (OPM), 140
parent-child, 48
and people skills, 73–74
pfc problems, 142
relaxation response, 59
relaxation techniques, 92, 105–07
diaphragmatic breathing, 102–04
guided imagery, 102
The Relaxation Response (Benson), 104
religious preoccupation, temporal lobe
dysfunction, 203, 208
resistance to treatment, 5, 6, 7
reverse psychology, 182
rhythms, movement in, 215, 288
Risperdal (risperidone), 113
Ritalin (methylphenidate), 143
for ADHD, 6, 33, 86, 88, 96, 151
and caffeine use, 250

effects on brain, 87–88
and head injuries, 134
for hyperactivity, 223
as non-addictive, 88
tics developed on, 149
Rivotril (clonazepam), 92
road rage, 161–62
romantic love, basal ganglia system in,
88–89
Russell, Harold, 149

St John's Wort, 80, 188
Salimbene (historian), 75
schizophrenia, 5, 118, 129–30
Schwartz, Jeffrey, 176
The Secret Life of the Unborn Child (Verny),
214
seizures, SPECT of, 17
self-hypnosis, 104–08, 271
sensationalism, antidepressants, 49
sensorimotor rhythm (SMR), 148
Serenity Prayer (Niebuhr), 180
serotonin
and dopamine, 96
see also dopamine
lack of in depression, 49, 83
and nutrition, 153–54, 190
and PMS, 54
and tryptophan, 81–82
Seroxat (paroxetine)
for cingulate system, 186
for intimate relationships, 281
and motivation, 97
for OCD, 164
for PMS, 54
sertraline see Lustral (sertraline)
sexuality
basal ganglia relational traits, 270
deep limbic system in, 42–43
losing spouse or lover, 46
loss of interest, 49, 182, 270
obsessive-compulsive disorder, 164
and smell, 42
see also pleasure/ecstasy
shallow breathing, 103
Shaw, Gordon, 213
shopping, compulsive, 165, 168–69
singing, benefits of, 211
single photon emission computed
tomography (SPECT), 3–8
in ADHD, 6–7, 120, 126, 128, 129, 151
for alcoholism, 238–43
alternatives to, 302
for Alzheimer's disease, 205, 206
and "bad behavior", 15

and basal ganglia, 85, 87, 92
cameras, 17
and cingulate system, 189
cysts, case history, 9–13, 303
day of scan, 301
defined, 16
and depression, 20
development of technology, 17
in differentiating between two
    problems with similar symptoms,
    22–23
displaying of studies, 17–18
dissemination of information on, 4
for early intervention, 18
eating disorders, 166
in eliciting understanding and
    compassion from patients'
    families, 21–22, 131
function, xi, 3
head injuries, 17, 134
in manic-depressive disorder, 52
marriages in difficulties, 265
medical uses, 18–24
need for SPECT study, 300–302
and nuclear medicine, 16–17
obsessive-compulsive disorder,
    29–30, 162, 164
oppositional defiant disorder, 170
other studies compared, 14, 17
in PMS, 27–28
post-traumatic stress disorder, 93
and prefrontal cortex, 117–18
in preventing future illnesses, 20–21
procedure, 301–02
and professional care, 295
recognition on medical community,
    302
side effects, lack of, 301
stalking, 231
for substance abuse, 236, 237, 240
    marijuana, 245
    and violence, 253
of temporal lobes, 22, 201, 217
Tourette's syndrome, 95
violent behavior, 23–24, 218, 219
    and substance abuse, 253
sleep
    deep limbic system in, 41, 45, 47
    and divorce, 47
    and empty nest syndrome, 48
    importance of, 216
    and physical exercise, 81
    prescriptions for, 105
smell and smells
    deep limbic system in, 41, 42

gender differences in, 43
great, surrounding yourself with,
    76–77
in intimate relationships, 42, 282
smoking, 216, 234, 249–50
SMR (sensorimotor rhythm), 148
social anxiety, 119
social connectedness see bonding
social isolation, 47, 124, 208
    social skills training, 202
social phobias, 109
Sonata for Two Pianos (Mozart), 213
spaciness, 52, 53, 228
    in sleep deprivation, 216
special time exercise, 71–72
SPECT see single photon emission
    computed tomography (SPECT)
spending, compulsive, 165, 168–69
Spiegel, David, 70
spiritual health, connection with
    mental health, 4
stalking, 230–31
stomach aches
    cingulate system in, 158
    temporal lobes in, 203
stress
    and ADHD, 30
    basal ganglia system in, 85–86
    cingulate system in, 158, 171–73
    medication for, 112
    paralysis by, 85
    post-traumatic stress disorder, 92–94
strokes, SPECT of, 17, 18, 20, 21
substance abuse, 4
    aggressiveness, 254–57
    amphetamines, 128
    and attention deficit disorder, 235
    brain, impact on, 232–52
    caffeine and nicotine in see caffeine;
        nicotine
    ceasing of abuse, effects, 237, 251
    cocaine in see cocaine
    decision-making problems, 261–62
    drug education poster, 251–52
    and head injuries, 243
    impact on brain function, 17
    inhalants in, 248–49
    marijuana in see marijuana
    methamphetamines in see
        methamphetamines
    and provocative behaviors, 261–62
    "scalloping effect" in, 234
    as self-medication for underlying
        brain problems, 257–59
    SPECT of, 236, 237, 240

strategies for dealing with, 262–64
in teenagers, 71
Valium, addiction to, 92
and violence, 253–64
suicidal tendencies
in ADHD, 123–24
brief nature of thoughts, 227
case histories, 6, 143
in children, 9, 13
and empty nest syndrome, 48
following death of pet, 47
gender differences in, 43
as leading cause of death, 50
in panic disorder, 293
pfc prescriptions, case study, 143
in psychoses, 131
suicide as modeled behavior, 229
in teenagers, 71
temporal lobes in, 199–200
violent behavior, 220, 227–30
supplements, nutritional, 83, 154
support groups, 70
Swedo, Susan, 165
Symmetrel (amantadine), 134
sympathetic nervous system, 44

teenagers, 71, 181, 297
Tegretol (carbamazepine), 113
for motor problems, 97
in PMS, 54
for post-traumatic stress disorder, 93
with Prozac, 230
for temporal lobes, 215
for violence, 220, 221, 222, 223, 224, 225
temper tantrums, in children, 110, 111
temporal lobes, 192–209
absence of one, 9
and aggressiveness, 9, 198–99, 201, 225
and biofeedback, 217
checklist for, 208–09
classical music, 212–14
in dementia, 21
dominant side, 192, 194, 195
problems with, 196
experiences, creating library of, 210
functions of, 9, 192–95
humming, 212
humming and toning for, 211–12
as interpretive cortex, 195
left abnormalities, 194, 200, 202
medications for, 215
musical instrument, learning to play, 214

nondominant side, 192–93, 195
problems with, 196, 202
and nutrition, 216–17
overactive/underactive, 35, 53, 241
partners of people with temporal lobe problems, 279
prescriptions for, 210–17
for partner, 288–89
for self, 287–88
problems with either or both, 196
and professional care, 291
relational traits, 278–80
rhythms, movement in, 215, 288
sections of, 193
singing for, 211
and sleep deprivation, 216
SPECT of, 22, 201, 217
and substance abuse, 246
toning, 212
vulnerability of, 197
workplace problems, 292
tension
basal ganglia system in, 87
cingulate system in, 158
and deep limbic system, 43
negative thoughts, 58
in workplace, 292
test anxiety, 119
thalamic structures, brain, 38n
theta brain waves, 148
thiamine, 238
thioridazine, 113
thoughtfulness, 117
thoughts and thinking
bad thoughts, as pollution, 60
delusional thinking, 51, 130
distorted, 131
future-oriented thinking, 156–57
inaccuracies of, 101
negative see negativeness: in thoughts
noticing effect on body, 59–60
positive thinking, strengthening, 56–83
as real, 58
repetitive see obsessive-compulsive disorder (OCD)
thinking with your feelings, 64, 66
training of, 61
see also automatic negative thoughts (ANTs)
3-D brain images, 18, 19
tic disorders see Tourette's syndrome (TS)
time management, 74

special time exercise, 71–72
Tofranil (imipramine), 112–13, 152
toning, 212
touch, importance of, 74–76
Tourette's syndrome (TS)
    basal ganglia system in, 87, 95–96
    as OCD spectrum disorder, 165
    SPECT of, 95
trauma
    deep limbic system in, 40, 41
    post-traumatic stress disorder, 92–94
    prefrontal cortex in, 133–34
treatment failures, 5, 6, 7
tremors, 87
trial-and-error diagnosis, xii
trichotillomania (hair pulling), 165
trust, 74
tryptophan, 81–82
Turner, R. M., 182
tyrosine, 83, 154

unstable atoms, nuclear medicine,
    16–17

valerian, 113
Valium (diazepam), 91, 112
    addiction to, 92
valproate semisodium see Depakote
    (valproate semisodium)
venlafaxine see Efexor (venlafaxine)
Verny, Thomas, 214
Vietnam War, and post-traumatic
    stress, 93–94
violence, 4
    brain differences in violent patients,
        218
    case histories, 219–24
    in children, 9, 13, 201
    complexity of, 218–31
    father-and-son study on, 226–27
    and head injuries, 35
    in PMS, 27–28
    profile of, 224–27
    SPECT of violent patient, 218, 219
    and stalking, 230–31
    strategies for dealing with, 262–64
    and substance abuse, 253–64
    suicidal tendencies, 220, 227–30
    in teenagers, 71
    and uses of SPECT, 23–24
    see also aggressiveness; anger
visual imagery, 102, 107–08
vitamin B, 83, 113, 190, 238
Volkow, Nora, 87–88

weight gain, 34
Windows into the ADD Mind (Amen), 126
Witzelsucht, 124
workaholics, 98
workplace see occupational setting,
    depression in
worrying
    in ADHD, 123
    and cingulate system, 158
    18/40/60 rule, 108–09
    overfocus issues see under cingulated
        system
    in PMS, 54
    and serotonin, lack of, 83
    thoughts of others, about self, 109

Xanax (alpraxolam), 112

Zametkin, Alan, 6
Zispin (mirtazapine), 164, 186
Zyban (bupropion), 22, 153, 269, 281

About the Author

Daniel G. Amen, M.D. is a clinical neuroscientist, psychiatrist, best-selling author and CEO and medical director of Amen Clinics, Inc., in Newport Beach and Fairfield, California, Tacoma, Washington and Reston, Virginia. He is a Distinguished Fellow of the American Psychiatric Association and Assistant Clinical Professor of Psychiatry and Human Behavior at the University of California, Irvine School of Medicine. Dr. Amen lectures to thousands of mental health professionals and lay people each year. His clinics have the world's largest database of brain images related to behavior.

Dr. Amen did his psychiatric training at the Walter Reed Army Medical Center in Washington, D.C. and his child psychiatry training in Hawaii. He has won writing and research awards from the American Psychiatric Association, the U.S. Army and the Baltimore-DC Institute for Psychoanalysis. He is the author of numerous professional and popular articles, 22 books and a number of audio and video programs. His books have been translated into 19 languages and include *Healing ADD, Healing the Hardware of the Soul, Healing Anxiety and Depression* (with Dr. Lisa Routh), *Preventing Alzheimer's Disease* (with Dr. Rod Shankle), *Making A Good Brain Great* (chosen as one of the best books in 2005 by Amazon.com and also won the prestigious Earphones Award for the audiobook) and *Sex on the Brain*.

Dr. Amen has appeared on the *Today Show, Good Morning America, The View, The Early Show*, CNN, HBO, and many other television and radio programs in the U.S.

Amen Clinics, Inc.

Amen Clinics, Inc. was established in 1989 by Daniel G. Amen, M.D. The clinics specialize in innovative diagnosis and treatment planning for a wide variety of behavioral, learning, emotional and cognitive problems for children, teenagers and adults. They have an international reputation for evaluating brain-behavior problems, such as of attention deficit hyperactivity disorder (ADHD), depression, anxiety, school failure, brain trauma, obsessive-compulsive disorders, aggressiveness, marital conflict, cognitive decline and brain toxicity from drugs or alcohol. Brain SPECT imaging is performed in the clinics. Amen Clinics, Inc. has the world's largest database of brain scans for behavioral problems.

The clinics welcome referrals from doctors, psychologists, social workers, marriage and family therapists, drug and alcohol counselors and individual clients.

Amen Clinics, Inc., Newport Beach
4019 Westerly Place, Suite 100
Newport Beach, CA 92660, USA
(949) 266-3700

Amen Clinics, Inc., Fairfield
350 Chadbourne Road
Fairfield, CA 9458, USA
(707) 429-7181

Amen Clinics, Inc., Northwest
3315 South 23rd Street
Tacoma, WA, USA
(253) 779-HOPE

Amen Clinics, Inc., DC
1875 Campus Commons Dr.
Reston, VA 20191, USA
(703) 860-5600

www.amenclinic.com

Amenclinic.com is an educational interactive brain website geared towards mental health and medical professionals, educators, students, and the general public. It contains a wealth of information to help you learn about our clinics and the brain. The site contains over 300 color brain SPECT images, thousands of scientific abstracts on brain SPECT imaging for psychiatry, a brain puzzle and much, much more. You can view over 300 astonishing color 3-D brain SPECT images on:

- Aggression
- Attention Deficit Hyperactivity Disorder, including the six subtypes
- Dementia and Cognitive Decline
- Drug Abuse
- PMS
- Anxiety Disorders
- Brain Trauma
- Depression
- Obsessive Compulsive Disorder
- Stroke
- Seizures